T0261586

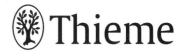

Ophthalmology

3rd Edition

Gerhard K. Lang, MD

Professor and Director
Department of Ophthalmology
University Eye Hospital
Ulm, Germany

600 illustrations

Thieme
Stuttgart · New York · Delhi · Rio de Janeiro

Library of Congress Cataloging-in-Publication Data

Lang, Gerhard K., author.
  [Augenheilkunde. English]
  Ophthalmology / Gerhard K. Lang ; translator: Gertrud G. Champe. -- 3rd edition.
     p. ; cm.

This book is an authorized translation of the 5th German edition published and copyrighted 2014 by Georg Thieme Verlag, Stuttgart. Title of the German edition: Augenheilkunde.

  ISBN 978-3-13-126163-2 -- ISBN 978-3-13-170223-4 (eISBN)
  I. Champe, Gertrud Graubart, translator. II. Title.
  [DNLM: 1. Eye Diseases. WW 140]
  RE48.9
  617.7--dc23
                                        2015025803

Important note: Medicine is an ever-changing science undergoing continual development. Research and clinical experience are continually expanding our knowledge, in particular our knowledge of proper treatment and drug therapy. Insofar as this book mentions any dosage or application, readers may rest assured that the authors, editors, and publishers have made every effort to ensure that such references are in accordance with **the state of knowledge at the time of production of the book.**

Nevertheless, this does not involve, imply, or express any guarantee or responsibility on the part of the publishers in respect to any dosage instructions and forms of applications stated in the book. **Every user is requested to examine carefully** the manufacturers' leaflets accompanying each drug and to check, if necessary in consultation with a physician or specialist, whether the dosage schedules mentioned therein or the contraindications stated by the manufacturers differ from the statements made in the present book. Such examination is particularly important with drugs that are either rarely used or have been newly released on the market. Every dosage schedule or every form of application used is entirely at the user's own risk and responsibility. The authors and publishers request every user to report to the publishers any discrepancies or inaccuracies noticed. If errors in this work are found after publication, errata will be posted at www.thieme.com on the product description page.

© 2016 Georg Thieme Verlag KG

Thieme Publishers Stuttgart
Rüdigerstrasse 14, 70469 Stuttgart, Germany
+49 [0]711 8931 421, customerservice@thieme.de

Thieme Publishers New York
333 Seventh Avenue, New York, NY 10001, USA
+1-800-782-3488, customerservice@thieme.com

Thieme Publishers Delhi
A-12, Second Floor, Sector-2, Noida-201301
Uttar Pradesh, India
+91 120 45 566 00, customerservice@thieme.in

Thieme Publishers Rio, Thieme Publicações Ltda.
Edifício Rodolpho de Paoli, 25° andar
Av. Nilo Peçanha, 50 – Sala 2508
Rio de Janeiro 20020-906 Brasil
+55 21 3172 2297 / +55 21 3172 1896

Cover design: Thieme Publishing Group
Typesetting by primustype Robert Hurler GmbH, Notzingen, Germany

Printed in China by Asia Pacific Offset Ltd,   5 4 3 2 1
Hong Kong
ISBN 9783131261632

Also available as an e-book:
eISBN 9783131702234

Some of the product names, patents, and registered designs referred to in this book are in fact registered trademarks or proprietary names even though specific reference to this fact is not always made in the text. Therefore, the appearance of a name without designation as proprietary is not to be construed as a representation by the publisher that it is in the public domain.

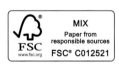

Contents

5 Cornea 68
Gerhard K. Lang

12 Retina 188

Gabriele E. Lang and Gerhard K. Lang

13 Optic Nerve 232

Oskar Gareis and Gerhard K. Lang

14 Visual Pathway.. 248
Oskar Gareis and Gerhard K. Lang

15 Orbital Cavity.. 258
Christoph W. Spraul and Gerhard K. Lang

18   Ocular Trauma 318
Gerhard K. Lang

19   Cardinal Symptoms 336
Stefan Lang and Gerhard K. Lang

20   Appendix 350

21   Glossary 364

Index 369

Prof. Gerhard K. Lang (born 1951) studied medicine in Erlangen, Germany. After residency and research work in Erlangen and at the Johns Hopkins Hospital in Baltimore, USA, he served as Co-Chairman at the Department of Ophthalmology at the University of Erlangen-Nuremberg. Since 1990 he has been Chairman of the Department of Ophthalmology at the University of Ulm.
The author's special interests lie in European and international ophthalmology, and in particular in the field of medical teaching.

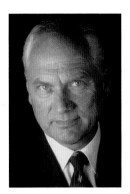

Preface to the 3rd Edition

The 2nd edition of this book was published in 2007 when the "revolution in the study room" was in full swing.

The use of electronic media was increasing and the financial resources of students were mainly decreasing due to the introduction of or rising course fees. Textbooks became less significant, especially in the smaller specialties, becoming replaced by things like scripts (schemata, material in note form) that require less effort at an even lower cost.

Set against this background, we authors were faced with the question of whether a textbook would still be remotely interesting to the current generation of students, especially a textbook in a larger format than 8 years earlier and completely different to scripts in its outward appearance. This book cannot be viewed as a script, nor does it intend to be one. It is a well-founded source of knowledge, a didactically sophisticated basis for a fast-moving specialty, and an attractive "picture book" in the best possible sense. It wants to put you in a position to understand ophthalmology and be able to make independent decisions, not just teach you facts. Thus, with the publication of the 3rd English edition, we are once again deliberately setting out on the "Textbook Venture."

We are pleased that we were able to recruit Professor Joachim Esser from the University Hospital in Essen and Dr. Stefan Lang from the University Eye Hospital in Freiburg as new contributors to our book.

Our thanks go to Dr. Jens Ulrich Werner at the University Eye Hospital in Ulm for the many new photographs. We are especially grateful to the students for their valuable input. Please continue to accompany us with your constructive criticism.
Finally, our thanks also go to the staff of Thieme Publishers for their motivating, professional, and unlimited support.

Prof. Gerhard K. Lang, MD

Contributors

Joachim Esser, MD
Professor
Department of Ophthalmology
University Hospital Essen
Essen, Germany

Oskar Gareis, MD
Ophthalmology Practice
Esslingen, Germany

Gabriele E. Lang, MD
Professor
Head of the Division of Medical Retina and Laser
Surgery
Department of Ophthalmology
University Eye Hospital
Ulm, Germany

Gerhard K. Lang, MD
Professor and Director
Department of Ophthalmology
University Eye Hospital
Ulm, Germany

Stefan J. Lang, MD
Department of Ophthalmology
University Eye Hospital
Freiburg, Germany

Doris Recker
Orthoptist
Department of Ophthalmology
University Eye Hospital
Ulm, Germany

Christoph W. Spraul, MD
Professor
Ophthalmology Practice
Augenärzte im Basteicenter
Ulm, Germany

Peter Wagner, MD
Chief of Medical Staff
Department of Ophthalmology
University Eye Hospital
Ulm, Germany

Chapter 1

The Ophthalmic Examination

1 The Ophthalmic Examination

Gabriele E. Lang and Gerhard K. Lang

1.1 Introduction

This chapter presents examination methods that the nonophthalmologist can apply, using simple equipment. Specific ophthalmologic methods are described in the following chapters.

1.2 Equipment

The **basic equipment** for an ophthalmic examination by a nonophthalmologist includes the following instruments:

- *Direct ophthalmoscope* for examining the fundus (▶ Fig. 1.1a).
- *Focused light* (▶ Fig. 1.1a) for examining the reaction of the pupil and the anterior chamber (**enlargement with a loupe**).
- *Aspheric lens* (▶ Fig. 1.1a) for examining the anterior chamber (see also ▶ Fig. 1.3).
- *Desmarres eyelid retractor* and glass rod or sterile cotton swab for eyelid eversion (ectropionizing) (▶ Fig. 1.1b).
- *Eye chart* for testing visual acuity at a distance of 5 meters (20 feet) (▶ Fig. 1.2).

▶ **Recommended medications**
- *Topical anesthetic* (such as oxybuprocaine 0.4% eye drops) to provide local anesthesia during removal of conjunctival and corneal foreign bodies and superficial anesthesia prior to flushing the conjunctival sac in chemical injuries.
- *Sterile buffer solution* for primary treatment of chemical injuries.
- *Antibiotic eye drops* for first aid treatment of injuries, *sterile eye compresses,* and a 1-cm *adhesive bandage* for protective bandaging.
- Pilocarpine 2% eye drops and acetazolamide tablets for first aid if a glaucoma attack is suspected.

> **Note**
> An ophthalmologist should be consulted following any emergency treatment of eye injuries.

1.3 History

A complete history includes four aspects:

- **Family history.** Many eye disorders are hereditary or of higher incidence in members of the same family. Examples include refractive errors, strabismus, cataract, glaucoma, retinal detachment, and retinal dystrophy.
- **Medical history.** As ocular changes may be related to systemic disorders, this possibility must be explored. Conditions affecting the eyes include diabetes mellitus, hypertension, infectious diseases, rheumatic disorders, skin diseases, and surgery. Eye disorders such as corticosteroid-induced glaucoma, corticosteroid-induced cataract, and chloroquine-induced maculopathy can occur as a result of treatment with medications such as steroids, chloroquine, amiodarone, or chlorpromazine (▶ Tables in Chapter 20).
- **Ophthalmic history.** The examiner should inquire about corrective lenses, strabismus or amblyopia, posttraumatic conditions, and surgery or eye inflammation.
- **Current history.** What symptoms does the patient present with? Does the patient have impaired vision, pain (sharp or dull, associated with eye movement), redness of the eye, or double vision? When did these symptoms occur? Are they unilateral or bilateral? Are injuries or associated generalized symptoms present? (See individual chapters for organization of this information.)

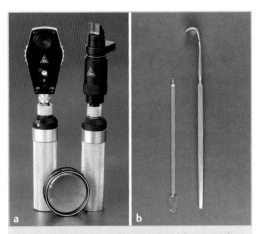

Fig. 1.1 Basic diagnostic instruments. (a) Direct ophthalmoscope, aspheric lens, and focused light. **(b)** Glass spatula and Desmarres lid retractor for eversion.

1.4 Visual Acuity

Visual acuity, the sharpness of near and distance vision, is tested separately for each eye. One eye is covered with a piece of paper or the palm of the hand placed lightly over the eye. The fingers should not be used to cover the eye because the patient will be able to see between them (▶ Fig. 1.3).

The **general practitioner** or **student** can perform an **approximate test of visual acuity**. The patient is first asked to identify certain visual symbols referred to as optotypes (see ▶ Fig. 1.2) at a distance of either 5 meters or 20 feet *(test of distance vision)*. These visual symbols are designed so that optotypes of a certain size can barely be resolved by the normal eye at a specified distance (this standard distance is specified in meters next to the respective symbol). The eye charts must be clean and well illuminated for the examination. The sharpness of vision measured is expressed as a fraction: Actual distance/Standard distance = Visual acuity **Normal visual acuity** is 5/5 (20/20), or 1.0 as a decimal number, where the actual distance equals the standard distance.

An example of **diminished visual acuity** (see ▶ Fig.1.2): the patient sees only the "4" and none of the smaller symbols on the left eye chart at a distance of 5 meters (or 20 feet) (actual distance). A normal-sighted person would be able to discern

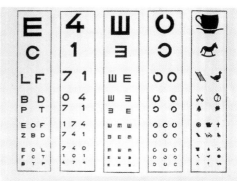

Fig. 1.2 Eye charts for testing visual acuity at a distance of 5 meters. *From left to right:* Snellen letter chart, Arabic number chart, E game, Landolt broken rings, and a children's pictograph. These eye charts are also used by nonophthalmologists such as pediatricians, occupational physicians, etc., to test visual acuity.

the "4" at a distance of 50 meters or 200 feet (standard distance). Accordingly, the patient has a visual acuity of 5/50 (or 20/200) or 0.1.

The **ophthalmologist** tests visual acuity after determining objective refraction using the integral lens system of a Phoroptor, or a box of individual lenses and an image projector that projects the visual symbols at a defined distance in front of the eye. Visual acuity is automatically calculated from

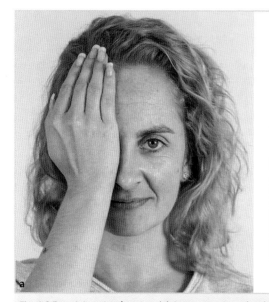
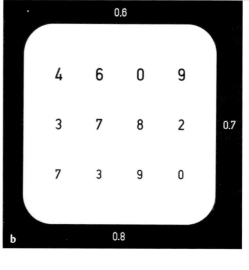

Fig. 1.3 Examining visual acuity. (a) One eye is covered with the palm of the hand without pressure, so that the far and near sight in the other eye can be tested separately. (b) Eye chart for testing visual acuity at a distance of 5 meters. The visual acuity is also shown on the chart. A patient who can read just the first line and none of the others has a visual acuity of 0.6.

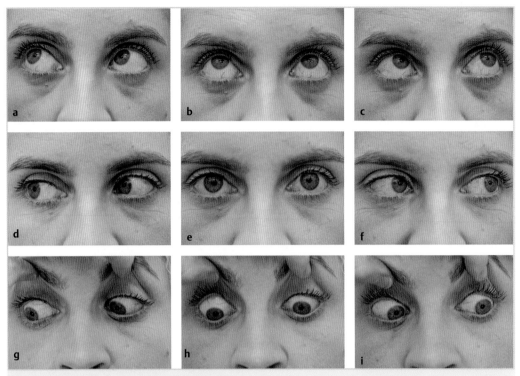

Fig. 1.4 (a–i) Evaluating the nine diagnostic positions of gaze. In doing this, the examiner notes the positions of the corneal reflexes of both eyes. If these light reflexes are not symmetrical, there is deviation or paresis in one or both eyes. See Chapter 17 on Ocular Motility and Strabismus (p. 296).

the fixed actual distance and is displayed as a decimal value. *Plus lenses* (convex lenses) are used for *farsightedness* (hyperopia or hypermetropia), *minus lenses* (concave lenses) for *nearsightedness* (myopia), and *cylindrical lenses* for *astigmatism*.

If the patient cannot discern the symbols on the eye chart at a distance of 5 meters (20 feet), the examiner shows the patient the chart at a distance of 1 meter or 3 feet (both the ophthalmologist and the general practitioner use eye charts for this examination). If the patient is still unable to discern any symbols, the examiner has the patient count fingers, discern the direction of hand motion, and discern the direction of a point light source.

1.5 Ocular Motility

The examiner gives the patient a brief explanation of the examination. Patient and examiner sit opposite each other, eye to eye.

With the patient's head immobilized, the examiner asks the patient to look at an object or a light source in each of the **nine diagnostic positions of gaze**: 1, straight ahead; 2, right; 3, upper right; 4, up; 5, upper left; 6, left; 7, lower left; 8, down; and 9, lower right (▶ Fig. 1.4). The examiner can diagnose strabismus, paralysis of ocular muscles, and gaze paresis from the position of the corneal reflex.

Evaluating the **six cardinal directions of gaze** (right, left, upper right, lower right, upper left, lower left) is sufficient when examining paralysis of one of the six extraocular muscles. The motion impairment of the eye resulting from paralysis of an ocular muscle will be most evident in these positions. Only one of the rectus muscles is involved in each of the left and right positions of gaze (lateral or medial rectus muscle). All other directions of gaze involve several muscles.

1.6 Binocular Alignment

The position of the eyes is tested with the **cover test** (at a distance and in the near field). Strabismus or latent strabismus (heterophoria, see p. 308) can be detected in this way. The examiner holds a point light source beneath his or her own eyes and observes the *light reflections in the patient's corneas* in the near field (40 cm) and at a distance (5 m). The

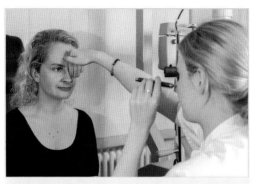

Fig. 1.5 Evaluation of binocular alignment. The examiner covers one eye of the patient with the hand to test if the uncovered eye makes a compensatory movement indicating the presence of tropia.

reflections are normally *in the center of each pupil.* If the corneal reflection is not in the center of the pupil in one eye, then a tropia is present in that eye. Then the examiner covers one eye with a hand or an occluder (► Fig. 1.5) and tests whether the *uncovered eye* makes a compensatory movement. Compensatory movement of the eye indicates the presence of tropia. However, there will also be a lack of compensatory movement if the eye is blind. The cover test is then repeated with the other eye.

If tropia is present in a newborn with extremely poor vision, the baby will not tolerate the good eye being covered.

1.7 Examination of the Eyelids and Nasolacrimal Duct

The *upper eyelid* covers the superior margin of the cornea. A few millimeters of the sclera will be visible above the *lower eyelid.* The *eyelids* are in direct contact with the eyeball. The lacrimal punctum should dip into the lacrimal lake.

Patency of the nasolacrimal duct is tested by instilling a 10% fluorescein solution in the conjunctival sac of the eye. If the dye is present in nasal mucus expelled into paper tissue after 2 minutes, the lacrimal duct is open. On this point, see also Chapter 3.2.2 on Evaluation of Tear Drainage (p. 34).

Note
Due to the danger of infection, any probing or irrigation of the nasolacrimal duct should only be performed by an ophthalmologist.

1.8 Examination of the Conjunctiva

The conjunctiva is examined by direct inspection. The bulbar conjunctiva is directly visible between the eyelids; the palpebral conjunctiva can only be examined by everting the upper or lower eyelid. The normal conjunctiva is smooth, shiny, and moist. The examiner should be alert to any reddening, secretion, thickening, scars, or foreign bodies.

▶ **Eversion of the lower eyelid.** The patient looks up while the examiner pulls the eyelid downward close to the anterior margin bilaterally (comparison of sides, ► Fig. 1.6a). This exposes the conjunctiva and the posterior surface of the lower eyelid.

▶ **Eversion of the upper eyelid**
▶ **Simple eversion** (► Fig. 1.6b). The patient is asked to look down. The patient should repeatedly be told to relax and to avoid tightly shutting the opposite eye. This relaxes the levator palpebrae superioris and orbicularis oculi muscles. The examiner grasps the eyelashes of the upper eyelid between the thumb and forefinger and everts the eyelid against a glass rod or swab used as a fulcrum. Eversion should be performed with a quick levering motion while applying slight traction. The palpebral conjunctiva can then be inspected and cleaned if necessary.

▶ **Double eversion.** To expose the superior fornix, the upper eyelid is fully everted around a Desmarres eyelid retractor (► Fig. 1.6c). This method is used solely by the ophthalmologist and is only discussed here for the sake of completeness. This eversion technique is required to remove foreign bodies or "lost" contact lenses from the superior fornix or to clean the conjunctiva of lime particles in a chemical injury with lime.

Note
Blepharospasm can render simple and full eversion very difficult, especially in the presence of chemical injury. In these cases, the spasm should first be eliminated by instilling a topical anesthetic such as oxybuprocaine hydrochloride eye drops.

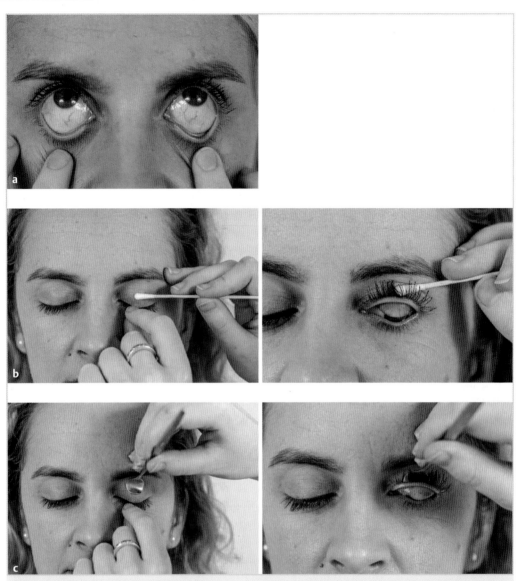

Fig. 1.6 Examination of the conjunctiva of the lower and upper lid as well as the upper and lower fornix conjuncti-vae. (a) The lower eyelid must be everted for this examination. The patient looks up while the examiner pulls the eyelid downward close to the anterior margin. (b) **Simple eversion for examination of the upper lid conjunctiva (i.e., the conjunctiva on the back surface of the tarsus).** The patient relaxes and looks down. The examiner places a swab or glass spatula superior to the tarsal region of the upper eyelid, grasps the eyelashes of the upper eyelid between the thumb and forefinger, and everts the eyelid using the swab as a fulcrum. (c) **Double eversion.** To examine the upper fornix in addition to the conjunctiva of the upper eyelid, the examiner must fold the eyelid twice over a Desmarres eyelid retractor.

1.9 Examination of the Cornea

The cornea is examined with a *point light source* and a *loupe* (▶ Fig.1.7). The cornea is *smooth, clear,* and *reflective with no blood vessels*. The reflection is distorted in the presence of corneal disorders. Epithelial defects, which are also very painful, will take on an intense green color after application of fluorescein dye; corneal infiltrates and scars are grayish-white. Evaluating corneal sensitivity is also important. Sensitivity is evaluated bilaterally to detect possible differences in the reaction of both eyes. The patient looks straight ahead during the examination. The examiner holds the upper eyelid to prevent reflexive closing and touches the cornea anteriorly (▶ Fig. 1.8). Decreased sensitivity can provide information about trigeminal or facial neuropathy, or may be a sign of a viral infection of the cornea.

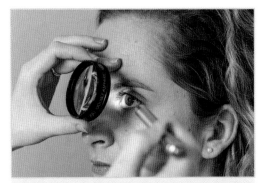

Fig. 1.7 Examination of the anterior portion of the eye. The examiner evaluates the eye using a focal light source and loupe magnification.

1.10 Examination of the Anterior Chamber

The anterior chamber is filled with clear aqueous humor. Cellular infiltration and collection of pus may occur (hypopyon). Bleeding in the anterior chamber is referred to as hyphema.

It is important to **evaluate the depth of the anterior chamber**. In a chamber of *normal depth*, the iris can be well illuminated by a lateral light source (▶ Fig. 1.9). In a *shallow anterior chamber* there will be a medial shadow on the iris. Pupillary dilation should be avoided in patients with shallow anterior chambers because of the risk of precipitating a glaucoma attack. Older patients with "small" hyperopic eyes are a particular risk group.

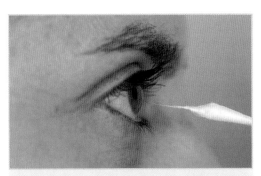

Fig. 1.8 Evaluation of corneal sensitivity with a distended cotton swab. The patient looks straight ahead while the examiner touches the cornea anteriorly.

> **Note**
> Dilation of the pupil with a mydriatic is *contraindicated* in patients with a shallow anterior chamber due to the risk of precipitating angle closure glaucoma.

1.11 Examination of the Lens

The ophthalmologist uses a **slit lamp** to examine the lens. The eye can also be examined with a **focused light** if necessary.

Direct illumination will produce a *red reflection of the fundus* if the lens is *clear* and *gray shadows* if lens opacities are present. With severe opacification of the lens, a gray coloration will be visible in the pupillary plane. Any such light-scattering opacity is referred to as a cataract.

1.12 Ophthalmoscopy

Indirect ophthalmoscopy (see p. 192) is usually performed by the ophthalmologist (see ▶ Fig. 12.4) and **produces a laterally reversed and upside-down image of the fundus.** Less experienced examiners will prefer **direct ophthalmoscopy**. Here, the ophthalmoscope is held as close to the patient as possible (▶ Fig. 1.10; see also ▶ Fig. 12.4a). Refractive errors in the patient's eye and the examiner's eye are corrected by selecting the ophthalmoscope lens (Rekoss disk with different plus and minus spherical lenses) required to bring the retina into focus. The examiner sees an *erect*, 16-power magnified image of the retina. The examination should be performed in a slightly darkened room with the patient's pupils dilated. Students should be able to identify the *optic disc*. In a normal eye, it is a sharply defined structure with vital coloration (i.e., yellowish-orange) at the level of the retina and may have a central excavation. The central vein lies lateral to the artery; venous diameter

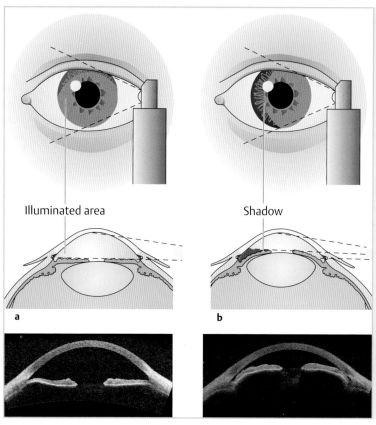

Illuminated area   Shadow

a   b

Fig. 1.9 Evaluation of the depth of the anterior chamber. **(a)** Normal anterior chamber depth: the iris can be well illuminated by a lateral light source. **(b)** Shallow anterior chamber: with lateral illumination there is a medial shadow on the iris. A variation in anterior chamber depth becomes particularly clear in optical coherence tomography (OCT) (see p. 198): deep anterior chamber in nearsighted (long) eyes, shallow anterior chamber in farsighted (short) eyes.

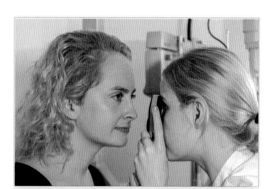

Fig. 1.10 Ophthalmoscopy (inspection of the fundus in an upright image with an electric ophthalmoscope). A direct ophthalmoscope produces an erect image of the fundus. The examiner views the patient's left eye with his or her own left eye so that their noses do not interfere with the examination. The examiner's left hand rests on the dial of the Rekoss disk of the ophthalmoscope to bring the retina into focus.

is normally 1.5 times greater than arterial diameter. Each vascular structure should be of uniform diameter, and there should be no vascular constriction where vessels overlap. A spontaneous *venous pulse* is normal; an *arterial pulse* is abnormal. Younger patients will have a foveal and macular light reflex, and the fundus will have a reddish color (see ▶ Fig. 12.8). An ophthalmologist should be consulted if there are any abnormal findings.

1.13 Confrontation Field Testing (Examination of the Visual Field)

Confrontation testing provides gross screening of the field of vision where perimetry tests (visual field tests) are not available (see p. 249).

The patient faces the examiner at a standard distance of 1 meter with his or her eyes at the same level as the examiner's (▶ Fig. 1.11). Both focus on the other's opposite eye (i.e., the patient's left eye focuses on the examiner's right eye) while covering their contralateral eye with the palm of the hand. The examiner moves an object such as a pen, cotton swab, or finger from the periphery toward the midline in all four quadrants (in the superior and inferior nasal fields and superior and inferior temporal fields). The patient indicates when he or she sees the object. A patient with a *normal field of vision* will see the object at the same time as the examiner; a patient with an *abnormal or restricted field of vision* will see the object later than the examiner.

Note
Confrontation testing is a gross method of assessing the field of vision. It can be used to diagnose a severely restricted field of vision such as homonymous hemianopsia or quadrant anopsia.

1.14 Measurement of Intraocular Pressure

With the patient's eyes closed, the examiner places his or her hands on the patient's head and palpates the eye through the upper eyelid with both index fingers (▶ Fig. 1.12). The test is repeated on the contralateral eye for comparison.

Note
A "rock-hard" eyeball occurs only in acute angle closure glaucoma. Slight increases in intraocular pressure, such as occur in chronic glaucoma, will not be palpable.

1.15 Eye Drops, Ointment, and Bandages

Eye drops and ointment should be administered posterior to the *everted lower eyelid* (▶ Fig. 1.13). One drop or strip of ointment approximately 1 cm long should be administered *laterally to the inferior*

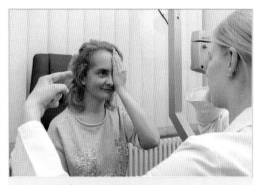

Fig. 1.11 Confrontation field testing. The patient faces the examiner at a distance of 1 m with his or her eyes at the same level as the examiner's. Each focuses on the other's opposite eye while covering their contralateral eye with the palm of the hand. The examiner moves his or her index finger from the periphery toward the midline in all four quadrants in the nasal and temporal fields and in the superior and inferior fields.

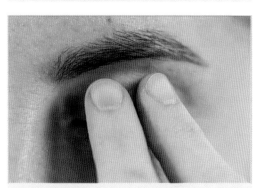

Fig. 1.12 Measurement of intraocular pressure. The examiner uses both index fingers to palpate the eye through the upper eyelid.

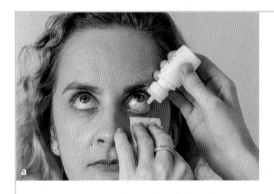

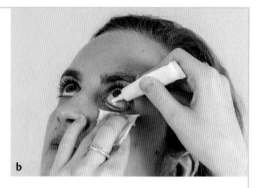

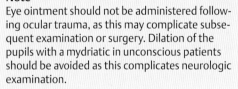

Fig. 1.13 Administration of eye drops and ointment. To avoid contamination or injury, the patient's eyelashes and eyes may not be touched while administering eye drops **(a)** and ointment **(b)**. Often patients must apply the eye drops themselves **(c)**. This is best done in the supine position or with the head tipped back.

conjunctival sac. To avoid injury to the eye, drops should be administered with the patient *supine* or seated with the *head tilted back and supported.* The person administering the medication places his or her hand on the patient's face for support. Bottles and tubes must not come into contact with the patient's eyelashes as they might otherwise become contaminated. Allow the drops or strip of ointment to drop into the conjunctival sac.

Note
Eye ointment should not be administered following ocular trauma, as this may complicate subsequent examination or surgery. Dilation of the pupils with a mydriatic in unconscious patients should be avoided as this complicates neurologic examination.

▶ **Eye bandage** (▶ Fig. 1.14). A sterile swab or commercially available bandage (two oval layers of bandage material with a layer of cotton between them) can be used. Care should be taken to avoid touching the side in contact with the eye. The bandage is fixed to the forehead and cheek with strips of adhesive tape.

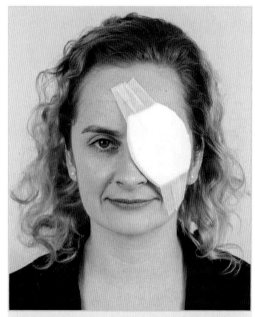

Fig. 1.14 Eye bandage. In case of an injury (corneal laceration), the eye should be covered with a sterile stable eye patch, fixed with a minimum of three adhesive tapes, with no pressure being put on the eye, and the nose and mouth being left uncovered.

Chapter 2

Eyelids (Palpebrae)

2 Eyelids (Palpebrae)

Peter Wagner and Gerhard K. Lang

2.1 Basic Knowledge

▶ **Protective functions of the eyelids.** The eyelids are folds of muscular soft tissue that lie anterior to the eyeball and protect it from injury. Their **shape** is such that the eyeball is completely covered when they are closed. Strong mechanical, optical, and acoustic stimuli (such as a foreign body, blinding light, or sudden loud noise) "automatically" elicit an **eye-closing reflex**. The cornea is also protected by an additional upward movement of the eyeball (**Bell's phenomenon**). **Regular blinking** (20–30 times/min) helps to uniformly distribute glandular secretions and tears over the conjunctiva and cornea, keeping them from drying out.

▶ **Structure of the eyelids.** The eyelids consist of superficial and deep layers (▶ Fig. 2.1).
- **Superficial layer** (supplied by N. V$_1$, N. V$_2$):
  - Thin, well-vascularized layer of **skin**.
  - Sweat glands.
  - Modified **sweat glands** (ciliary glands or **glands of Moll**) and **sebaceous glands** (**glands of Zeis**) in the vicinity of the eyelashes.
  - Striated muscle fibers of the **orbicularis oculi muscle**, which actively closes the eye (supplied by the facial nerve).
  - Striated muscle fibers of the **levator palpebrae muscle**, which actively opens the eye (supplied by the oculomotor nerve).
- **Deep layer:**
  - The **tarsal plate** gives the eyelid firmness and shape.

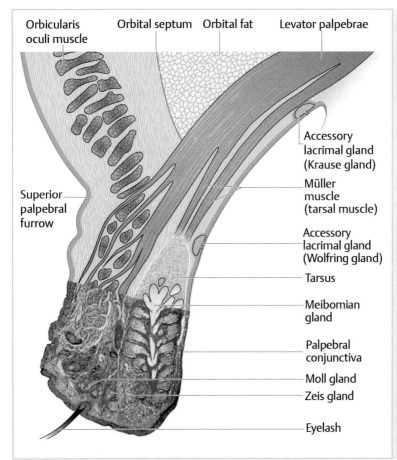

Orbicularis oculi muscle · Orbital septum · Orbital fat · Levator palpebrae

Superior palpebral furrow

Accessory lacrimal gland (Krause gland)

Müller muscle (tarsal muscle)

Accessory lacrimal gland (Wolfring gland)

Tarsus

Meibomian gland

Palpebral conjunctiva

Moll gland

Zeis gland

Eyelash

Fig. 2.1 Sagittal section through the upper eyelid. The superficial layer of the eyelid consists of the skin, glands of Moll and of Zeis, and the orbicularis oculi and levator palpebrae muscles. The deep layer consists of the tarsal plate, tarsal muscle, palpebral conjunctiva, and meibomian glands.

○ Smooth musculature of the levator palpebrae that inserts into the tarsal plate (**tarsal muscle**). The tarsal muscle is supplied by the sympathetic nervous system and regulates the width of the palpebral fissure. High sympathetic tone contracts the tarsal muscle and widens the palpebral fissure; low sympathetic tone relaxes the tarsal muscle and narrows the palpebral fissure.

○ The **palpebral conjunctiva** is firmly attached to the tarsal plate. It forms an articular layer for the eyeball. Every time the eye blinks, it acts like a windshield wiper and uniformly distributes glandular secretions and tears over the conjunctiva and cornea.

○ **Sebaceous glands (tarsal or meibomian glands)** are tubular structures in the cartilage of the eyelid that lubricate the margin of the eyelid. Their function is to prevent the escape of tear fluid past the margins of the eyelids and build the superficial oily layer of the tear film, preventing it from evaporating. The fibers of Riolan's muscle at the inferior aspect of these sebaceous glands squeeze out the ducts of the tarsal glands every time the eye blinks.

The **eyelashes** project from the anterior aspect of the margin of the eyelid. On the upper eyelid, approximately 150 eyelashes are arranged in three or four rows; on the lower eyelid, there are about 75 in two rows. Like the **eyebrows**, the eyelashes help prevent dust and sweat from entering the eye. The orbital septum is located between the tarsal plate and the margin of the orbit. It is a membranous sheet of connective tissue attached to the margin of the orbit that retains the orbital fat.

2.2 Examination Methods

The eyelids are examined by direct inspection under a bright light. A slit lamp can be used for this purpose. **Bilateral inspection of the eyelids** includes the following aspects:

• *Eyelid position.* Normally, the margins of the eyelids are in contact with the eyeball and the puncta are submerged in the lacus lacrimalis.

• *Width of the palpebral fissure.* When the eye is open and looking straight ahead, the upper lid should cover the superior margin of the cornea by about 2 mm. Occasionally a thin strip of sclera will be visible between the cornea and the margin of the lower lid. The width of the palpebral fissure is normally 6 to 10 mm, and the distance between the lateral and medial angles of the eye is 28 to 30 mm (▶ Fig. 2.2). Varying widths of the gaps between the eyelids may be a sign of protrusion of the eyeball, enophthalmos, or eyeballs of varying size (▶ Table 2.1).

• *Skin of the eyelid.* The skin of the eyelid is thin with only a slight amount of subcutaneous fatty tissue. Allergic reaction and inflammation can rapidly cause extensive edema and swelling. In older patients, the skin of the upper eyelid may become increasingly flaccid (cutis laxa senilis). Occasionally, it can even hang down over the eyelashes and restrict the field of vision (dermatochalasis or blepharochalasis).

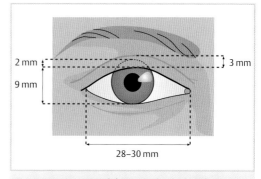

Fig. 2.2 Dimensions of the normal palpebral fissure. The width of the palpebral fissure is an important indicator for a number of pathologic changes in the eye (see ▶ Table 2.1).

Table 2.1 Possible causes of abnormal width of the palpebral fissure

Increased palpebral fissure	Decreased palpebral fissure
• Peripheral facial paresis (lagophthalmos) • Graves's disease • Perinaud's syndrome • Buphthalmos • High-grade myopia • Retrobulbar tumor	• Congenital ptosis • Ptosis in oculomotor nerve palsy • Ptosis in myasthenia gravis • Sympathetic ptosis (see p. 15) (with Horner's syndrome) • Progressive ophthalmoplegia (Graefe's sign) • Microphthalmos • Enophthalmos • Shrinkage of the orbital fat (as in senile enophthalmos)

The palpebral conjunctiva is examined by **simple eversion of the eyelid** (see ▶ Fig. 1.6 b). The normal palpebral conjunctiva is smooth and shiny without any scar strictures or papilliform projections.

Full eversion of the upper eyelid with a Desmarres eyelid retractor (see ▶ Fig. 1.6 c) allows examination of the **superior fornix** (for normal appearance, see palpebral conjunctiva).

2.3 Developmental Anomalies

2.3.1 Coloboma

Definition
A normally unilateral triangular eyelid defect with its base at the margin of the eyelid occurring most often in the upper eyelid (▶ Fig. 2.3).

▶ **Epidemiology and etiology.** Colobomas are *rare* defects resulting from a reduction malformation (defective closure of the optic cup). They are only rarely the result of an injury.

▶ **Diagnostic considerations.** The disorder is often accompanied by additional deformities such as dermoid cysts or a microphthalmos. Congenital defects of the first embryonic branchial arch that can result in coloboma include Franceschetti's syndrome (mandibulofacial dysostosis) or Goldenhar's syndrome (oculoauriculovertebral dysplasia). Depending on the extent of the coloboma, desiccation symptoms on the conjunctiva and cornea with incipient ulceration may arise from the lack of regular and uniform moistening of the conjunctiva and cornea.

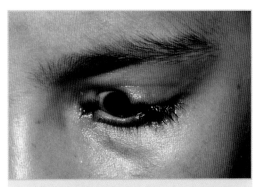

Fig. 2.3 Congenital coloboma. The triangular eyelid defect with its base at the margin of the eyelid results from a reduction malformation during closure of the optic cup in the embryonic stage.

▶ **Treatment.** Defects are closed by direct approximation or plastic surgery with a skin flap.

2.3.2 Epicanthal Folds

The epicanthal fold is a crescentic fold of skin usually extending bilaterally between the upper and lower eyelids and covering the medial angle of the eye. This *rare congenital anomaly* is *harmless* and is typical in the population of Eastern Asia. However, it also occurs with Down syndrome (trisomy 21 syndrome). Thirty percent of newborns have epicanthal folds until the age of 6 months. Where one fold is more pronounced, it can simulate esotropia. The nasal bridge becomes more pronounced as the child grows, and most epicanthal folds disappear by the age of 4 years.

2.3.3 Blepharophimosis

This refers to **shortening of the horizontal palpebral fissure without pathologic changes in the eyelids.** The palpebral fissure, normally 28 to 30 mm wide, may be reduced to half that width. Blepharophimosis is a *rare* disorder that is either *congenital* or *acquired* (for example, from scar contracture or aging). As long as the center of the pupil remains unobstructed despite the decreased size of the palpebral fissure, *surgical enlargement* of the palpebral fissure (by canthotomy or plastic surgery) has a purely cosmetic purpose.

2.3.4 Ankyloblepharon

This refers to **horizontal shortening of the palpebral fissure with fusion of the eyelids at the lateral and medial angles of the eye.** Usually, the partial or total fusion between the upper and lower eyelids will be bilateral, and the palpebral fissure will be partially or completely occluded as a result. Posterior to the eyelids, the eyeball itself will be deformed or totally absent. Ankyloblepharon is frequently associated with other skull deformities.

2.4 Deformities

2.4.1 Ptosis Palpebrae

Definition
Paralysis of the levator palpebrae muscle with resulting drooping of one or both upper eyelids (from the Greek *ptosis*, a falling). The following forms are differentiated according to their origin (see also Etiology):
- **Congenital ptosis** (▶ Fig. 2.4).
- **Acquired ptosis:**
  - Paralytic ptosis.
  - Sympathetic ptosis.
  - Myotonic ptosis.
  - Traumatic ptosis.

▶ **Epidemiology.** Ptosis is a rare disorder.

▶ **Etiology.** Ptosis may be congenital or acquired.

▶ **Congenital ptosis.** The disorder is usually hereditary and is primarily autosomal-dominant as opposed to recessive. The cause is frequently *aplasia* in the *core of the oculomotor nerve* (neurogenic) that supplies the levator palpebrae muscle; less frequently it is attributable to an *underdeveloped levator palpebrae muscle* (myogenic).

▶ **Acquired ptosis**
- Neurogenic causes:
  - Oculomotor palsy (*paralytic ptosis*).
  - Lesions in the sympathetic nerve (*sympathetic ptosis*) in Horner's palsy (ptosis, miosis, and enophthalmos).

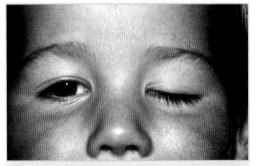

Fig. 2.4 Congenital ptosis. Congenital ptosis of the levator palpebrae muscle causes the upper eyelid to droop; usually the deformity is unilateral. Amblyopia will result if the center of the pupil is covered.

- Myotonic ptosis: myasthenia gravis and myotonic dystrophy.
- *Traumatic ptosis* can occur after injuries.

▶ **Symptoms.** The drooping of the upper eyelid may be *unilateral* (usually a sign of a *neurogenic* cause) or *bilateral* (usually a sign of a *myogenic* cause). A characteristic feature of the *unilateral form* is that the patient attempts to increase the palpebral fissure by frowning (contracting the frontalis muscle). **Congenital ptosis** (▶ Fig. 2.4) generally affects one eye only; bilateral symptoms are observed far less frequently (7%).

▶ **Diagnostic considerations**
▶ **Congenital ptosis.** The affected eyelid in general is underdeveloped. The skin of the upper eyelid is smooth and thin; the superior palpebral furrow is absent or ill-defined. A typical symptom is "lid lag," in which the upper eyelid does not move when the patient glances down. *This important distinguishing symptom excludes acquired ptosis in differential diagnosis.* In about 3% of cases, congenital ptosis is associated with epicanthal folds and blepharophimosis (Waardenburg's syndrome).

Congenital ptosis can occur in varying degrees of severity and may be complicated by the presence of additional eyelid and ocular muscle disorders such as strabismus.

> **Note**
> Congenital ptosis in which the upper eyelid droops over the center of the pupil always involves an increased risk of amblyopia. In bilateral congenital ptosis, the child tilts the head back so that both eyes can see. In this case, there is no risk of amblyopia.

▶ **Acquired ptosis**
- *Paralytic ptosis* in oculomotor palsy is usually unilateral with the drooping eyelid covering the whole eye. For additional information regarding oculomotor palsy see page 314. Often there will be other signs of palsy in the area supplied by the oculomotor nerve. In *external oculomotor palsy*, only the extraocular muscles are affected (mydriasis will not be present), whereas in *complete oculomotor palsy*, the inner ciliary muscle and the sphincter pupillae muscle are also affected (internal ophthalmoplegia with loss of accommodation, mydriasis, and complete loss of pupillary light reflexes).
- *Myasthenia gravis* (myogenic ptosis that is often bilateral and may be asymmetrical) is associated with abnormal fatigue of the striated extraocular

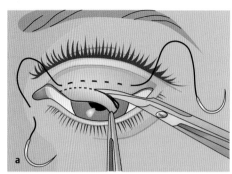

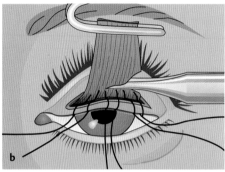

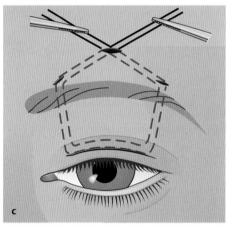

Fig. 2.5 Methods of surgical retraction of the upper eyelid. (a) The **Fasanella–Servat** procedure, indicated for correction of minimal ptosis, involves resection of a portion of the tarsus (2 mm or less) to vertically shorten the eyelid. **(b)** The amount of muscle removed in a **levator resection** depends on levator function (ranging from approximately 10 mm with slight ptosis, up to 22 mm with moderate ptosis). **(c)** Where levator function is poor (less than 5 mm), the upper eyelid can be connected to tissue in the eyebrow region. The **frontalis suspension** technique may employ autogenous fascia lata or synthetic material.

muscles. Ptosis typically becomes more severe as the day goes on.
• *Sympathetic ptosis* occurs in Horner's palsy (ptosis, miosis, and enophthalmos).

Note
Rapidly opening and closing the eyelids provokes ptosis in myasthenia gravis and simplifies the diagnosis.

▶ **Treatment** (▶ Fig. 2.5 a, b)
• **Congenital ptosis.** This involves surgical retraction of the upper eyelid, which should be undertaken as quickly as possible when there is a risk of the affected eye developing a visual impairment as a result of the ptosis.
• **Acquired ptosis.** Treatment depends on the cause. As palsies often *resolve spontaneously,* the patient should be observed before resorting to surgical intervention. Conservative treatment with special eyeglasses may be sufficient even in irreversible cases.

Because of the risk of overcorrecting or undercorrecting the disorder, several operations may be necessary.

▶ **Prognosis and complications.** Prompt surgical intervention in congenital ptosis can prevent *amblyopia.* Surgical overcorrection of the ptosis can lead to desiccation of the conjunctiva and cornea with *ulceration,* as a result of incomplete closure of the eyelids.

2.4.2 Entropion

Definition
Entropion is characterized by inward rotation of the eyelid margin. The margin of the eyelid and eyelashes or even the outer skin of the eyelid are in contact with the globe instead of only the conjunctiva. The following forms are differentiated according to their origin (see Etiology):
• Congenital entropion (▶ Fig. 2.6).
• Senile entropion (▶ Fig. 2.7).
• Cicatricial entropion.

▶ **Epidemiology.** Congenital entropion occurs frequently among Asians but is rare among people of European descent, in whom the senile and cicatricial forms are more commonly encountered (see also Chapter 18 on connective tissue injury, p. 320).

▶ **Etiology**
- **Congenital entropion.** This results from fleshy thickening of the skin and orbicularis oculi muscle near the margin of the eyelid. *Usually the lower eyelid is affected.* This condition may persist into adulthood.
- **Senile entropion.** This *affects only the lower eyelid.* A combination of several pathogenetic factors of varying severity is usually involved:
  - The structures supporting the lower eyelid (palpebral ligaments, tarsus, and eyelid retractor) may become lax with age, causing the tarsus to tilt inward.
  - This causes the fibers of the orbicularis oculi muscle to override the normally superior margin of the eyelid, intensifying the blepharospasm resulting from the permanent contact between the eyelashes and the eyeball.
  - Senile enophthalmos, usually occurring in old age as a result of atrophy of the orbit fatty tissue, further contributes to instability of the lower eyelid.
- **Cicatricial entropion.** This form of entropion is frequently the result of postinfectious or post-traumatic tarsal contracture (such as trachoma [see p. 55]; burns and chemical injuries). Causes can also include allergic and toxic reactions (pemphigus, Stevens–Johnson syndrome, and Lyell's syndrome).

▶ **Symptoms and diagnostic considerations (see also Etiology).** Constant rubbing of the eyelashes against the eyeball (trichiasis) represents a permanent foreign-body irritation of the conjunctiva which causes a blepharospasm (eyelid spasm, see p. 19) that in turn exacerbates the entropion. The chronically irritated conjunctiva is reddened, and the eye fills with tears. Only congenital entropion is usually asymptomatic.

▶ **Treatment**
- **Congenital entropion.** To the extent that any treatment is required, it consists of measured, semicircular resection of skin and orbicularis oculi muscle tissue that can be supplemented by everting sutures where indicated.
- **Senile entropion.** Surgical management must be tailored to the specific situation. Usually treatment combines several techniques such as shortening the eyelid horizontally combined with weakening or diverting the pretarsal fibers of the orbicularis oculi muscle and shortening the skin vertically.

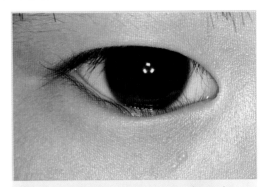

Fig. 2.6 Congenital entropion. Congenital inward rotation of the margins of the upper and lower eyelids is a frequent finding in Asian populations and is usually asymptomatic.

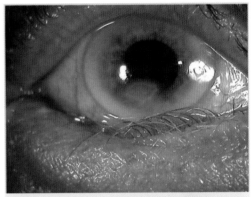

Fig. 2.7 Senile entropion. Displaced fibers of the orbicularis oculi muscle cause the eyelashes of the lower eyelid to turn inward. This causes damage to the corneal epithelium (= so-called corneal erosion, visualized by application of fluorescein). Surgical intervention is indicated to correct the laxity of the lower eyelid.

- **Cicatricial entropion.** The surgical management of this form is identical to that of senile entropion.

Note
An adhesive bandage can be applied to increase tension on the eyelid for temporary relief of symptoms prior to surgery.

▶ **Prognosis and complications**

>
>
> **Note**
> Congenital entropion is usually asymptomatic and often resolves within the first few months of life.

- **Senile entropion.** The prognosis is favorable with prompt surgical intervention, although the disorder may recur. Left untreated, senile entropion entails a risk of damage to the corneal epithelium with superinfection which may progress to the complete clinical syndrome of a serpiginous corneal ulcer (see p. 75).
- **Cicatricial entropion.** The prognosis is favorable with prompt surgical intervention (i. e., before any corneal changes occur).

2.4.3 Ectropion

Definition
Ectropion refers to the condition in which the margin of the eyelid is turned away from the eyeball. This condition almost exclusively affects the lower eyelid. The following forms are differentiated according to their origin (see also Etiology):
- Congenital ectropion.
- Senile ectropion.
- Paralytic ectropion.
- Cicatricial ectropion.

▶ **Epidemiology.** Senile ectropion is the most prevalent form; the paralytic and cicatricial forms occur less frequently. Congenital ectropion is very rare and is usually associated with other developmental anomalies of the eyelid and face such as Franceschetti's syndrome.

▶ **Etiology**
- **Congenital ectropion:** see Epidemiology.
- **Senile ectropion:** the palpebral ligaments and tarsus may become lax with age, causing the tarsus to sag outward (▶ Fig. 2.8).
- **Paralytic ectropion:** this is caused by facial paralysis with resulting loss of function of the orbicularis oculi muscle that closes the eyelid.
- **Cicatricial ectropion:** like cicatricial entropion, this form is usually a sequela of infection or injury.

▶ **Symptoms and diagnostic considerations.** Left untreated, incomplete closure of the eyelids can lead to symptoms associated with desiccation of

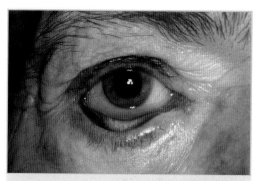

Fig. 2.8 Senile ectropion. The structures supporting the eyelid are lax, causing the lower eyelid to sag outward.

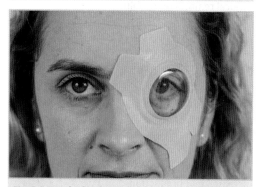

Fig. 2.9 Watch glass bandage for paralytic ectropion. In patients with lagophthalmos resulting from facial paralysis, a watch glass bandage creates a moist chamber that protects the cornea against desiccation.

the cornea including ulceration from lagophthalmos. At the same time, the eversion of the punctum causes tears to flow down across the cheek instead of draining into the nose. Wiping away the tears increases the ectropion. This results in chronic conjunctivitis and blepharitis.

▶ **Treatment**
- **Congenital ectropion:** surgery.
- **Senile ectropion:** surgery is indicated. A proven procedure is to tighten the lower eyelid via a tarsal wedge resection followed by horizontal tightening of the skin.
- **Paralytic ectropion:** depending on the severity of the disorder, artificial tear solutions, eyeglasses with an anatomic lateral protective feature, or a "watch glass" bandage (▶ Fig. 2.9) may be sufficient to prevent desiccation of the cornea. In severe or irreversible cases, the lagophthalmos is treated surgically via a lateral tarsorrhaphy.
- **Cicatricial ectropion:** plastic surgery is often required to correct the eyelid deformity.

▶ **Prognosis.** The prognosis is favorable when the disorder is treated promptly. Sometimes several operations are required. Surgery is more difficult when scarring is present.

2.4.4 Trichiasis

Trichiasis refers to the rare **postinfectious or post-traumatic inward turning of the eyelashes.** The deformity causes the eyelashes to run against the conjunctiva and cornea, causing a permanent foreign-body sensation, increased tear secretion, and chronic conjunctivitis. The eyelash follicles can be obliterated by electrolysis. The disorder may also be successfully treated by cryocautery epilation or surgical removal of the follicle bed.

2.4.5 Blepharospasm

> **Definition**
> This refers to an involuntary spasmodic contraction of the orbicularis oculi muscle supplied by the facial nerve.

▶ **Etiology.** In addition to photosensitivity and increased tear production, blepharospasm will also accompany *inflammation* or *irritation of the anterior chamber.* (Photosensitivity, epiphora, and blepharospasm form a triad of reactive clinical symptoms.) Causes of the disorder include *extrapyramidal disease* such as encephalitis or multiple sclerosis. *Trigeminal neuralgia* or *psychogenic causes* may also be present.

▶ **Symptoms.** Clinical symptoms include spasmodically narrowed or closed palpebral fissures and lowered eyebrows.

▶ **Treatment.** Treatment depends on the cause of the disorder. *Mild cases* can be controlled well with muscle relaxants. *Severe cases* may require transection of the fibers of the facial nerve supplying the orbicularis oculi muscle. The disorder may also be successfully treated with repeated local injections of botulinum toxin.

▶ **Prognosis.** The prognosis is *good* where a *cause-related* treatment is possible. *Essential* blepharospasm *does not respond well* to treatment.

2.5 Disorders of the Skin and Margin of the Eyelid

2.5.1 Contact Eczema

▶ **Epidemiology.** Light-skinned patients and patients susceptible to allergy are frequently affected.

▶ **Etiology.** Contact eczema is caused by an antigen–antibody reaction in patients with intolerance to certain noxious substances. *Cosmetics, adhesive bandages*, or *eye drops and eye ointments* are often responsible, particularly the *preservatives* used in them, such as benzalkonium chloride.

▶ **Symptoms.** Reddening, swelling, lichenification, and severe itching of the skin of the eyelid occur initially, followed by scaling of the indurated skin with a sensation of tension (▶ Fig. 2.10).

▶ **Treatment.** Treatment consists of eliminating the causative agent. (Allergy testing may be necessary.) Limited use of corticosteroids usually brings quick relief of symptoms.

▶ **Prognosis.** The prognosis is good if the cause can be identified.

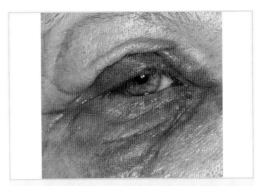

Fig. 2.10 Contact eczema. This disorder is frequently caused by preservatives such as those used in eye drops. They cause typical reddening, swelling, and lichenification of the skin of the eyelid.

Table 2.2 Differential diagnosis of eyelid edema

Criteria	Inflammatory eyelid edema	Noninflammatory eyelid edema
Symptoms	• Swelling	• Swelling
	• Reddening	• Pale skin
	• Sensation of heat	• Cool skin
	• Painful	• Painless
	• Usually unilateral	• Usually bilateral
Possible causes	• Hordeolum (see p. 24)	• Systemic disorder:
	• Abscess (see p. 22)	– Heart
		– Kidneys
	• Erysipelas	– Thyroid gland
	• Eczema	
	• Associated with:	• Allergy such as Quincke's edema
	○ Paranasal sinus disorders	
	○ Orbital cellulitis (see p. 263)	
	○ Dacryoadenitis (see p. 41)	
	○ Dacryocystitis (see p. 34)	

2.5.2 Eyelid Edema

Definition
This refers to swelling of the eyelid due to abnormal collection of fluid in the subcutaneous tissue.

▶ **Epidemiology.** Eyelid edema is a frequently encountered clinical symptom.

▶ **Etiology.** The skin of the eyelid is affected intensively by infectious and allergic processes. With the upper eyelid's relatively thin skin and the loose structure of its subcutaneous tissue, water can easily accumulate and cause eyelid edema.

▶ **Symptoms.** The intensity of swelling in the eyelid will vary depending on the cause (▶ Table 2.2). The location of swelling is also influenced by gravity and can vary in intensity. For example, it may be more intense in the early morning after the patient rises than in the evening (▶ Fig. 2.11).

  ▶ Table 2.2 shows the causes and **differential diagnosis** for inflammatory and noninflammatory eyelid edemas.

▶ **Treatment.** This depends on the cause of the disorder.

▶ **Clinical course and prognosis.** This depends on the underlying disorder.

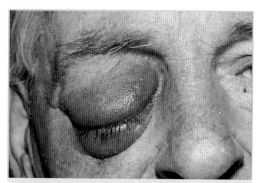

Fig. 2.11 Eyelid edema. With its relatively thin skin and its subcutaneous tissue that contains little fat, the upper eyelid is particularly susceptible to rapid fluid accumulations from pathologic processes.

2.5.3 Seborrheic Blepharitis

Definition
This relatively frequent disorder is characterized by scaly inflammation of the margins of the eyelids. Usually both eyes are affected.

▶ **Etiology.** There are often *several contributing causes.* The constitution of the skin, seborrhea, refractive anomalies, hypersecretion of the eyelid glands, and external stimuli such as dust, smoke, and dry air in air-conditioned rooms often contribute to persistent chronic inflammation.

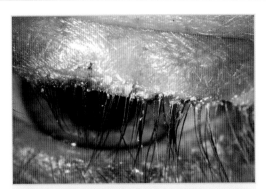

Fig. 2.12 Seborrheic blepharitis. The margins of the eyelids are slightly reddened, with adhesion of the eyelashes. Scaly deposits form along the margins of the eyelids.

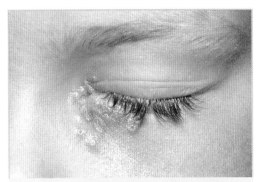

Fig. 2.13 Herpes simplex of the eyelid. Painful vesicles filled with serous fluid erupt in clusters at the angle of the eye.

▶ **Symptoms and diagnostic considerations.** The margins of the eyelids usually exhibit *slight inflammatory changes* such as thickening. The eyelashes adhere due to the increased secretion from the glands of the eyelids, and *scaly deposits* form (▶ Fig. 2.12). The disorder will often be accompanied by chronic conjunctivitis.

▶ **Treatment.** Treatment depends on the cause of the disorder (see Etiology). The scales and crusts can usually be softened with *warm olive oil* and then easily removed with a cotton-tipped applicator. In more severe cases, recommended treatment includes expressing the glands of the eyelid and local application of *antibiotic ointment*. Treatment with *topical steroids* may be indicated under certain conditions.

▶ **Prognosis.** The prognosis is good, although the clinical course of the disorder is often quite protracted.

2.5.4 Herpes Simplex of the Eyelids

Definition
An acute, usually unilateral eyelid disorder accompanied by skin and mucous membrane vesicles.

▶ **Etiology.** Infection of the skin of the eyelids results when latent herpes simplex viruses present in the tissue are activated by *ultraviolet radiation.* The virus spreads along sensory nerve fibers from the trigeminal ganglion to the surface of the skin.

▶ **Symptoms.** Typical *clustered eruptions* of painful *vesicles* filled with serous fluid frequently occur at the junction of mucous membranes and skin (▶ Fig. 2.13). Later the vesicles dry and crusts form. Lesions heal without scarring. The disorder is usually unilateral.

▶ **Treatment.** Topical use of virostatic agents is indicated. The patient should avoid intense ultraviolet radiation as a prophylactic measure against recurrence.

▶ **Prognosis.** The prognosis is good, although the disorder frequently recurs.

2.5.5 Herpes Zoster Ophthalmicus

Definition
Facial rash caused by the varicella-zoster virus (human herpesvirus 3).

▶ **Epidemiology.** The disorder usually affects immunocompromised persons between the ages of 40 and 60 years who have underlying disorders.

▶ **Etiology.** The disorder is caused by the varicella-zoster virus, which initially manifests itself as chickenpox. If activation or reinfection occurs, the latent neurotropic viruses present in the body can lead to the clinical syndrome of herpes zoster ophthalmicus (▶ Fig. 2.14).

▶ **Symptoms and diagnostic considerations.** The incubation period is 7 to 18 days, after which *severe pain* occurs in the area supplied by the first branch

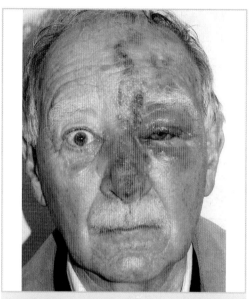

Fig. 2.14 Herpes zoster ophthalmicus. The facial rash of herpes zoster is caused by the neurotropic varicella-zoster virus. After the clear watery vesicles burst, brownish scabs form, which are later shed. Of special prognostic significance are efflorescences reaching the tip of the nose, indicating an involvement of the nasociliaris nerve (Hutchinson's sign, with an increased likelihood of ocular involvement).

of the trigeminal nerve (the ophthalmic nerve with its frontal, lacrimal, and nasociliary branches). *Prodromal symptoms* of erythema, swelling, photosensitivity, and lacrimation may occur before the characteristic *clear watery vesicles* appear. The vesicles burst and brownish scabs form, which are later shed. *Blepharitis* is also present in 50 to 70% of cases (see p. 20). As herpes zoster usually affects immunocompromised persons, the patient should be examined for a possible underlying disorder.

Note
The skin sensitivity at the tip of the nose should be evaluated on both sides in the initial stage of the disorder. Decreased sensitivity to touch suggests involvement of the nasociliary branch of the ophthalmic nerve, which can lead to severe intraocular inflammation.

▶ **Treatment.** This includes topical virostatic agents and systemic acyclovir, brivudin, famciclovir, or valacyclovir.

▶ **Complications.** Involvement of the nasociliary branch of the ophthalmic nerve can lead to severe intraocular inflammation.

▶ **Prognosis.** The skin lesions heal within 3 to 4 weeks; scars may remain. Often neuralgiform pain and hypesthesia may persist.

2.5.6 Eyelid Abscess

Definition
Circumscribed collection of pus with severe inflammation, swelling, and subsequent fluctuation.

▶ **Etiology.** An abscess of the upper or lower eyelid can form as a sequela of minor trauma, insect sting, or spread of inflammation from the paranasal sinuses.

▶ **Symptoms.** The severe inflammation and swelling often make it impossible actively to open the eye (▶ Fig. 2.15). The contents of the abscess can fluctuate during the clinical course of the disorder. Spontaneous perforation with pus drainage can occur.

▶ **Treatment.** Oral or intravenous antibiotics and dry heat are indicated. A stab incision can relieve tension at the onset of fluctuation.

▶ **Prognosis.** The prognosis is generally good.

Note
Orbital cellulitis or cavernous sinus thrombosis can occasionally occur as a sequela of eyelid abscess, especially when located at the medial angle of the eye. This represents a life-threatening complication.

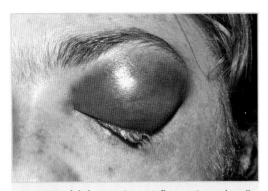

Fig. 2.15 Eyelid abscess. Severe inflammation and swelling make it impossible to open the eye actively.

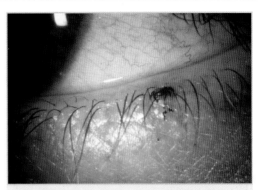

Fig. 2.16 Tick infestation of the lower eyelid. If the tick has attached, it must be removed mechanically.

2.5.7 Tick Infestation of the Eyelids

Ticks have been known to infest the eyelids (▶ Fig. 2.16). They are thought to be vectors of borreliosis and can cause encephalitis. Treatment consists of mechanical removal of the parasites.

2.5.8 Louse Infestation of the Eyelids

This refers to **infestation of the margin of the eyelid with crab lice** as a result of poor hygienic conditions. The small oval nits frequently hang from the eyelashes (▶ Fig. 2.17), causing inflammation of the margin of the eyelid with severe itching. *Mechanical removal with forceps* is a time-consuming but effective treatment. *Application of a 2% mercury precipitate ointment* over an extended period is also effective.

2.5.9 Hair Follicle Mite

With increasing age, almost everyone can be diagnosed with hair follicle mites (*Demodex folliculorum*) (▶ Fig. 2.18). However, the hair follicle mite only leads to diseases like chronic inflammation of the palpebral margins or dry eye in certain cases. The patients principally affected are those already suffering from seborrheic dermatitis or rosacea.

Demodex mites attack the hair follicles of the eyelashes and form a cuff of scales at the base of the cilia. They can also occlude the meibomian sebaceous glands, so that the oily layer of the lacrimal film is compromised. This results in the onset of dry eye symptoms like burning, redness, itching, and a grainy feeling.

Therapeutically, in addition to regular massage of the eyelid borders with 50% tea tree oil, local application of antibiotics such as erythromycin or metronidazole has proven efficacious.

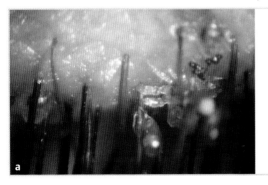

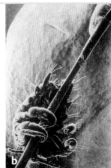

Fig. 2.17 Louse infestation of the eyelids. (a) In poor hygienic conditions, crab lice can infest the bases of the eyelashes. (b) Scanning electron microscopy (SEM) image, showing a louse and a deposited nit on the eyelash.

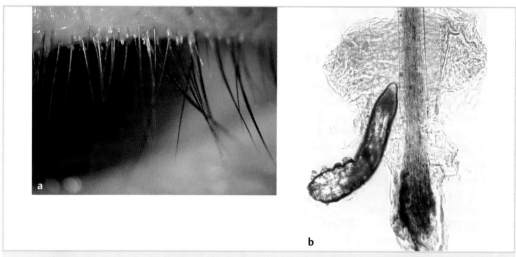

Fig. 2.18 Hair follicle mites. **(a)** Hair follicle mites form a cuff of scales at the base of the eyelashes. **(b)** Plucked eyelash with mite: immediate verification under the light microscope.

2.6 Disorders of the Eyelid Glands

2.6.1 Hordeolum

Definition
A hordeolum is the result of an acute bacterial infection of one or more *eyelid glands*. If several glands are affected at the same time, it is called hordeolosis.

▶ **Epidemiology and etiology.** *Staphylococcus aureus* is a common cause of hordeolum. **External hordeolum** involves infection of the glands of Zeis or Moll. **Internal hordeolum** arises from infection of the meibomian glands. Hordeolum is often associated with diabetes, gastrointestinal disorders, or acne.

▶ **Symptoms and diagnostic considerations.** Hordeolum presents as *painful nodules with a central core of pus*. **External hordeolum** appears on the *margin of the eyelid* where the sweat glands are located (▶ Fig. 2.19). **Internal hordeolum** of a sebaceous gland is usually *only revealed by everting the eyelid* and usually accompanied by a more severe reaction such as conjunctivitis or chemosis of the bulbar conjunctiva. Pseudoptosis and swelling of the preauricular lymph nodes may also occur.

▶ **Differential diagnosis.** Chalazion (tender to palpation) and inflammation of the lacrimal glands (rarer and more painful).

▶ **Treatment.** Antibiotic ointments and application of dry heat (red heat lamp) will rapidly heal the lesion.

▶ **Clinical course and prognosis.** After eruption and drainage of the pus, the symptoms will rapidly disappear. The prognosis is good. An underlying internal disorder should be excluded in cases in which the disorder frequently recurs (see Etiology).

2.6.2 Chalazion

Definition
Firm nodular bulb within the tarsus.

▶ **Epidemiology and etiology.** Chalazia occur relatively frequently and are caused by a chronic granulomatous inflammation due to build-up of secretion from the meibomian gland.

▶ **Symptoms.** The firm painless nodule develops very slowly. Aside from the cosmetic flaw, it is usually asymptomatic (▶ Fig. 2.20).

▶ **Differential diagnosis.** Hordeolum (tender to palpation) and adenocarcinoma (see p. 28).

▸ **Treatment.** Surgical incision is usually unavoidable.

Note
After the chalazion clamp has been introduced, the lesion is incised either medially, perpendicular to the margin of the eyelid, or laterally, perpendicular to the margin of the eyelid (this is important to avoid cicatricial ectropion). The fatty contents are then removed with a curet.

▸ **Prognosis.** Good, except for the chance of local recurrence.

2.7 Tumors

2.7.1 Benign Tumors

Ductal Cysts (Hidrocystomas)

The **round cysts** of the glands of Moll are **usually located in the angle of the eye**. Their contents are clear and watery and can be transilluminated. Gravity can result in ectropion (▸ Fig. 2.21). *Therapy* consists of marsupialization (see p. 62). The *prognosis* is good.

Xanthelasma

Definition
Local fat metabolism disorder that produces lipoprotein deposits. These are usually bilateral in the medial canthus.

▸ **Epidemiology.** Postmenopausal women are most frequently affected. A higher incidence has also been observed in patients with diabetes, increased levels of plasma lipoprotein, or bile duct disorders.

▸ **Symptoms.** The soft yellow-white plaques are sharply demarcated. They are usually bilateral and distributed symmetrically (▸ Fig. 2.22). Aside from the cosmetic flaw, patients are asymptomatic.

▸ **Treatment and prognosis.** The plaques can only be removed surgically. The incidence of recurrence is high.

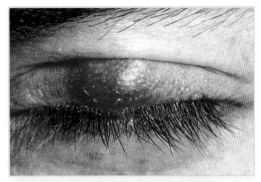

Fig. 2.19 External hordeolum. A painful inflamed hordeolum is usually caused by *Staphylococcus aureus* infection of an eyelid gland.

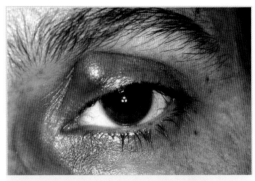

Fig. 2.20 Chalazion. Painful to palpation, the chalazion is caused by a chronic build-up of secretions from the meibomian glands. Compare with this ▸ Fig. 2.29, showing sebaceous gland carcinoma, which in its early stages can look so similar that it is mistaken for a chalazion.

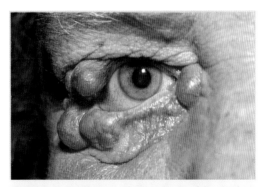

Fig. 2.21 Hidrocystoma. The round cysts of the glands of Moll are usually located in the angle of the eye. The weight causes temporary ectropion.

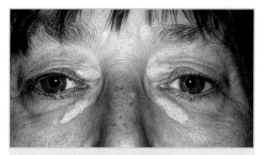

Fig. 2.22 Xanthelasma. The fatty deposits are often symmetrically distributed in the medial canthus.

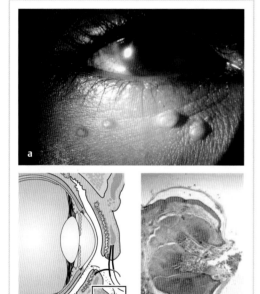

Fig. 2.23 Molluscum contagiosum. (a) The pinhead-sized molluscum lesions have typical central depressions. (b) As a result of expression of virus particles out of the molluscum lesion and displacement of them into the conjunctival sac viral conjunctivitis develops. (c) Histologic appearance of the molluscum contagiosum crater (detail from b).

Molluscum Contagiosum

This **noninflammatory contagious infection** is caused by DNA viruses. The disease usually affects *children and teenagers* and is transmitted by direct contact. The *pinhead-sized lesions have typical central depressions* and are scattered near the upper and lower eyelids (▶ Fig. 2.23). These lesions are removed with a curet. (In children this is done under short-acting anesthesia.)

Cutaneous Horn

The **yellowish-brown cutaneous protrusions** consist of keratin (▶ Fig. 2.24). Older patients are more frequently affected. The cutaneous horn should be surgically removed as 25% of keratosis cases can develop into *malignant squamous cell carcinomas* years later.

Keratoacanthoma

A rapidly growing **tumor with a central keratin mass that opens on the skin surface**, which can sometimes be expressed (▶ Fig. 2.25). The tumor may resolve spontaneously, forming a small sunken scar.

Differential diagnosis should exclude a *basal cell carcinoma* (see p. 28); the margin of a keratoacanthoma is characteristically avascular. Likewise, a *squamous cell carcinoma* can only be excluded by a biopsy.

Hemangioma

Definition
Congenital benign vascular anomaly resembling a neoplasm that is most frequently noticed in the skin and subcutaneous tissues.

▶ **Epidemiology.** Girls are most often affected (approximately 70% of cases). Facial lesions most commonly occur in the eyelids (▶ Fig. 2.26).

▶ **Symptoms.** Hemangiomas include capillary or superficial, cavernous, and deep forms.

▶ **Diagnostic considerations.** Hemangiomas can be compressed, and the skin will then appear white.

▶ **Differential diagnosis.** *Nevus flammeus:* this is characterized by a sharply demarcated bluish-red mark or "port-wine" stain) resulting from vascular expansion under the epidermis (not a growth or tumor).

▶ **Treatment.** A watch-and-wait approach is justified in light of the high rate of *spontaneous remission* (approximately 70%). Where there is increased

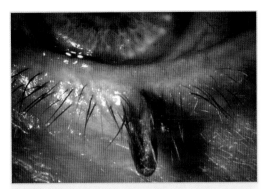

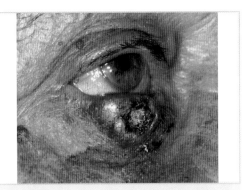

Fig. 2.24 Cutaneous horn. The yellowish-brown cutaneous protrusions consist of keratin. They frequently (in 25 % of cases) develop into a malignant squamous cell carcinoma in later years if they are not surgically removed.

Fig. 2.25 Keratoacanthoma. The rapidly growing benign tumor has a central keratin mass that opens onto the surface of the skin (histologically confirmed keratoacanthoma). It is possible to mistake it for a basalioma (▶ Fig. 2.28).

risk of amblyopia due to the size of the lesion, Beta blockers appear to be highly effective and well tolerated. Additional therapeutic alternatives are cryotherapy, intralesional steroid injections, or radiation therapy, which can accelerate regression of the hemangioma.

▶ **Prognosis.** Generally good.

Neurofibromatosis (Recklinghausen's Disease)

Definition
A congenital developmental defect of the neuroectoderm gives rise to neural tumors and pigment spots (*café au lait* spots).

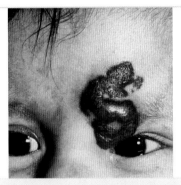

Fig. 2.26 Cavernous hemangioma. This congenital vascular anomaly occurs as a facial lesion most commonly in the eyelids. The lesion regresses spontaneously in approximately 70 % of cases.

Neurofibromatosis is regarded as a *phacomatosis* (a developmental disorder involving the simultaneous presence of changes in the skin, central nervous system, and ectodermal portions of the eye).

▶ **Symptoms and diagnostic considerations.** The numerous tumors are soft, broad-based, or pediculate, and occur either in the skin or in subcutaneous tissue, usually in the vicinity of the upper eyelid.

They can reach monstrous proportions and present as *elephantiasis of the eyelids* (▶ Fig. 2.27).

▶ **Treatment.** Smaller fibromas can be easily removed by surgery. Larger tumors always entail a risk of postoperative bleeding and recurrence. On the whole, treatment is *difficult*.

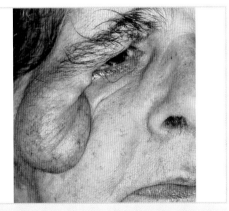

Fig. 2.27 Neurofibroma. Larger fibromas can lead to elephantiasis of the eyelids.

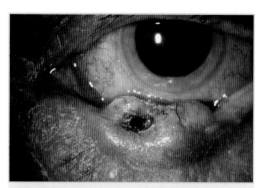

Fig. 2.28 Basal cell carcinoma. A halo resembling a string of beads, superficial vascularization, and a central crater with a tendency to bleed are characteristic signs of this moderately malignant tumor.

2.7.2 Semimalignant and Malignant Tumors

Basal Cell Carcinoma

Definition
Basal cell carcinoma is a frequent, moderately malignant, fibroepithelial tumor that can cause severe local tissue destruction but very rarely metastasizes.

▶ **Epidemiology.** Approximately 90% of malignant eyelid tumors are basal cell carcinomas. Their incidence increases with age. In approximately 60% of cases they are localized on the *lower eyelid*. Morbidity in sunny countries is 110 cases per 100,000 persons (in Central Europe, approximately 20 per 100,000 persons). *Dark-skinned people* are *affected significantly less often.* Gender is not a predisposing factor.

▶ **Etiology.** Causes of basal cell carcinoma may include a genetic disposition. *Increased exposure to the sun's ultraviolet radiation, carcinogenic substances* (such as arsenic), and *chronic skin damage* can also lead to an increased incidence. Basal cell carcinomas arise from the basal cell layers of the epidermis and the sebaceous gland hair follicles, where their growth locally destroys tissue.

▶ **Symptoms.** Typical characteristics include a firm, slightly raised margin (*a halo resembling a string of beads*) with a *central crater* and *superficial vascu-*

larization with an increased tendency to bleed (▶ Fig. 2.28).

Ulceration with "gnawing" peripheral proliferation is occasionally referred to as an *ulcus rodens*; an *ulcus terebrans* refers to deep infiltration with invasion of cartilage and bone.

▶ **Diagnostic considerations.** The diagnosis can very often be made on the basis of clinical evidence. A biopsy is indicated if there is any doubt.

Note
Loss of the eyelashes in the vicinity of the tumor always suggests malignancy.

▶ **Treatment.** The lesion is treated by surgical excision within a margin of healthy tissue. This is the safest method. If a radical procedure is not feasible, the only remaining options are radiation therapy or cryotherapy with liquid nitrogen.

▶ **Prognosis.** The chances of successful treatment by surgical excision are very good. Frequent follow-up examinations are indicated.

Note
The earlier a basal cell carcinoma is detected, the easier it is to remove.

Squamous Cell Carcinoma

This is the *second most frequently encountered* malignant eyelid tumor. The carcinoma arises from the epidermis, grows rapidly, and destroys tissue. It can metastasize into the regional lymph nodes. Distant metastases are rarer. The **treatment of choice** is complete surgical removal.

Adenocarcinoma

The *rare* adenocarcinoma arises from the meibomian glands or the glands of Zeis. The **firm, painless swelling** is usually located in the **upper eyelid** and is mobile with respect to the skin but not with respect to the underlying tissue (▶ Fig. 2.29). In its early stages it can be *mistaken easily for a chalazion* (see p. 24). The lesion can metastasize into local lymph nodes.

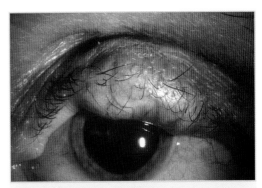

Note
An apparent chalazion that cannot be removed by the usual surgical procedure always suggests a suspected adenocarcinoma.

The **treatment of choice** is complete surgical removal.

Fig. 2.29 Adenocarcinoma of the upper lid. The lesion may be quite similar to a chronic chalazion.

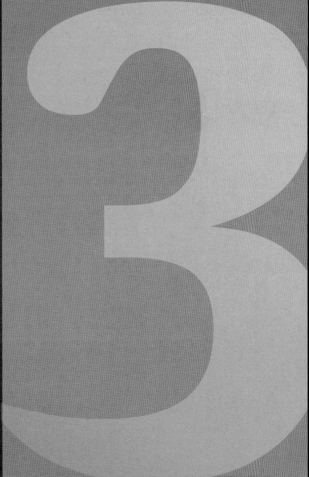

Chapter 3

Lacrimal System

3 Lacrimal System

Peter Wagner and Gerhard K. Lang

3.1 Basic Knowledge

The lacrimal system (▶ Fig. 3.1) consists of two sections:

- Structures that secrete tear fluid.
- Structures that facilitate tear drainage.

▶ **Position, structure, and nerve supply of the lacrimal gland.** The **lacrimal gland** is about the *size of a walnut*; it lies beneath the superior temporal margin of the orbital bone in the lacrimal fossa of the frontal bone and is *neither visible nor palpable.* A palpable lacrimal gland is usually a sign of a pathologic change such as dacryoadenitis. The tendon of the levator palpebrae muscle divides the lacrimal gland into a *larger orbital part* (two-thirds) and a *smaller palpebral part* (one-third). Several tiny **accessory lacrimal glands (glands of Krause and Wolfring)** located in the superior fornix secrete additional serous tear fluid.

The lacrimal gland receives its **sensory supply** from the *lacrimal nerve*. Its parasympathetic secretomotor nerve supply comes from the *nervus inter-medius*. The sympathetic fibers arise from the superior cervical sympathetic ganglion and follow the course of the blood vessels to the gland.

▶ **Tear film.** The tear film (▶ Fig. 3.2) that moistens the conjunctiva and cornea is composed of **three layers**:

1. The **outer oily layer** (approximately 0.1 µm thick) is a product of the *meibomian glands* and the *sebaceous glands and sweat glands of the margin of the eyelid.* The primary function of this layer is to stabilize the tear film. With its hydrophobic properties, like those of an extremely thin layer of wax, it prevents rapid evaporation.
2. The **middle watery layer** (approximately 8 µm thick) is produced by the *lacrimal gland* and the *accessory lacrimal glands* (glands of Krause and Wolfring). Its task is to clean and protect the surface of the cornea and ensure mobility of the palpebral conjunctiva over the cornea and a smooth corneal surface *for high-quality optical images.*

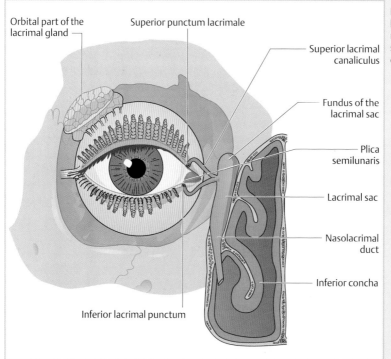

Orbital part of the lacrimal gland

Superior punctum lacrimale

Superior lacrimal canaliculus

Fundus of the lacrimal sac

Plica semilunaris

Lacrimal sac

Nasolacrimal duct

Inferior concha

Inferior lacrimal punctum

Fig. 3.1 Anatomy of the lacrimal system. The lacrimal system consists of tear secretion structures and tear drainage structures.

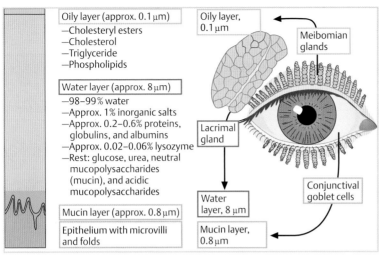

Oily layer (approx. 0.1 µm)
—Cholesteryl esters
—Cholesterol
—Triglyceride
—Phospholipids

Water layer (approx. 8 µm)
—98–99% water
—Approx. 1% inorganic salts
—Approx. 0.2–0.6% proteins, globulins, and albumins
—Approx. 0.02–0.06% lysozyme
—Rest: glucose, urea, neutral mucopolysaccharides (mucin), and acidic mucopolysaccharides

Mucin layer (approx. 0.8 µm)

Epithelium with microvilli and folds

Oily layer, 0.1 µm

Meibomian glands

Lacrimal gland

Water layer, 8 µm

Mucin layer, 0.8 µm

Conjunctival goblet cells

Fig. 3.2 Structure of the tear film. The tear film consists of the lipid layer (prevents rapid evaporation), the watery layer (promotes clean, smooth, and thus optimally transparent cornea), and the mucous layer (like the lipid layer, stabilizes the tear film).

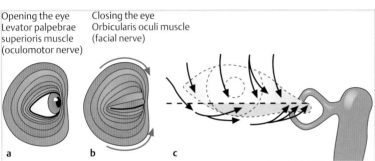

Opening the eye
Levator palpebrae superioris muscle (oculomotor nerve)

Closing the eye
Orbicularis oculi muscle (facial nerve)

a   b   c

Fig. 3.3 (a–c) Combined function of the orbicularis oculi muscle and the lower lacrimal system. As the eyelids close, they act like a windshield wiper to move the tear fluid medially across the eye toward the puncta and lacrimal canaliculi.

3. The **inner mucin layer** (approximately 0.8 µm thick) is secreted by the *goblet cells of the conjunctiva* and the *lacrimal gland*. It is hydrophilic with respect to the microvilli of the corneal epithelium, which also helps to *stabilize the tear film*. It prevents the watery layer from beading up on the cornea, thus promoting even distribution of the watery layer over the cornea and the conjunctiva.

Lysozyme, beta-lysin, lactoferrin, and gamma globulin (IgA) are **tear-specific proteins** that give the tear fluid *antimicrobial characteristics* among other properties.

▶ **Tear drainage.** The shinglelike arrangement of the **fibers of the orbicularis oculi muscle** (supplied by the facial nerve) causes the eye to close progressively from lateral to medial instead of the eyelids simultaneously closing along their entire length. This *windshield wiper motion* moves the tear fluid medially across the eye toward the medial canthus (▶ Fig. 3.3a–c).

The **superior and inferior puncta lacrimales** collect the tears, which then drain through the superior and inferior **lacrimal canaliculi** into the **lacrimal sac**. From there they pass through the **nasolacrimal duct** into the **inferior concha** (see ▶ Fig. 3.1).

3.2 Examination Methods

3.2.1 Evaluation of Tear Formation

▶ **Schirmer tear testing.** This test (▶ Fig. 3.4) provides information about the **quantity of watery component in tear secretion.**
- *Test:* a strip of litmus paper is inserted into the conjunctival sac of the temporal third of the lower eyelid.
- *Normal:* after about 5 minutes, at least 15 mm of the paper should turn blue due to the alkalinity of tear fluid.
- *Abnormal:* values less than 5 mm are abnormal (although they will not necessarily be associated with clinical symptoms).

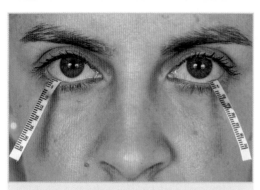

Fig. 3.4 Measuring tear secretion with Schirmer tear testing. A strip of litmus paper is folded over and inserted into the conjunctival sac of the temporal third of the lower eyelid. Normally, at least 15 mm of the paper should turn blue within 5 minutes.

The same method is used after application of a topical anesthetic to **evaluate normal secretion without irritating the conjunctiva.**

▶ **Tear break-up time (TBUT).** This test evaluates the **stability of the tear film**. *Test:* fluorescein dye (10 µL of a 0.125% fluorescein solution) is added to the precorneal tear film. The examiner observes the eye under 10- to 20-power magnification with a slit lamp and cobalt blue filter and notes when the first signs of drying occur, initially *without the patient closing the eye* and then with the patient *keeping the eye open as he or she would normally.*
• *Normal:* TBUT of *at least* 10 seconds is normal.

▶ **Rose bengal test.** Rose bengal **dyes dead epithelial cells and mucin.** This test has proven particularly useful in evaluating *dry eyes* (keratoconjunctivitis sicca, see p. 40 as it reveals conjunctival and corneal symptoms of desiccation.

▶ **Impression cytology.** A Millipore filter is fastened to a tonometer and pressed against the superior conjunctiva with 20 to 30 mm Hg of pressure for 2 seconds. The **density of goblet cells** is estimated under a microscope (*normal density* is 20–45 goblet cells per square millimeter of epithelial surface). The number of mucus-producing goblet cells is reduced in various disorders such as keratoconjunctivitis sicca, ocular pemphigoid, and xerophthalmia.

3.2.2 Evaluation of Tear Drainage

▶ **Conjunctival fluorescein dye test.** Normal **tear drainage** can be demonstrated by having the patient blow his or her nose into a facial tissue following application of a 2% fluorescein sodium solution to the inferior fornix.

▶ Probing and irrigation. These examination methods are used to **locate stenoses**. After application of a topical anesthetic, a conical probe is used to dilate the punctum. Then the lower lacrimal system is flushed with a physiologic saline solution introduced through a blunt cannula (▶ Fig.3.5). If the passage is *unobstructed,* the solution will drain freely into the nose.

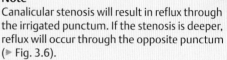

Note
Canalicular stenosis will result in reflux through the irrigated punctum. If the stenosis is deeper, reflux will occur through the opposite punctum (▶ Fig. 3.6).

A probe can be used to determine the site of the stricture, and possibly to eliminate obstructions (▶ Fig. 3.7).

▶ **Radiographic contrast studies.** Radiographic contrast medium is instilled in the same manner as the saline solution. These studies demonstrate the **shape**, **position**, **and size** of the passage and possible **obstructions to drainage.**

▶ **Digital subtraction dacryocystography.** These studies demonstrate only the contrast medium and image the lower lacrimal system without superimposed bony structures. They are particularly useful as preoperative diagnostic studies (▶ Fig. 3.6e).

▶ **Lacrimal duct endoscopy** (▶ **Fig. 3.8**). Fine endoscopes now permit **direct visualization of the internal mucous surface of the lacrimal duct system.** Until recently, endoscopic examination of the lacrimal system was not a routine procedure.

3.3 Disorders of the Lower Lacrimal System

3.3.1 Dacryocystitis

Inflammation of the lacrimal sac is the *most frequent* disorder of the lower lacrimal system. It is usually the result of obstruction of the nasolacrimal duct and is *unilateral in most cases.*

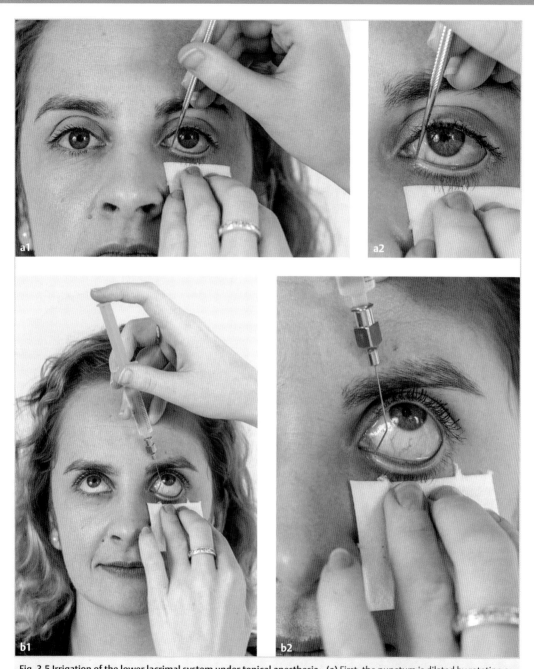

Fig. 3.5 Irrigation of the lower lacrimal system under topical anesthesia. (a) First, the punctum is dilated by rotating a conical probe. **(b)** Then the lacrimal passage is flushed with a physiologic saline solution. The examiner should be particularly alert to good drainage or possible reflux.

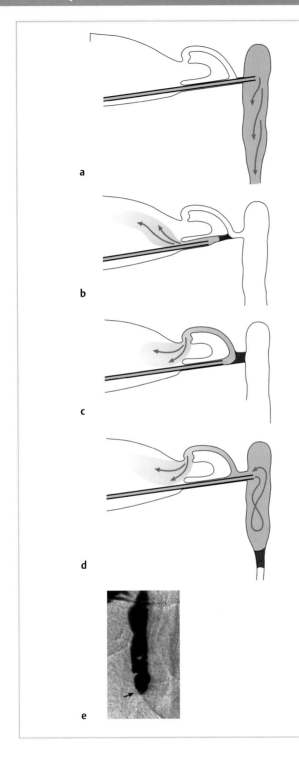

a

b

c

d

e

Fig. 3.6 Localizing an obstruction by irrigating the lower lacrimal system. The lower lacrimal system should be irrigated with care by an experienced ophthalmologist. Failure to locate the passage will inflate the eyelid and provide no diagnostic information. **(a)** No obstruction. **(b)** Stenosis of the inferior canaliculus. Reflux through the irrigated punctum. **(c)** Stenosis of the canaliculus communis. Reflux through the opposite punctum. **(d)** Stenosis within the lacrimal sac. Reflux through the opposite punctum, often associated with gelatinous purulent retention of the lacrimal sac. It should be noted that irrigation requires a larger amount of fluid in comparison with **(c)**. **(e)** Radiographic image of the lower lacrimal system. Digital subtraction dacryocystography images the lower lacrimal system and can demonstrate a possible stenosis (arrow) without superimposed bony structures. This method provides valuable information about the size of the lacrimal sac for the planning of a surgical approach (see ▶ Fig. 3.8).

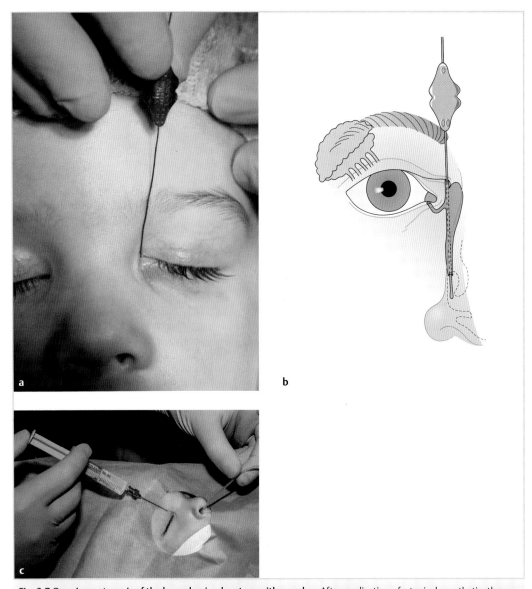

Fig. 3.7 Opening a stenosis of the lower lacrimal system with a probe. After application of a topical anesthetic, the probe is carefully introduced into the lacrimal system. **(a,b)** The puncta are dilated and then the valve of Hasner is opened. **(c)** A dye solution can then be introduced to verify patency of the lacrimal system. In infants aged 6 months or older, the procedure is best carried out with short-acting general anesthesia.

Acute Dacryocystitis

▶ **Epidemiology.** The disorder most frequently affects adults between the ages of 50 and 60 years.

▶ **Etiology.** The cause is usually a *stenosis within the lacrimal sac*. The retention of tear fluid leads to

infection from staphylococci, pneumococci, *pseudomonads*, or other pathogens.

▶ **Symptoms.** Clinical symptoms include highly inflamed, painful *swelling in the vicinity of the lacrimal sac* (▶ Fig. 3.9), which may be accompanied by *malaise, fever*, and *involvement of the regional lymph nodes*. The pain may be referred as far as the fore-

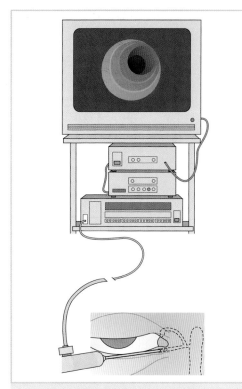

Fig. 3.8 Lacrimal duct endoscopy. The endoscope is introduced to the inferior canaliculus. The endoscopic image is viewed on the monitor.

head and teeth. An *abscess in the lacrimal sac* may form in advanced disorders; it can spontaneously rupture the skin and form a *draining fistula*.

> **Note**
> Acute inflammation that has spread to the surrounding tissue of the eyelids and cheek entails a risk of sepsis and cavernous sinus thrombosis, which is a life-threatening complication.

▶ **Diagnostic considerations.** Radiographic contrast studies or digital subtraction dacryocystography can visualize the obstruction for preoperative planning (but this is to be avoided in the acute phase of the disease, because there is a risk of pathogen dissemination).

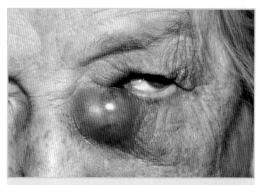

Fig. 3.9 Acute dacryocystitis. Typical symptoms include highly inflamed, painful swelling in the vicinity of the lacrimal sac.

> **Note**
> Diagnostic or therapeutic lacrimal duct irrigation in the acute phase is to be avoided (risk of pathogen dissemination).

▶ **Differential diagnosis.** Hordeolum (small, circumscribed, nonmobile inflamed swelling).
• Orbital cellulitis (usually associated with reduced motility of the eyeball).

▶ **Treatment**
▶ **Acute cases.** Acute cases are treated with *local and systemic antibiotics* according to the specific pathogens detected. *Disinfectant compresses,* such as a 1:1,000 aminoacridine solution (e.g., Rivanol, Alasulf) can also positively influence the clinical course of the disorder. Pus from *a fluctuating abscess* is best drained through a *stab incision* following cryoanesthesia with a refrigerant spray.

▶ **Treatment after acute symptoms have subsided.** For durable success, operative treatment is often necessary (Toti's dacryocystorhinostomy, see ▶ Fig. 3.10). Also known as a lower system bypass, this operation either involves opening the lateral wall of the nose and bypassing the nasolacrimal duct to create a direct connection between the lacrimal sac and the nasal mucosa (Toti operation) or an endoscopic approach via the nose in case of a large lacrimal sac (West operation).

Chronic Dacryocystitis

▶ Etiology. Obstruction of the nasolacrimal duct is often secondary to chronic inflammation of the connective tissue or nasal mucosa.

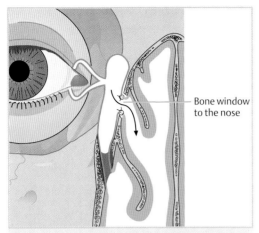

— Bone window
to the nose

Fig. 3.10 Dacryocystorhinostomy. The principle of dacryocystorhinostomy is to create a new drainage route for the tear fluid that bypasses the nasolacrimal duct. Via a bone window, the mucosa of the lacrimal sac and the nasal mucosa are sutured together to keep the shunt open. This can be done using an outside approach over a skin incision (Toti operation) or—in case of a large lacrimal sac—endoscopically via the nose (West operation).

▶ Symptoms and diagnostic considerations. The *initial characteristic* of chronic dacryocystitis is *increased lacrimation*. Signs of inflammation are not usually present. Applying pressure to the inflamed lacrimal sac causes *large quantities of transparent mucoid pus* to regurgitate through the punctum.

> **Note**
> Chronic inflammation of the lacrimal sac can lead to a serpiginous corneal ulcer.

▶ **Treatment.** Surgical intervention is the only effective treatment in the vast majority of cases. This involves either a dacryocystorhinostomy (creation of a direct connection between the lacrimal sac and the nasal mucosa; ▶ Fig. 3.10) or removal of the lacrimal sac.

Neonatal Dacryocystitis

▶ **Etiology.** Approximately 6% of newborns have a stenosis of the mouth of the nasolacrimal duct due to a *persistent mucosal fold* (lacrimal fold or valve of Hasner). The resulting retention of tear fluid provides ideal growth conditions for bacteria, particularly staphylococci, streptococci, and pneumococci.

▶ **Symptoms and diagnostic considerations.** Shortly after birth (usually within 2–4 weeks), *pus is secreted from the puncta.* The disease continues subcutaneously and pus collects in the palpebral fissure. The *conjunctiva* is *not usually involved.*

▶ **Differential diagnosis**
- Gonococcal conjunctivitis and inclusion conjunctivitis (▶ Table 4.2).
- Silver catarrh (harmless conjunctivitis with slimy mucoid secretion following Credé's method of prophylaxis with silver nitrate).

▶ **Treatment. During the first few weeks** the infant should be monitored for *spontaneous opening of the stenosis.* During this period, *antibiotic and anti-inflammatory eye drops and nose drops* (such as erythromycin and xylometazoline 0.5% for infants) are administered.

    If symptoms persist, *irrigation or probing* under short-acting general anesthesia may be indicated (▶ Fig. 3.7a–c).

> **Note**
> Often, massaging the region several times daily while carefully applying pressure to the lacrimal sac will be sufficient to open the valve of Hasner and eliminate the obstruction.

3.3.2 Canaliculitis

> **Definition**
> Canaliculitis usually involves inflammation of only one canaliculus.

▶ **Epidemiology and etiology.** *Genuine canaliculitis is rare.* Usually a stricture will be present and the actual *inflammation proceeds from the conjunctiva.* Actinomycetes (fungoid bacteria) often cause persistent purulent granular concrements (drusen, "sulfur granules") that are difficult to express.

▶ **Symptoms and diagnostic considerations.** The canaliculus region is swollen, reddened, and often tender to palpation. Pus or granular concrements can be expressed.

▶ **Treatment.** The disorder is treated with antibiotic eye drops and ointments according to the specific pathogens detected in cytologic smears. Surgical incision can occasionally become necessary for a definitive cure.

3.3.3 Tumors of the Lacrimal Sac

▶ **Epidemiology.** Tumors of the lacrimal sac are *rare* but are *primarily malignant* when they do occur. They include papillomas, carcinomas, and sarcomas.

▶ **Symptoms and diagnostic considerations.** Usually the tumors cause unilateral painless swelling followed by dacryostenosis.

▶ **Diagnostic considerations.** The irregular and occasionally bizarre form of the structure in radiographic contrast studies is typical. Ultrasound, CT, MRI, and biopsy all contribute to confirming the diagnosis.

▶ **Differential diagnosis.** Chronic dacryocystitis (see p. 38), mucocele of the ethmoid cells.

▶ **Treatment.** The entire tumor should be removed.

3.4 Lacrimal System Dysfunction

3.4.1 Keratoconjunctivitis Sicca

Definition
Noninfectious keratopathy characterized by reduced moistening of the conjunctiva and cornea (dry eyes).

▶ **Epidemiology.** Keratoconjunctivitis sicca as a result of dry eyes is one of the most common eye problems between the ages of 40 and 50 years. As a result of hormonal changes in menopause, *women are far more frequently affected* (86%) than *men*. There are also indications that keratoconjunctivitis sicca is more prevalent in regions with higher levels of environmental pollution.

▶ **Etiology.** Keratoconjunctivitis sicca results from dry eyes, which may be due to one of two causes:
- **Reduced tear production** (hypovolemic) associated with certain systemic disorders (such as Sjögren's syndrome and rheumatoid arthritis) or as a result of atrophy or destruction of the lacrimal gland.

- **Altered composition of the tear film**. The composition of the tear film can alter due to vitamin A deficiency, medications (such as oral contraceptives and retinoids), or certain environmental influences (such as nicotine, smog, or air conditioning). The tear film breaks up too quickly and causes (hyperevaporative) corneal drying.

Dry eyes can represent a **disorder in and of itself**.

▶ **Symptoms.** Patients complain of burning, reddened eyes, and excessive lacrimation (reflex lacrimation) from only slight environmental causes such as wind, cold, low humidity, or reading for an extended period of time. A foreign-body sensation is also present. These symptoms may be accompanied by intense pain. Eyesight is usually minimally compromised if at all.

▶ **Diagnostic considerations.** Often there is a discrepancy between the *minimal clinical findings* that the ophthalmologist can establish and the *intense symptoms reported by the patient*. Results from **Schirmer tear testing** usually show reduction of the watery component of tears, and the **tear break-up** time (see p. 34) is reduced (the tear break-up time provides information about the mucin content of the tear film, important for its stability). Values of at least 10 seconds are normal; the tear break-up time in keratoconjunctivitis sicca is less than 5 seconds.

Slit lamp examination will reveal dilated conjunctival vessels and minimal pericorneal injection. A tear film meniscus cannot be demonstrated on the lower eyelid margin, and the lower eyelid will push the conjunctiva along in folds in front of it.

In *severe cases* the eye will be reddened, and the tear film will contain thick mucus and small filaments that proceed from a superficial epithelial lesion (filamentary keratitis; see ▶ Fig. 5.15). The corneal lesion can be demonstrated with **fluorescein dye**. In less severe cases the eye will only be reddened, although application of fluorescein dye will reveal corneal lesions (superficial punctate keratitis, see p. 81). The **rose bengal test** (see p. 34) and **impression cytology** (see p. 34) are additional diagnostic tests that are useful in evaluating persistent cases.

▶ **Treatment.** Depending on the severity of findings, **artificial tear solutions** in varying viscosities are prescribed. These range from eye drops to high-viscosity long-acting gels that may be applied every hour or every half hour, depending on the severity of the disorder. In persistent cases, the

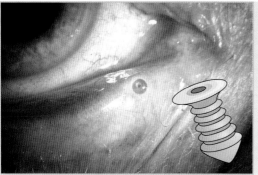

Fig. 3.11 Treatment of dry eyes. Treatment can be promoted by temporarily closing the puncta with silicone punctal plugs.

puncta can be temporarily closed with silicone **punctal plugs** (▶ Fig. 3.11) to at least retain the few tears that are still produced. **Surgical obliteration of the puncta** may be indicated in severe cases.

Patients should also be informed about the possibility of installing an **air humidifier** in the home and redirecting blowers in automobiles to avoid further drying of the eyes. Dry eyes in women may also be due to hormonal changes, and a **gynecologist should be consulted** regarding the patient's hormonal status.

▶ **Prognosis.** The prognosis is good for those treatments discussed here. However, the disorder cannot be completely healed.

3.4.2 Illacrimation

Illacrimation or epiphora may be due to hypersecretion from the lacrimal gland. However, it is more often caused by obstructed drainage through the lower lacrimal system.

▶ **Causes of hypersecretion**
- Emotional distress (crying).
- *Increased irritation of the eyes* (by smoke, dust, foreign bodies, injury, or intraocular inflammation) leads to excessive lacrimation in the context of the defensive triad of blepharospasm, photosensitivity, and epiphora.

▶ **Causes of obstructed drainage**
- Stricture or stenosis in the lower lacrimal system.
- Eyelid deformity, e.g., eversion of the punctum lacrimale, ectropion (see p. 18), or entropion (see p. 16).

3.5 Disorders of the Lacrimal Gland

3.5.1 Acute Dacryoadenitis

Definition
Acute inflammation of the lacrimal gland is a *rare* disorder characterized by intense inflammation and extreme tenderness to palpation.

▶ **Etiology.** The disorder is often attributable to pneumococci and staphylococci, and less frequently to streptococci. There may be a relationship between the disorder and infectious diseases such as mumps, measles, scarlet fever, diphtheria, and influenza.

▶ **Symptoms and diagnostic considerations.** Acute dacryoadenitis usually occurs *unilaterally.* The inflamed *swollen gland* is especially *tender to palpation.*

Note
The upper eyelid exhibits a characteristic **S**-curve (▶ Fig. 3.12).

▶ **Differential diagnosis**
- Internal hordeolum (smaller and circumscribed).
- Eyelid abscess (fluctuation).
- Orbital cellulitis (usually associated with reduced motility of the eyeball).

▶ **Treatment.** This will depend on the *underlying disorder. Moist heat, disinfectant compresses* (Rivanol [ethacridine lactate], Alasulf [allantoin, aminoacridine hydrochloride, sulfanilamide]), and local *antibiotics* are helpful.

▶ **Clinical course and prognosis.** Acute inflammation of the lacrimal gland is characterized by a rapid clinical course and *spontaneous healing within 8 to 10 days.* The prognosis is good, and complications are not usually to be expected.

3.5.2 Chronic Dacryoadenitis

▶ **Etiology.** The chronic form of inflammation of the lacrimal gland may be the result of an incompletely healed *acute* dacryoadenitis. Diseases such as tuberculosis, sarcoidosis, leukemia, or lymphogranulomatosis can be causes of chronic dacryoadenitis.

> **Note**
> Bilateral chronic inflammation of the lacrimal and salivary glands is referred to as Mikulicz's syndrome.

▶ **Symptoms and diagnostic considerations.** Usually there is no pain. The symptoms are less pronounced than in the acute form. However, the **S**-curve deformity of the palpebral fissure resulting from swelling of the lacrimal gland is readily apparent (see ▶ Fig. 3.12).

▶ **Differential diagnosis**
• Periostitis of the upper orbital rim (rare).
• Lipodermoid (no signs of inflammation).

▶ **Treatment.** This will depend on the *underlying disorder. Systemic corticosteroids* may be effective in treating unspecific forms.

▶ **Prognosis.** The prognosis for chronic dacryoadenitis is good when the underlying disorder can be identified.

3.5.3 Tumors of the Lacrimal Gland

▶ **Epidemiology.** Tumors of the lacrimal gland account for 5 to 7 % of orbital neoplasms. Lacrimal gland tumors are *much rarer in children* (approximately 2% of orbital tumors). The ratio of benign to malignant tumors of the lacrimal gland specified in the literature is 10:1. The **most frequent benign epithelial lacrimal gland tumor** is the *pleomorphic adenoma.* **Malignant tumors** include the *adenoid cystic carcinoma* and *pleomorphic adenocarcinoma* (▶ Fig. 3.13).

▶ **Etiology.** The WHO classification of 1980 divides lacrimal gland tumors into the following categories:
• Epithelial tumors.
• Tumors of the hematopoietic or lymphatic tissue.
• Secondary tumors.
• Inflamed tumors.
• Other and unclassified tumors.

▶ **Symptoms.** Tumors usually *grow very slowly.* After a while, they displace the eyeball inferiorly and medially, which can cause double vision.

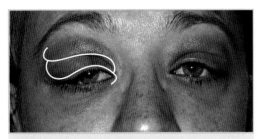

Fig. 3.12 Bilateral acute dacryoadenitis (more pronounced on the right than the left) with the characteristic S-shaped curve of the upper eyelids.

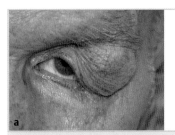 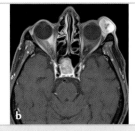 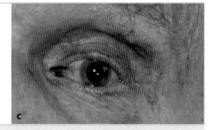

Fig. 3.13 Lacrimal gland tumor. (a) Clinical diagnosis of a noninflammatory, pressure-indolent, mobile lacrimal gland tumor with displacement of the optical axis. (b) MRI study of the tumor with contrast medium. (c) Postoperative diagnosis after excision. *Histologic diagnosis:* pleomorphic adenoma of the lacrimal gland.

▶ **Diagnostic considerations.** Testing **motility** provides information about the infiltration of the tumor into the extraocular muscles or mechanical changes in the eyeball resulting from tumor growth. The echogenicity of the tumor in **ultrasound studies** is an indication of its consistency. **CT** and **MRI** studies show the exact location and extent of the tumor. A biopsy will confirm whether it is malignant and what type of tumor it is.

▶ **Treatment.** To the extent that this is possible, the entire tumor should be removed; orbital exenteration (removal of the entire contents of the orbit) may be required. Systemic administration of corticosteroids is indicated for unspecific tumors.

▶ **Prognosis.** This depends on the degree of malignancy of the tumor. Adenoid cystic carcinomas have the least favorable prognosis.

Chapter 4

Conjunctiva

4 Conjunctiva

Gerhard K. Lang and Gabriele E. Lang

4.1 Basic Knowledge

▶ **Structure of the conjunctiva.** The conjunctiva is a thin vascular mucous membrane that is normally of shiny appearance (▶ Fig. 4.1). It forms the conjunctival sac together with the surface of the cornea. The **bulbar conjunctiva** is loosely attached to the sclera and is more closely attached to the limbus of the cornea. There the conjunctival epithelium fuses with the corneal epithelium. The **palpebral conjunctiva** lines the inner surface of the eyelid and is firmly attached to the tarsus. The loose palpebral conjunctiva forms a fold in the **conjunctival fornix**, where it joins the bulbar conjunctiva. A half-moon–shaped fold of mucous membrane, the plica semilunaris, is located in the medial corner of the palpebral fissure. This borders on the lacrimal caruncle, which contains hairs and sebaceous glands.

▶ **Function of the conjunctival sac.** The conjunctival sac has three main tasks:
1. **Motility of the eyeball.** The loose connection between the bulbar conjunctiva and the sclera and the "spare" conjunctival tissue in the fornices allows the eyeball to move freely in every direction of gaze.
2. **Articulating layer.** The surface of the conjunctiva is smooth and moist to allow the mucous membranes to glide easily and painlessly across each other. The tear film acts as a lubricant.
3. **Protective function.** The conjunctiva must be able to protect against pathogens. Follicle-like aggregations of lymphocytes and plasma cells (the lymph nodes of the eye) are located beneath the palpebral conjunctiva and in the fornices. Antibacterial substances, immunoglobulins, interferon, and prostaglandins help protect the eye.

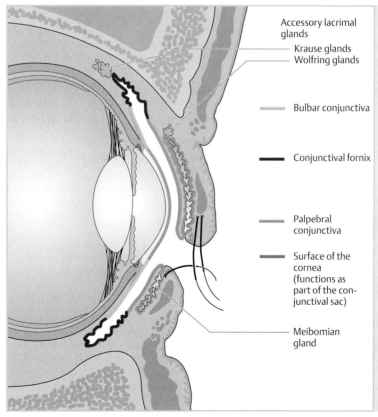

Accessory lacrimal glands

Krause glands
Wolfring glands

Bulbar conjunctiva

Conjunctival fornix

Palpebral conjunctiva

Surface of the cornea (functions as part of the conjunctival sac)

Meibomian gland

Fig. 4.1 Anatomy of the conjunctiva. The conjunctiva consists of the bulbar conjunctiva, the conjunctival fornices, and the palpebral conjunctiva. The surface of the cornea functions as the floor of the conjunctival sac.

4.2 Examination Methods

▶ **Inspection.** The **bulbar conjunctiva** can be evaluated by direct inspection under a focused light. Normally it is shiny and transparent. The **other parts of the conjunctiva** will not normally be visible. They can be inspected by everting the upper or lower eyelid (see Eyelid eversion below).

▶ **Dye staining.** Defects and tears in the conjunctiva or cornea can be visualized by applying a drop of fluorescein dye and inspecting the eye under illumination with a cobalt blue filter (see ▶ Fig. 5.15). The dye rose bengal (see p. 34) makes dead epithelial cells of the conjunctiva and cornea and mucus visible, especially in dry eye syndrome.

▶ **Eyelid eversion.** Even the nonophthalmologist must be familiar with the technique of everting the upper or lower eyelid. This is an important examination method in cases in which the conjunctival sac requires cleaning or irrigation, such as removing a foreign body or rendering first aid after a chemical injury. See eversion of the lower (p. 5) or upper lid (p. 5) for a detailed description of the examination method.

4.3 Conjunctival Degeneration and Aging Changes

4.3.1 Pinguecula

Definition
Harmless grayish-yellow thickening of the conjunctival epithelium in the palpebral fissure.

▶ **Epidemiology.** Pingueculae are the most frequently observed conjunctival changes.

▶ **Etiology.** The harmless thickening of the conjunctiva is due to *hyaline degeneration* of the subepithelial collagen tissue. Advanced age and exposure to sun, wind, and dust foster the occurrence of the disorder.

▶ **Symptoms.** Pingueculae do not cause any symptoms.

▶ **Diagnostic considerations.** Inspection will reveal grayish-yellow thickening at the 3 o'clock and 9 o'clock positions on the limbus. The base of the triangular thickening (often located medially)

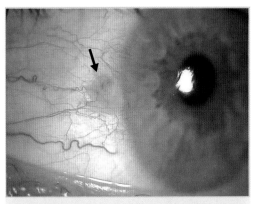

Fig. 4.2 Pinguecula. A harmless triangular pinguecula, the base of which is parallel to the cornea (arrow).

will be parallel to the limbus of the cornea; the tip will be directed toward the angle of the eye (▶ Fig. 4.2).

▶ **Differential diagnosis.** A pinguecula is an unequivocal finding.

▶ **Treatment.** No treatment is necessary.

4.3.2 Pterygium

Definition
A triangular fold of conjunctiva that usually grows from the medial portion of the palpebral fissure toward the cornea. The apex of the triangle is known as the head of the pterygium, the base is known as the body.

▶ **Epidemiology.** Pterygium is especially prevalent in southern countries due to increased exposure to intense sunlight.

▶ **Etiology.** Histologically, a pterygium is identical to a pinguecula. However, it differs in that it can grow onto the cornea; the gray head of the pterygium will grow gradually toward the center of the cornea (▶ Fig. 4.3a). This progression is presumably the result of a *disorder of Bowman's layer of the cornea*, which provides the necessary growth substrate for the pterygium.

▶ **Symptoms and diagnostic considerations.** A pterygium only produces symptoms when its head threatens the center of the cornea and with it the visual axis (▶ Fig. 4.3b). Tensile forces acting on the cornea can cause severe corneal astigmatism. A

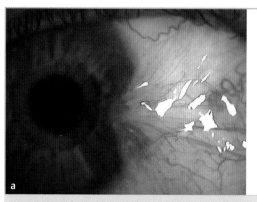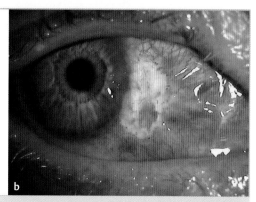

Fig. 4.3 Pterygium. (a) A triangular fold of conjunctiva growing from the medial portion of the palpebral fissure toward the cornea. **(b)** Same image as **(a)** after removal of the pterygium and replacement with a free conjunctival graft with multiple 10–0 vicryl sutures.

steadily advancing pterygium that includes scarred conjunctival tissue can also gradually impair ocular motility; the patient will then experience double vision in abduction.

▶ **Differential diagnosis.** A pterygium is an unequivocal finding.

▶ **Treatment.** Treatment is only necessary when the pterygium produces the symptoms discussed above. Surgical removal is indicated in such cases. The head and body of the pterygium are largely removed, and the scleral defect is covered with a free conjunctival graft. The cornea is smoothed with a diamond reamer or an excimer laser (a special laser that operates in the ultraviolet range at a wavelength of 193 nm) (▶ Fig. 4.3b).

▶ **Clinical course and prognosis.** Pterygia tend to recur. An eccentric lamellar keratoplasty (see p. 89) is indicated in such cases to replace the diseased Bowman's layer with normal tissue. Otherwise the diseased Bowman's layer will continue to provide a growth substrate for a recurrent pterygium.

4.3.3 Pseudopterygium

A pseudopterygium due to conjunctival scarring differs from a pterygium in that there are *adhesions* between the scarred conjunctiva and the cornea and sclera. Causes include corneal injuries and/or chemical injuries and burns. Pseudopterygia cause pain and double vision. Treatment consists of lysis of the adhesions, excision of the scarred conjunctival tissue, and coverage of the defect (this can be achieved with a free conjunctival graft harvested from the temporal aspect).

4.3.4 Subconjunctival Hemorrhage

Extensive bleeding under the conjunctiva (▶ Fig. 4.4) frequently occurs with conjunctival injuries (see p. 320). Subconjunctival hemorrhaging will also often occur spontaneously in elderly patients (as a result of compromised vascular structures in arteriosclerosis), or it may occur after coughing, sneezing, pressing, bending over, or lifting heavy objects. Although these findings are often very unsettling for the patient, they are usually *harmless* and resolve spontaneously within 2 weeks. The patient's blood pressure and coagulation status need only be checked to exclude hypertension or coagulation disorders when subconjunctival hemorrhaging occurs repeatedly.

4.3.5 Calcareous Infiltration

A foreign-body sensation in the eye is often caused by white punctate concrements on the palpebral conjunctiva. These concrements are the *calcified contents* of goblet cells, accessory conjunctival and lacrimal glands, or meibomian glands where there is insufficient drainage of secretion. These calcareous infiltrates can be removed with a scalpel under topical anesthesia.

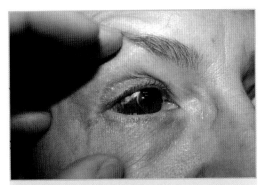

Fig. 4.4 **Subconjunctival hemorrhage.** Extensive bleeding under the conjunctiva.

4.3.6 Conjunctival Xerosis

Definition
Desiccation of the conjunctiva due to a vitamin A deficiency.

▶ **Epidemiology.** Due to the high general standard of nutrition, this disorder is very rare in the developed world. However, it is one of the most frequent causes of blindness in developing countries.

▶ **Etiology.** Vitamin A deficiency results in keratinization of the superficial epithelial cells of the eye. Degeneration of the goblet cells causes the surface of the conjunctiva to lose its luster (▶ Fig. 4.5a). The keratinized epithelial cells die and are swept into the palpebral fissure by blinking, where they accumulate and create characteristic white Bitot's spots (▶ Fig. 4.5b). Xerosis bacteria frequently are involved.

▶ **Treatment and prognosis.** The changes disappear after local and systemic vitamin A substitution. Without vitamin A substitution, the disorder will lead to blindness within a few years.

For details on keratoconjunctivitis sicca (dry eyes) see Chapter 3.

4.4 Conjunctivitis

4.4.1 General Notes on the Causes, Symptoms, and Diagnosis of Conjunctivitis

Definition
Conjunctivitis is an inflammatory process involving the surface of the eye and characterized by vascular dilatation, cellular infiltration, and exudation. Two forms of the disorder are distinguished:
- **Acute conjunctivitis.** Onset is abrupt and initially unilateral with inflammation of the second eye within 1 week. Duration is less than 4 weeks.
- **Chronic conjunctivitis.** Duration is longer than 3 to 4 weeks.

▶ **Epidemiology.** Conjunctivitis is one of the most frequent eye disorders.

▶ **Etiology.** The causes of conjunctivitis fall into two broad categories:
- **Infectious**
  ○ Bacterial.
  ○ Viral.
  ○ Parasitic.
  ○ Mycotic.

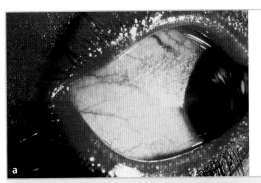
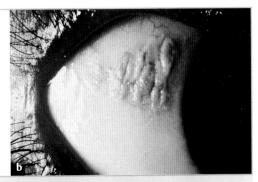

Fig. 4.5 **Conjunctival xerosis due to vitamin A deficiency.** (a) Keratinization of the superficial epithelial cells causes the surface of the conjunctiva to lose its luster. (b) The keratinized epithelial cells die and produce characteristic Bitot's spots in the palpebral fissure.

- **Noninfectious** (see ▸ Table 4.3)
  - From a persistent irritation (such as lack of tear fluid or uncorrected refractive error; see ▸ Table 4.3).
  - Allergic.
  - Toxic (due to irritants such as smoke, dust, etc.).
  - As a result of another disorder (such as Stevens–Johnson syndrome).

▸ **Symptoms.** Typical symptoms exhibited by all patients include **reddened eyes** and **sticky eyelids** in the morning due to *increased secretion*. Any conjunctivitis also causes **swelling of the eyelid**, which will appear partially closed *(pseudoptosis)*. **Foreign-body sensation**, a **sensation of pressure**, and a **burning sensation** are usually present, although these symptoms may vary between individual patients. Intense itching always suggests an allergic reaction. **Photophobia** and **lacrimation** (epiphora) may also be present but can vary considerably. Simultaneous presence of **blepharospasm** suggests corneal involvement (keratoconjunctivitis).

▸ **Diagnostic considerations.** There are many causes of conjunctivitis, and the clinical picture and symptoms can vary considerably between individual patients. This makes it all the more important to note certain characteristic findings that permit an accurate diagnosis, such as the type of exudation, conjunctival findings, or swollen preauricular lymph nodes (▸ Table 4.1).

▸ **Hyperemia.** Reddened eyes are a typical sign of conjunctivitis. The conjunctival injection is due to increased filling of the conjunctival blood vessels, which occurs most prominently in the conjunctival fornices. Hyperemia is present in all forms of conjunctivitis. However, the visibility of the hyperemic vessels and their location and size are important criteria for differential diagnosis. One can also distinguish conjunctivitis from other disorders such as scleritis or keratitis according to the injection (▸ Fig. 4.6).

The following types of injection are distinguished:
- *Conjunctival injection* (bright red, clearly visible distended vessels that move with the conjunctiva, decreasing toward the limbus; ▸ Fig. 4.7).
- *Pericorneal injection* (superficial vessels, circular or circumscribed in the vicinity of the limbus).
- *Ciliary injection* (not clearly discernible, brightly colored nonmobile vessels in the episclera near the limbus).
- *Composite injection* (frequent).

▸ **Discharge.** The quantity and nature of the exudate (mucoid, purulent, watery, stringy, or bloody) depend on the etiology (see ▸ Table 4.1).

▸ **Chemosis.** This may range from the absence of any conjunctival thickening to a white glassy edema and swelling of the conjunctiva projecting from the palpebral fissure (chemosis this severe occurs with bacterial and allergic conjunctivitis) (▸ Fig.4.8).

▸ **Epiphora (excessive tearing).** Illacrimation should be distinguished from exudation. Illacrimation is usually reflex lacrimation in reaction to a conjunctival or corneal foreign body or toxic irritation.

▸ **Follicle.** Lymphocytes in the palpebral and bulbar conjunctiva accumulate in punctate masses of lymph tissue cells that have a granular appearance. Follicles occur typically in viral and chlamydial infections (▸ Fig. 4.9).

▸ **Papillae.** Papillae appear as polygonal "cobblestone" conjunctival projections with a central network of finely branching vessels. They are a typical sign of allergic conjunctivitis (▸ Fig. 4.10).

▸ **Membranes and pseudomembranes.** These are conjunctival reactions to severe infectious or toxic conjunctivitis. They form from necrotic epithelial tissue and can either be easily removed without bleeding (pseudomembranes) or leave behind a bleeding surface when they are removed (membranes; ▸ Fig. 4.11).

▸ **Swollen lymph nodes.** Lymph from the eye region drains through the preauricular and submandibular lymph nodes. Swollen lymph nodes are an important and frequently encountered diagnostic sign of viral conjunctivitis.

▸ **Pannus formation.** Pannus is conjunctival or vascular ingrowth between Bowman's layer and the corneal epithelium in the upper circumference.

> **Note**
> The combination and severity of individual symptoms usually provide essential information that helps to identify the respective presenting form of conjunctivitis.

▸ **Granulomas.** Granulomas are inflamed nodes of conjunctival stroma with circumscribed areas of

Table 4.1 Symptoms and findings in conjunctivitis as they relate to various forms of the disorder

Symptom or finding	Bacterial conjunctivitis	Chlamydial conjunctivitis	Viral conjunctivitis	Allergic conjunctivitis	Toxic conjunctivitis
Itching	–	–	±	++	–
Hyperemia (reddened eye)	++	+	+	+	+
Bleeding	+	–	+	–	–
Discharge	Purulent; yellow crusts	Mucopurulent	Watery	Ropy white, viscous	–
Chemosis	++	–	±	++	±
Lacrimation (epiphora)	+	+	++	+	+
Follicles	–	++	+	+	+
Papillae	+	±	–	+	–
Pseudomembranes, membranes	±	–	±	–	–
Swollen lymph nodes	+	+	++	–	–
Pannus formation	–	+	–	–	±
Concurrent keratitis	±	+	±	–	±
Fever or angina	±	–	±	–	–
Results of cytologic smear	Granulocytes, bacteria	Intracytoplasmic inclusions in epithelial cells, leukocytes, plasma cells, lymphocytes	Lymphocytes, monocytes	Eosinophilic granulocytes, lymphocytes	Epithelial cells, granulocytes, lymphocytes

Note: ++, severe; +, moderate; ±, occasional; –, rare or absent.

reddening and vascular injection. They can occur with systemic disorders such as tuberculosis or sarcoidosis or may be exogenous, such as postoperative suture granulomas or other foreign-body granulomas. Granulomas occur in conjunction with swollen preauricular and submandibular lymph nodes in disorders such as Parinaud's oculoglandular syndrome (see p. 61). Granulomas are not a sign of conjunctivitis in the strict sense and for that reason have not been included as symptoms or findings in ▶ Table 4.1.

▶ **Examination methods.** The symptoms and findings mentioned above are worked up by the following means:

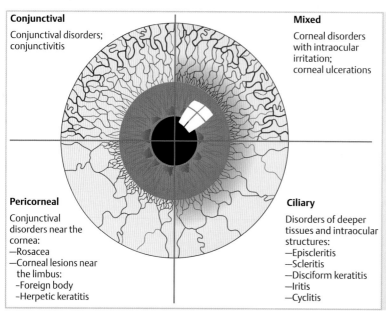

Conjunctival

Conjunctival disorders; conjunctivitis

Mixed

Corneal disorders with intraocular irritation; corneal ulcerations

Pericorneal

Conjunctival disorders near the cornea:
–Rosacea
–Corneal lesions near the limbus:
 –Foreign body
 –Herpetic keratitis

Ciliary

Disorders of deeper tissues and intraocular structures:
–Episcleritis
–Scleritis
–Disciform keratitis
–Iritis
–Cyclitis

Fig.4.6 Forms of conjunctival injection.

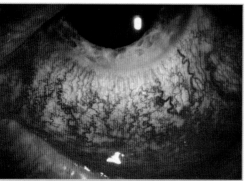

Fig. 4.7 Conjunctival injection. Clearly visible bright red, distended conjunctival vessels, decreasing toward the limbus of the cornea.

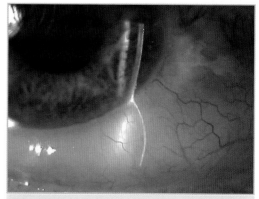

Fig. 4.8 Conjunctival chemosis. White, glassy edema and swelling of the conjunctiva.

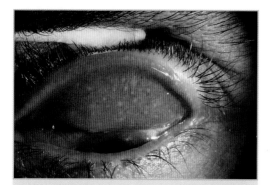

Fig. 4.9 Follicular conjunctivitis. Punctate masses of lymph tissue cells with a granular appearance.

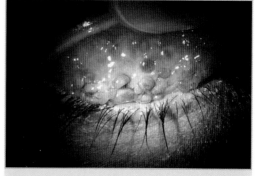

Fig. 4.10 Papillary conjunctivitis. Eversion of the upper eyelid reveals "cobblestone" conjunctival projections.

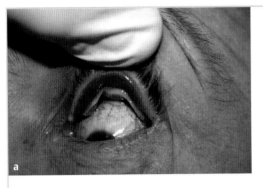
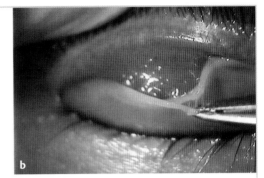
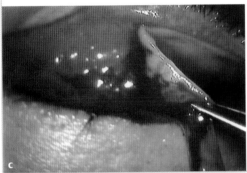

Fig. 4.11 Highly infectious membranous conjunctivitis (a). Genuine membranes leave behind a bleeding surface when they are removed (b,c).

▶ **Slit lamp examination** The nature and extent of vascular injections, discharge, conjunctival swelling, etc. are evaluated using a slit lamp.

▶ **Eyelid eversion.** This is performed to examine the upper and lower eyelids for the presence of follicles, papillae, membranes, and foreign bodies.

▶ **Conjunctival smear.** If the diagnosis is uncertain or what appears to be bacterial conjunctivitis does not respond to antibiotics, a *conjunctival smear* (▶ Fig. 4.12) should be obtained for microbiological examination to identify the pathogen. Cotton swabs with sterile shipping tubes are commercially available; special test kits with specific cultures are available for detecting chlamydiae.

Note
An antibiotic that is not effective in treating what appears to be bacterial conjunctivitis should be discontinued. A conjunctival smear should then be obtained 24 hours later. Microbiological examination to identify the pathogen is indicated for any conjunctivitis in children.

▶ **Epithelial smear.** This is used to detect chlamydiae in particular and to more clearly identify the pathogen in general. A scraping of conjunctival epithelium is smeared on a slide and dyed with Giemsa and Gram stain. Cytologic findings provide important information about the etiology of the conjunctivitis.
- Bacterial conjunctivitis: granulocytes with polymorphous nuclei and bacteria.
- Viral conjunctivitis: lymphocytes and monocytes.
- Chlamydial conjunctivitis (special form of bacterial conjunctivitis): composite findings of lymphocytes, plasma cells, and leukocytes; characteristic intracytoplasmic inclusion bodies in epithelial cells may also be present.
- Allergic conjunctivitis: findings primarily include eosinophilic granulocytes and lymphocytes.
- Mycotic conjunctivitis (very rare): the Giemsa or Gram stain will reveal the hyphae.

▶ **Irrigation.** Conjunctivitis will occur occasionally in asymptomatic dacryocystitis (see p. 34) or canaliculitis (see p. 39) as a result of continuous scattered spread of bacteria. The lower lacrimal system

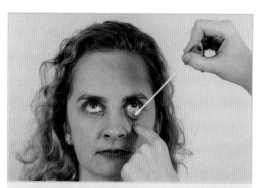

Fig. 4.12 Conjunctival smear for microbiological examination. The lower eyelid is slightly everted, and a smear from the conjunctival secretion is obtained with a cotton swab.

should always be irrigated in the presence of inflammation that recurs or resists treatment to verify or exclude that it is the source of the inflammation.

4.4.2 Infectious Conjunctivitis

The normal conjunctiva contains microorganisms. Inflammation usually occurs as a result of infection from *direct contact with pathogens* (such as from a finger, towel, or swimming pool) but also from *complicating factors* (such as a compromised immune system or injury). There are significant regional differences in the spectrum of pathogens. ▶ Table 4.3 provides an overview of pathogens, symptoms, and treatments.

Bacterial Conjunctivitis

▶ **Epidemiology.** Bacterial conjunctivitis is very frequently encountered.

▶ **Etiology.** Staphylococcal, streptococcal, and pneumococcal infections are most common in temperate countries.

▶ **Symptoms.** Typical symptoms include severe reddening, swelling of the conjunctiva, and purulent discharge that leads to formation of yellowish crusts.

▶ **Diagnostic considerations.** Bacterial conjunctivitis can usually be reliably diagnosed from the presence of typical symptoms. Laboratory tests (conjunctival smear) are usually only necessary when the conjunctivitis fails to respond to antibiotic treatment.

> **Note**
> Bacterial conjunctivitis is diagnosed on the basis of clinical symptoms. Smears are obtained only in severe, uncertain, or persistent cases.

▶ **Treatment.** Bacterial conjunctivitis usually responds very well to antibiotic treatment. A wide range of well-tolerated, highly effective **antibiotic agents** is available today. Most of these are supplied as ointments (which are longer acting and suitable for overnight therapy) and as eye drops for *topical therapy.* Substances include gentamicin, tobramycin, chlortetracycline (Aureomycin), chloramphenicol, neomycin, polymyxin B in combination with bacitracin and neomycin, oxytetracycline (Terramycin), kanamycin, fusidic acid, ofloxacin, and azidamfenicol; see Chapters 20.1 and 20.2 for side effects of gentamicin and chloramphenicol.

Preparations that combine an antibiotic and cortisone can more rapidly alleviate subjective symptoms when findings are closely monitored. These include medications such as gentamicin and dexamethasone; neomycin, polymyxin B, and dexamethasone; or tetracycline, polymyxin B, and hydrocortisone.

In severe, uncertain, or persistent cases requiring microbiological examination to identify the pathogen, treatment with broad-spectrum antibiotics or topical antibiotic combination preparations that cover the full range of gram-positive and gram-negative pathogens should begin immediately. This method is necessary because microbiological identification of the pathogen and resistance testing of the antibiotic are not always successful and may require several days. It is not advisable to leave the conjunctivitis untreated for this period.

> **Note**
> In the presence of severe, uncertain, or persistent conjunctivitis, treatment with broad-spectrum antibiotics or topical antibiotic combination preparations should be initiated immediately, even before the laboratory results are available.

▶ **Clinical course and prognosis.** Bacterial conjunctivitis usually responds well to antibiotic treatment and remits within a few days.

Chlamydial Conjunctivitis

Chlamydiae are gram-negative bacteria.

Inclusion Conjunctivitis

▶ **Epidemiology.** Inclusion conjunctivitis is *very frequent* in temperate countries. The incidence in Western industrialized countries ranges between 1.7% and 24% of sexually active adults depending on the specific population studied.

▶ **Etiology.** Oculogenital infection (*Chlamydia trachomatis* serotypes D–K) is also caused by direct contact. In the newborn (see Neonatal Conjunctivitis, p. 56), this occurs at birth through the cervical secretion. In adults, it is primarily transmitted during sexual intercourse, and rarely from infection in poorly chlorinated swimming pools.

▶ **Clinical symptoms.** The eyes are only moderately red and slightly sticky from viscous discharge.

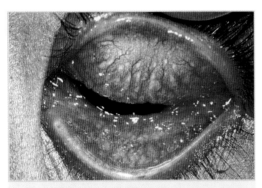

Fig. 4.13 Trachoma (stage II–III). Prominent tarsal follicles and papillae on the upper and lower eyelids.

▶ **Diagnostic considerations.** Tarsal follicles are observed typically on the upper and lower eyelids, and pannus will be seen to spread across the limbus of the cornea. As this is an oculogenital infection, it is essential to determine whether the mother has any history of vaginitis, cervicitis, or urethritis if there is clinical suspicion of neonatal infection. Gynecologic or urologic examination is indicated in appropriate cases. Chlamydia can be detected in conjunctival smears, by immunofluorescence, or in tissue cultures. Typical cytologic signs include basophilic cytoplasmic inclusion bodies.

▶ **Treatment.** In adults, the disorder is treated with tetracycline or erythromycin eye drops or ointment over a period of 4 to 6 weeks. The oculogenital mode of infection entails a risk of reinfection. Therefore, patients and sexual partners of treated patients should all be treated simultaneously with oral tetracycline. *Children* should be treated with erythromycin instead of tetracycline (see Chapters 20.1 and 20.2 for side effects of medications).

▶ **Clinical course and prognosis.** The prognosis is good when the sexual partner is included in therapy.

Trachoma

Trachoma (*Chlamydia trachomatis* serotype A–C) is rare in temperate countries. In endemic regions (with warm climates, poor standard of living, and poor hygiene), it is among the most frequent causes of blindness. Left untreated, the disorder progresses through four stages (▶ Fig. 4.13):
- **Stage I.** Hyperplasia of the lymph follicles on the upper tarsus.

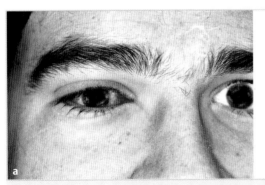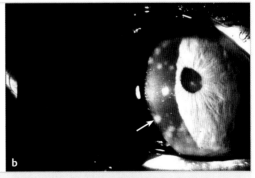

Fig. 4.14 Epidemic keratoconjunctivitis (viral conjunctivitis). **(a)** Acute unilateral reddening of the conjunctiva accompanied by pseudoptosis. **(b)** After 8 to 10 days, coinlike infiltrates (keratitis nummularis or Dimmer's keratitis) appear in the superficial corneal stroma. These may persist for months or years.

- **Stage II.** Papillary hypertrophy of the upper tarsus, subepithelial corneal infiltrates, pannus formation, follicles on the limbus.
- **Stages III and IV.** Increasing scarring and symptoms of keratoconjunctivitis sicca. The progression is entropion, trichiasis, keratitis, superinfection, ulceration, perforation, and finally loss of the eye.

▶ **Treatment.** Administration of erythromycin or tetracycline, depending on stage either local (2–3 weeks) or systemic (at least 3 weeks).

Viral Conjunctivitis

▶ **Epidemiology.** The incidence of **epidemic keratoconjunctivitis** is high in general, and it is by far the most frequently encountered viral conjunctivitis.

▶ **Etiology.** This highly contagious conjunctivitis is usually caused by type 18 or 19 adenovirus and is spread by direct contact (▶ Fig. 4.14a, b) (also see prophylaxis below). The incubation period is 8 to 10 days.

▶ **Symptoms.** Onset is usually unilateral. Typical signs include severe illacrimation and itching accompanied by a watery mucoid discharge. The eyelid and often the conjunctiva are swollen. Patients often also have a moderate influenza infection.

▶ **Diagnostic considerations.** Characteristic findings include reddening and swelling of the plica semilunaris and lacrimal caruncle, and nummular keratitis (▶ Fig. 4.14b) after 8 to 15 days, during the healing phase.

▶ **Treatment.** The disease runs a well-defined clinical course that is nearly impossible to influence and resolves after 2 weeks. No specific therapy is possible. Treatment with artificial tears and cool compresses helps relieve symptoms. Cortisone eye drops should usually be avoided as they can compromise the immune system and prolong the clinical symptoms.

▶ **Prophylaxis.** This is particularly important. Because the disease is spread by contact, patients should refrain from rubbing their eyes despite a severe itching sensation and should avoid direct contact with other people such as shaking hands, sharing tools, or using the same towels or wash cloths, etc.

Special **hygiene precautions** should be taken when examining patients with epidemic keratoconjunctivitis in ophthalmologic care facilities and doctors' offices to minimize the risk of infecting other patients. Patients with epidemic keratoconjunctivitis should not be seated in the same waiting room as other patients. They should not be greeted with a handshake, and they should be requested to refrain from touching objects where possible. Examination should be by indirect means only, avoiding applanation tonometry, contact lens examination, or gonioscopy. After examination, the examiner should clean his or her hands and the work site with a surface disinfectant.

Neonatal Conjunctivitis

▶ **Epidemiology.** Approximately 10% of the newborn contract conjunctivitis.

▶ **Etiology.** The most frequent pathogens are *Chlamydiae*, followed by gonococci (▶ Table 4.2). Neonatal conjunctivitis is less frequently attributable to *other bacteria*—such as *Pseudomonas aeruginosa, Haemophilus, Staphylococcus aureus,* and *Streptococcus pneumoniae*—or to herpes simplex. The infection occurs at birth. Chlamydia infections are particularly important because they are among the most common undetected maternal genital diseases in Europe, affecting 5% of pregnant women. Neonatal conjunctivitis sometimes occurs as a result of Credé's method of prophylaxis with silver nitrate, which in Europe is no longer required by law but still often recommended to prevent *bacterial* infection.

▶ **Symptoms.** Depending on the pathogen, the inflammation will manifest itself between the 2nd and 14th day of life (▶ Table 4.2). The spectrum ranges from mild conjunctival irritation to life-threatening infection (especially with gonococcal infection). Conjunctivitis as a result of Credé's method of prophylaxis appears within hours, but leads only to mild conjunctival irritation.

Note
Acute purulent conjunctivitis in the newborn (gonococcal conjunctivitis) is considered a medical emergency. The patient should be referred to an ophthalmologist for specific diagnosis.

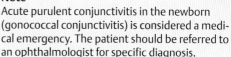

▶ **Diagnostic considerations.** The tentative clinical diagnosis is made on the basis of the onset of

Table 4.2 Differential diagnosis of neonatal conjunctivitis (ophthalmia neonatorum)

Cause	Onset	Findings	Cytology and laboratory tests
Toxic (AgNO₃: silver nitrate; Credé's prophylaxis)	Within hours	• Hyperemia • Slight watery to mucoid discharge	Negative culture
Gonococci (gonococcal conjunctivitis)	2nd–4th day of life	• Acute purulent conjunctivitis	Intracellular gram-negative diplococci; positive culture on blood agar and chocolate agar
Other bacteria (*Pseudomonas aeruginosa, Staphylococcus aureus, Streptococcus pneumoniae, Haemophilus*)	4th–5th day of life	• Mucopurulent conjunctivitis	Gram-positive or gram-negative organisms; positive culture on blood agar
Chlamydia (inclusion conjunctivitis)	5th–14th day of life	• Mucopurulent conjunctivitis, less frequently purulent • Viscous mucus	Giemsa-positive cytoplasmic inclusion bodies in epithelial cells; negative culture
Herpes simplex virus	5th–7th day of life	• Watery blepharoconjunctivitis • Corneal involvement • Systemic manifestations	Multinucleated giant cells, cytoplasmic inclusion bodies; negative culture

the disease (▶ Table 4.2) and the clinical symptoms. For example, gonococcal infections (gonococcal conjunctivitis) are typified by particularly severe accumulations of pus (▶ Fig. 4.15). The newborn's eyelids are tight and swollen because the pus accumulates under them. When the baby's eyes are opened, the pus can squirt out under pressure and cause dangerous conjunctivitis in the examiner's own eyes.

Note
The examiner should always wear eye protection in the presence of suspected gonococcal conjunctivitis to guard against infection from pus issuing from the newborn's eyes. Gonococci can penetrate the eye even in the absence of a corneal defect and lead to loss of the eye.

The diagnosis should be confirmed by cytologic and microbiological studies. However, these studies often fail to yield unequivocal results, so that treatment must proceed on the basis of clinical findings.

▶ **Differential diagnosis.** The onset of the disease is crucial to differential diagnosis (▶ Table 4.2). Neonatal conjunctivitis must be distinguished from neonatal dacryocystitis (see p. 39). This disorder differs from the specific forms of conjunctivitis and it only becomes symptomatic 2 to 4 weeks after birth, with reddening and swelling of the region of the lacrimal sac and purulent discharge from the puncta. It can be readily distinguished

from neonatal conjunctivitis because of these symptoms.

▶ **Treatment**
▶ **Toxic conjunctivitis (Credé's method of prophylaxis).** When the eye is regularly flushed and the eyelids cleaned, symptoms will abate spontaneously within 1 or 2 days.

▶ **Gonococcal conjunctivitis.** Topical administration of broad-spectrum antibiotics (gentamicin eye drops every hour) and systemic penicillin (penicillin G IV 2 million IU daily) or cephalosporin in the presence of penicillinase-producing strains.

▶ **Chlamydial conjunctivitis.** Systemic erythromycin and topical erythromycin eye drops five times daily. There is a risk of recurrence where the dosage or duration of treatment is insufficient. It is essential to examine the parents and include them in therapy.

▶ **Herpes simplex conjunctivitis.** Therapy involves application of acyclovir ointment to the conjunctival sac and eyelids as herpes vesicles will usually be present there, too. Systemic acyclovir therapy is only required in severe cases.

▶ **Prophylaxis. Credé's method of prophylaxis** (application of 1% silver nitrate solution) prevents bacterial inflammation but not chlamydial or herpes infection. Prophylaxis of chlamydial infection consists of regular examination of the woman

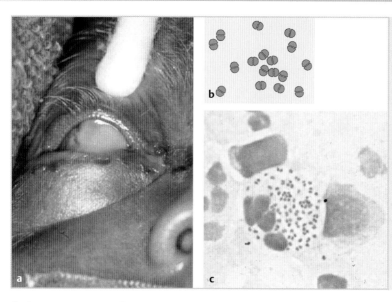

Fig. 4.15 Neonatal conjunctivitis (gonococcal conjunctivitis). (a) Highly infectious conjunctivitis with swelling of the eyelids and a creamy purulent discharge issuing from the palpebral fissure. **(b,c)** Gram staining of the conjunctival smear reveals characteristic gram-negative intracellular diplococci (gonococci).

during pregnancy and treatment in appropriate cases.

Parasitic and Mycotic Conjunctivitis

Parasitic and mycotic forms of conjunctivitis are less important in temperate climates. They are either *very rare* or occur primarily as comorbidities associated with a primary corneal disorder, such as mycotic infections of corneal ulcers.

4.4.3 Noninfectious Conjunctivitis

▶ Table 4.3 provides an overview of pathogens, symptoms, and treatments of noninfectious conjunctivitis.

Acute conjunctivitis is frequently attributable to a series of external irritants or to dry eyes (conjunctivitis sicca). The disorder is *unpleasant but benign*. Primary symptoms include foreign-body sensation, reddening of the eyes of varying severity, and epiphora. Therapy should focus on eliminating the primary irritant and treating the symptoms.

Acute conjunctivitis should be distinguished from the group of **allergic forms of conjunctivitis**, which can be due to seasonal influences and often affect the nasal mucosa. Examples include *allergic conjunctivitis* (hay fever; ▶ Fig. 4.16) and *vernal conjunctivitis*. In *giant papillary conjunctivitis*, the inflammation is triggered by a foreign body (hard or soft contact lenses.) There may also be an additional chronic microbial irritation such microbial contamination of contact lenses. *Phlyctenular keratoconjunctivitis* is a *delayed allergic reaction* to

microbial proteins or toxins (staphylococcal inflammation). This disease occurs frequently in atopic individuals and is promoted by poor hygiene. The cardinal rule in allergic conjunctivitis is to avoid the causative agent. Desensitization should be performed as a *prophylactic measure* by a dermatologist or allergist. Long-term treatment includes cromoglycic acid eye drops, lodoxamide, olopatadine, azelastine, antazoline, or levocabastine to prevent mast cell degranulation. *Treatment of acute allergic conjunctivitis* consists of administering cooling compresses, artificial tears with preservatives, astringent eye drops (tetryzoline and naphazoline), and, if necessary, surface-acting cortisone eye drops (fluorometholone).

Oculomucocutaneous syndromes such as *Stevens–Johnson syndrome* (erythema multiforme), *Lyell's syndrome* (toxic epidermal necrolysis), and

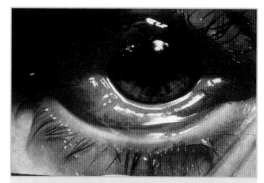

Fig. 4.16 Seasonal allergic conjunctivitis. Conjunctival swelling (chemosis) in a patient with hay fever.

Table 4.3 Overview of noninfectious conjunctivitis

Cause and form of conjunctivitis		Clinical course	Symptoms and findings	Other characteristic features	Treatment
Irritant	Acute conjunctivitis	Acute to chronic	Foreign-body sensation, conjunctival reddening, epiphora, blepharitis	• Lack of tears (keratoconjunctivitis sicca)	• Artificial tears
				• External irritants: smoke, heat, cold, wind (car window or open convertible top), ultraviolet light (welding, high-altitude sunlight)	• Avoiding specific irritants
				• Positional anomalies of the eyelids or eyelashes	• Correction of anomaly or eyelash epilation
				• Uncorrected refractive error (usually hyperopia)	• Eyeglasses
				• Dysfunction of binocular vision (uncompensated heterophoria)	• Prism lenses
				• Improperly centered eyeglasses or wrong correction	• Center or replace eyeglass lenses
				• Overexertion, lack of sleep (burnout syndrome)	• Rest
Allergy	Allergic conjunctivitis (hay fever)	Acute (seasonal)	Severe tearing, chemosis (can be extremely severe), watery discharge, foreign-body sensation, sneezing	Typically accompanied by rhinitis; seasonal allergy to pollen, grasses, and plant allergens	• Desensitization • Astringent eye drops (tetryzoline, naphazoline), if necessary with surface-acting cortisone eye drops (fluorometholone)
	Vernal conjunctivitis	Acute (seasonal)	• *Tarsal and conjunctival form:* "cobblestone" conjunctival projections on the palpebral conjunctiva of the upper eyelid, pseudoptosis, foreign-body sensation, epiphora • *Limbic form:* Swelling of the bulbar conjunctiva is the primary symptom, accompanied by a ring of nodules on the limbus of the cornea, foreign-body sensation, and epiphora	Occurs in boys and male adolescents during spring, either isolated in the eyes or in combination with generalized asthma; IgE-mediated reaction	• Brief treatment with cortisone eye drops to control swelling • Acetylcysteine gel to liquefy the mucus • Cromoglycic acid eye drops as prophylaxis during the asymptomatic interval • Levocabastine hydrochloride

Table 4.3 Overview of noninfectious conjunctivitis (continued)

Cause and form of conjunctivitis		Clinical course	Symptoms and findings	Other characteristic features	Treatment
			• *Corneal involvement:* Widespread corneal erosion to which mucus adheres (plaques), defensive triad of pain, blepharospasm, and epiphora		
	Giant papillary conjunctivitis	Chronic	Conjunctival reddening and irritation with pronounced papillary hypertrophy, similar to the findings and symptoms in vernal conjunctivitis	Frequently due to overwearing contact lenses (especially soft lenses); microbial component is probable (smear should be obtained)	Use of contact lenses should be discontinued until the inflammation abates. Contact lenses should be replaced or refitted; if the disorder recurs, they should be discontinued
	Phlyctenular keratoconjunctivitis	Chronic	Discrete nodular areas of inflammation of the cornea or conjunctiva (phlyctenules), photophobia, epiphora, itching, rarely foreign body sensation, no pain	Usually occurs in children and young adults living in poor hygienic conditions and in countries characterized by a high rate of tuberculosis. The disease is uncommon in Western countries	Topical broad-spectrum antibiotics combined with cortisone or cortisone eye drops alone provide rapid relief of symptoms
Oculomucocutaneous syndrome	Stevens–Johnson syndrome (erythema multiforme)	Chronic	Allergic, membranous conjunctivitis with blistering and increasing symblepharon; often the skin is also involved	Toxic immunologic disorder, usually generalized as a reaction to medications (generally an antibiotic); life-threatening	• Bland ointment therapy (such as dexpanthenol) • Rarely cortisone eye ointment • Clean conjunctiva of fibrin daily • Lysis of symblepharon
	Toxic epidermal necrolysis (Lyell's syndrome)	Hyperacute	Generalized blistering and shedding of necrotic skin, mucous membrane, and conjunctivitis	Extremely acute, life-threatening disorder	Stevens-Johnson and Lyell's syndromes have a similar clinical course and similar treatment as well

	Ocular pemphigoid	Chronic	Chronic bilateral conjunctivitis persisting for years; leads to increased scarring, symblepharon, and increasingly shallow conjunctival fornix that may progress to total obliteration of the conjunctival sac between the bulbar conjunctiva and the palpebral conjunctiva	Autoimmune process with chronic episodic course; eye drops and preservatives used in them exacerbate the process	• *Symptomatic:* Artificial tears without preservatives
					  ○ *Topical broad-spectrum antibiotics* in case of bacterial superinfection
					  ○ *Topical steroid therapy* relieves symptoms. Note: this increases intraocular pressure (risk of cataract)
					  ○ *Systemic steroids* in an acute episode
					  ○ *Immunosuppressive agents:* cyclosporine

ocular pemphigoid (progressive shrinkage of the conjunctiva) are clinical syndromes that involve multiple toxic and immunologic causative mechanisms. The clinical course of the disorder is severe, therapeutic options are limited, and the prognosis for eyesight is poor (▶ Fig. 4.17).

Conjunctival irritation symptoms can occur with *Graves's orbitopathy, gout, rosacea, neurodermatitis, erythema multiforme, Sjögren's syndrome,* and *Reiter's syndrome* (triad: conjunctivitis or iridocyclitis, urethritis, and polyarthritis). **Parinaud's oculoglandular syndrome** describes a clinical syndrome of widely varied etiology. *Granulomatous conjunctivitis always occurs unilaterally* and in conjunction with swollen preauricular and submandibular lymph nodes in the presence of tuberculosis, syphilis, viruses, bacteria, fungi, and parasites. The excisional biopsy of the conjunctival granuloma is itself part of the *treatment of granulomatous conjunctivitis*. The specific medications will depend on the underlying disorder.

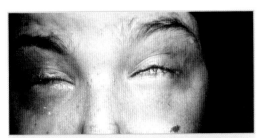

Fig. 4.17 Stevens–Johnson syndrome (erythema multiforme). After several years, the conjunctival sac has fused completely (total symblepharon), effectively causing blindness.

4.5 Tumors

Primary benign conjunctival tumors (nevi, dermoids, lymphangiomas, hemangiomas, lipomas, and fibromas) occur *frequently,* as do tumorlike inflammatory changes (viral papillomas, granulomas such as suture granulomas after surgery to correct strabismus, cysts, and lymphoid hyperplasia). **Malignant conjunctival tumors** (carcinomas in situ, carcinomas, Kaposi's sarcomas, lymphomas, and primary acquired melanosis) are *rare.* **Benign lesions may become malignant**; for example, a nevus or acquired melanosis may develop into a malignant melanoma. This section presents only the most important tumors.

4.5.1 Epibulbar Dermoid

Epibulbar dermoid is a round dome-shaped grayish-yellow or whitish *congenital* tumor. It is generally located on the limbus of the cornea, extending into the corneal stroma to a varying depth. Epibulbar dermoids can occur as *isolated lesions* or as a *symptom of oculoauriculovertebral dysplasia* (Goldenhar's syndrome). Additional symptoms of that disorder include outer ear deformities and preauricular appendages (▶ Fig. 4.18a, b). Dermoids can contain hair and minor skin appendages. Ophthalmologists are often asked to remove them for cosmetic reasons. Surgical excision should remain strictly superficial; complete excision may risk perforating the globe as dermoids often extend through the entire wall of the eyeball.

4.5.2 Conjunctival Hemangioma

Conjunctival hemangiomas are small, cavernous proliferations of blood vessels. They are congenital anomalies and usually resolve spontaneously by

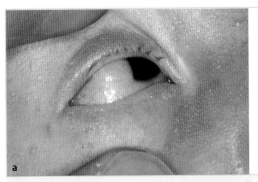
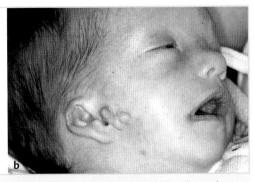

Fig. 4.18 Epibulbar dermoid in oculoauriculovertebral dysplasia (Goldenhar's syndrome). (a) Epibulbar dermoid on the limbus of the cornea. **(b)** Additional preauricular appendages.

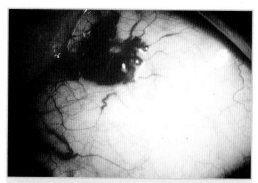

Fig. 4.19 Conjunctival hemangioma. Small cavernous proliferations of blood vessels on the conjunctiva.

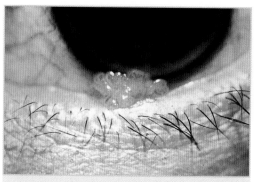

Fig. 4.21 Conjunctival papilloma. A broad-based papilloma originating from the surface of the palpebral conjunctiva.

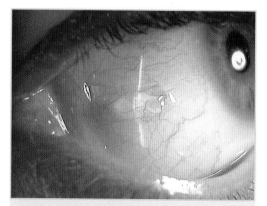

Fig. 4.20 Conjunctival cyst. Small, clear, fluid-filled inclusions of conjunctival epithelium (slit lamp examination).

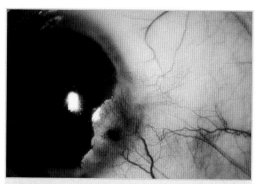

Fig. 4.22 Conjunctival squamous cell carcinoma. Typical features include the whitish, raised, thickened area of epithelial tissue.

the age of 7 years. Where this is not the case, they can be surgically removed (▶ Fig. 4.19).

4.5.3 Epithelial Conjunctival Tumors

Conjunctival Cysts

Conjunctival cysts are *harmless and benign*. Occurrence is most often postoperative (for example, after surgery to correct strabismus), posttraumatic, or spontaneous. They usually take the form of small clear fluid-filled inclusions of conjunctival epithelium whose goblet cells secrete into the cyst and not onto the surface (▶ Fig. 4.20). Cysts can lead to a foreign-body sensation and are removed surgically by marsupialization (removal of the upper half of the cyst).

Conjunctival Papilloma

Papillomas are of viral origin (human papillomavirus) and may develop from the bulbar or palpebral conjunctiva. They are *benign and do not turn malignant*. As in the skin, conjunctival papillomas can occur as *branching pediculate* tumors or as *broad-based* lesions on the surface of the conjunctiva (▶ Fig. 4.21). Papillomas produce a permanent foreign-body sensation that is annoying to the patient, and the entire lesion should be surgically removed.

Conjunctival Carcinoma

Conjunctival carcinomas are usually whitish, raised, thickened areas of epithelial tissue whose surface forms a plateau. These lesions are usually keratinizing squamous cell carcinomas that develop from epithelial dysplasia (precancer) and progress to a carcinoma in situ (▶ Fig. 4.22). Conjunctival carcinomas must be excised and a cytologic diagnosis obtained, and the patient must undergo postoperative radiation therapy to prevent growth deep into the orbit.

4.5.4 Melanocytic Conjunctival Tumors

Conjunctival Nevus

Birthmarks can occur on the conjunctiva as on the skin. They are usually located near the limbus in the temporal portion of the palpebral fissure, less frequently on the lacrimal caruncle. These *benign*, slightly raised epithelial or subepithelial tumors are *congenital*. Fifty percent of nevi contain hollow cystic spaces (pseudocysts) consisting of conjunctival epithelium and goblet cells. Conjunctival nevi may be pigmented (▶ Fig. 4.23a) or unpigmented (▶ Fig. 4.23b), and they may increase in size as the patient grows older. Increasing pigmentation of the nevus as a result of hormonal changes during pregnancy or puberty or from exposure to sunlight can simulate an increase in the size of the nevus, as can proliferation of the pseudocysts. *Conjunctival nevi*

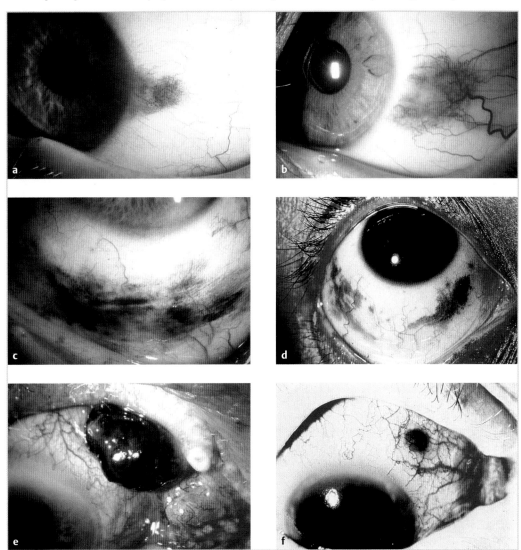

Figs. 4.23 Differential diagnosis of pigmented conjunctival changes. (a) Pigmented conjunctival nevus. **(b)** Unpigmented conjunctival nevus. **(c)** Primary acquired melanosis. **(d)** Congenital melanosis. **(e)** Malignant conjunctival melanoma. **(f)** Malignant melanoma of the ciliary body penetrating through the sclera beneath the conjunctiva.

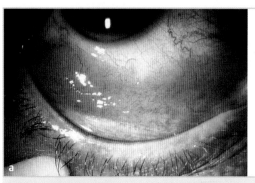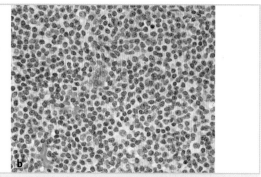

Fig. 4.24 Conjunctival lymphoma. (a) Typical salmon-colored conjunctival tumor in the inferior fornix. (b) Histologic examination shows that this is a MALT (Mucosa Associated Lymphoid Tissue) non-Hodgkin lymphoma.

can degenerate into conjunctival melanomas (50% of conjunctival melanomas develop from a nevus). Therefore, complete excision and histologic diagnostic studies are indicated if the nevus significantly increases in size or shows signs of inflammation (► Fig. 4.23e, ► Fig. 4.23f).

> **Note**
> Photographs should always be taken during follow-up examinations of conjunctival nevi. Small, clear, watery inclusion cysts are always a sign of a conjunctival nevus.

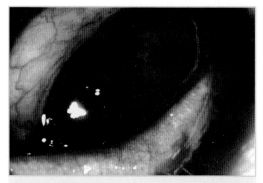

Fig. 4.25 Kaposi's sarcoma. A prominent dark red tumor in the conjunctival fornix in a patient with AIDS.

Conjunctival Melanosis

Definition
Conjunctival melanosis is a pigmented thickening of the conjunctival epithelium (► Fig. 4.23c).

Synonym: Primary acquired conjunctival melanosis

► **Epidemiology.** Conjunctival melanosis is rare like all potentially malignant or malignant tumors of the conjunctiva.

► **Etiology.** Unclear.

► **Symptoms.** Acquired conjunctival melanosis usually occurs after the age of 40 years. Typical symptoms include irregular diffuse pigmentation and thickening of the epithelium that may "come and go."

► **Diagnostic considerations.** Acquired conjunctival melanosis is mobile with the conjunctiva (an important characteristic that distinguishes it from congenital melanosis). It requires close observation with follow-up examinations every 6 months as it can develop into a malignant melanoma.

► **Differential diagnosis.** This disorder should be distinguished from *benign congenital melanosis* (see below), which remains stable throughout the patient's lifetime and appears more bluish-gray than brownish. In contrast to acquired melanosis, it is not mobile with the conjunctiva.

► **Treatment.** Because the disorder occurs diffusely over a broad area, treatment is often difficult. Usually it combines excision of the prominent deeply pigmented portions (for histologic confirmation of the diagnosis) with cryocoagulation of the adjacent melanosis and in some cases with postoperative radiation therapy.

► **Clinical course and prognosis.** About 50% of conjunctival melanomas develop from conjunctival

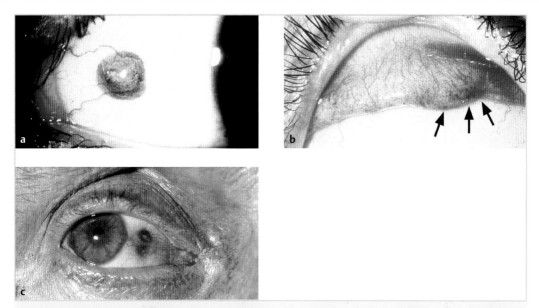

Fig. 4.26 Differential diagnosis of pigmented conjunctival changes. (a) A metallic foreign body that has healed into the conjunctiva. (b) Iron deposits from makeup (mascara). (c) Ochronosis (alkaptonuria).

melanosis (the other 50% develop from conjunctival nevi; see above). Conjunctival melanomas are not usually as aggressively malignant as skin melanomas. The radical resection required to remove the tumor can be a problem. Multiple recurrences will produce significant conjunctival scarring that can result in symblepharon with fusion of the eyelid skin and conjunctiva. Where the tumor has invaded the eyelids or the deeper portions of the orbit, orbital exenteration will be unavoidable to completely remove the tumor.

Congenital Ocular Melanosis

Benign congenital melanosis (▶ Fig. 4.23d) is subepithelial in the episclera. The conjunctival epithelium is *not* involved. Pigmentation is bluish-gray. In contrast to acquired melanosis, congenital melanosis remains *stable* and *stationary* throughout the patient's lifetime. In contrast to nevi and acquired melanosis, congenital melanosis remains stationary when the conjunctiva above it is moved with forceps. Congenital ocular melanosis can occur as an *isolated anomaly of the eye* or *in association with skin pigmentations* (oculodermal melanosis or Ota's nevus). Although the tumor is benign, evidence suggests that malignant melanomas in the choroid occur more frequently in patients with congenital melanosis.

4.5.5 Conjunctival Lymphoma

Prominent areas of salmon-colored conjunctival thickening frequently occurring in the inferior fornix (▶ Fig. 4.24) are often the first sign of lymphatic disease. Identifying the specific forms and degree of malignancy requires biopsy and histologic examination. Lesions may range from benign lymphoid hyperplasia to malignant lymphomas that are moderately to highly malignant. Because lymphomas respond to radiation, a combination of radiation therapy and chemotherapy is usually prescribed according to the specific histologic findings.

4.5.6 Kaposi's Sarcoma

This is a prominent, light to dark red tumor in the conjunctival fornix or proceeding from the palpebral conjunctiva. It consists of malignant spindle cells and nests of atypical endothelial cells. Today Kaposi's sarcomas are rare and are seen most frequently as opportunistic disease in patients with acquired immune deficiency syndrome (AIDS). The ophthalmologist can make a tentative diagnosis of AIDS on the basis of typical clinical signs on the conjunctiva and order further diagnostic studies (▶ Fig. 4.25). Recently there has been evidence that herpesvirus (HHV-8) is involved in the development of Kaposi's sarcoma.

4.6 Conjunctival Deposits

These can occur in both the conjunctiva and cornea. Some, like some tumors, lead to pigmented changes in the conjunctiva. However, their typical appearance usually readily distinguishes them from tumors (▶ Fig. 4.26). The following conjunctival and corneal deposits and discolorations may occur.

▶ **Adrenochrome deposit.** Prolonged use of epinephrine eye drops (as in glaucoma therapy) produces brownish pigmented changes in the inferior conjunctival fornix and on the cornea as a result of epinephrine oxidation products (adrenochrome). This can simulate a melanocytic conjunctival tumor. The physician should therefore always ascertain whether the patient has a history of prolonged use of epinephrine eye drops. No therapy is indicated.

▶ **Iron deposits.** In women, iron deposits from eye makeup and mascara are frequently seen to accumulate in the conjunctival sac (▶ Fig. 4.26b). No therapy is indicated.

▶ **Argyrosis conjunctivae.** Prolonged used of silver-containing eye drops can produce brownish-black silver deposits in the conjunctiva.

▶ **Ochronosis (alkaptonuria: an inherited autosomal-recessive deficiency of the enzyme homogentisate 1,2-dioxygenase).** Approximately 70% of patients with ochronosis exhibit brownish pigmented deposits in the skin of the eyelids, conjunctiva, sclera, and limbus of the cornea (▶ Fig. 4.26c). The deposits increase with time. The disorder cannot be treated in the eye.

▶ **Metallic foreign bodies in the conjunctiva.** A metallic foreign body that is not removed immediately will heal into the conjunctiva, where it will simulate a pigmented change in the conjunctiva (▶ Fig. 4.26a). Obtaining a meticulous history (the examiner should always enquire about ocular trauma) will quickly reveal the cause of the anomaly. The foreign body can be removed under topical anesthesia. For details, see Chapter 18.4.4, page 321.

▶ **Jaundice.** Jaundice will lead to yellowing of the conjunctiva and sclera.

Chapter 5

Cornea

5

5 Cornea

Gerhard K. Lang

5.1 Basic Knowledge

▶ **Fundamental importance of the cornea for the eye.** The cornea is the eye's optical window that makes it possible for humans to see. The ophthalmologist is only able to discern structures in the interior of the eye because the cornea is transparent. At 43 diopters, the cornea is the *most important refractive medium in the eye.*

▶ **Shape and location.** The cornea's *curvature is greater than the sclera's curvature.* It fits into the sclera like a *watchglass* with a shallow sulcus (the limbus of the cornea) marking the junction of the two structures.

▶ **Embryology.** The corneal tissue consists of *five layers.* The cornea and the sclera are formed during the second month of embryonic development. The epithelium develops from ectoderm, and the deeper corneal layers develop from mesenchyme.

▶ **Morphology and healing (▶ Fig. 5.1):**
- The **surface** of the cornea is formed by **stratified nonkeratinized squamous epithelium** that regenerates quickly when injured. Within 1 hour, epithelial defects are closed by cell migration and rapid cell division. However, this assumes that the **limbus stem cells** in the limbus of the cornea are undamaged. Regular corneal regeneration will no longer be possible when these cells are compromised. An intact epithelium protects

against infection; a defect in the epithelium makes it easy for pathogens to enter the eye.
- A thin **basement membrane anchors** the basal cells of the stratified squamous epithelium to **Bowman's layer**. This layer is highly resistant but cannot regenerate. As a result, injuries to Bowman's layer usually produce corneal scarring.
- Beneath Bowman's layer, many lamellae of collagen fibrils form the **corneal stroma**. The stroma is a highly bradytrophic tissue. As avascular tissue, it only regenerates slowly. However, its avascularity makes it an *immunologically privileged site* for grafting. Routine corneal transplants can be performed without prior tissue typing. An increased risk of rejection need only be feared where the *recipient's cornea is highly vascularized,* as may be the case following chemical injury or inflammation. Such cases require either a tissue-typed donor graft or immunosuppressive therapy with cyclosporine.
- Descemet's membrane and the corneal endothelium lie on the posterior surface of the corneal stroma adjacent to the anterior chamber. Descemet's membrane is a relatively strong membrane. It will continue to define the shape of the anterior chamber (e.g., as the result of an inflammation) even where the corneal stroma has completely melted (so-called descemetocele, see p. 75). Because it is a genuine basement *membrane,* lost tissue is regenerated by functional endothelial cells. The **corneal endothelium** is responsible for the *transparency* of the

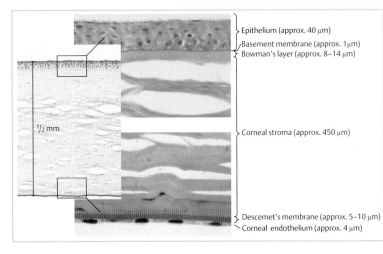

Epithelium (approx. 40 μm)
Basement membrane (approx. 1μm)
Bowman's layer (approx. 8–14 μm)

½ mm

Corneal stroma (approx. 450 μm)

Descemet's membrane (approx. 5–10 μm)
Corneal endothelium (approx. 4 μm)

Fig. 5.1 Anatomy of the cornea. See text for discussion.

cornea (see also Transparency, below). A high density of epithelial cells is necessary to achieve this. The corneal endothelium does not regenerate; defects in the endothelium are closed by cell enlargement and cell migration.

▶ **Diameter.** The **normal average diameter of the adult cornea** is 11.5 mm (10–13 mm). A congenitally small cornea (**microcornea**, diameter less than 10.0 mm) or a congenitally large cornea (**megalocornea**, diameter from 13 to 15 mm) is always an abnormal finding (see Chapter 5.3.2).

▶ **Nourishment.** The five layers of the cornea have few cells and are unstructured and avascular. Like the lens, sclera, and vitreous body, the cornea is a bradytrophic tissue structure. Its metabolism is slow, which means that healing is slow. The cornea is nourished with nutritive metabolites (amino acids and glucose) from three sources:
1. Diffusion from the **capillaries at its edge**.
2. Diffusion from the **aqueous humor**.
3. Diffusion from the **tear film**.

▶ **Significance of the tear film for the cornea.** The three-layer precorneal tear film ensures that the surface of the cornea remains smooth and helps to nourish the cornea (see above). Without a tear film, the surface of the epithelium would be rough, and the patient would see a blurred image. The enzyme lysozyme contained in the tear film also protects the eye against infection (see Chapter 3, p. 32 for composition of the tear film).

▶ **Transparency.** This is due to two factors.
1. The **uniform arrangement of the lamellae of collagen fibrils in the corneal stroma** and the smooth endothelial and epithelial surface produced by the intraocular pressure.
2. The **water content of the corneal stroma, which remains constant at 70%**. The combined action of the epithelium and endothelium maintains a constant water content; the epithelium seals the stroma off from the outside, while the endothelium acts as an ion pump to remove water from the stroma. This requires a *sufficiently high density of endothelial cells*. Endothelial cell density is age-dependent; normally it is approximately 2,500 cells/mm^2. At cell densities below 300 endothelial cells/mm^2, the endothelium is no longer able to pump water out of the cornea, resulting in edema of the corneal stroma and epithelium. The epithelial as well as endothelial layers act as barriers and regulate the exchange between cornea, tear film and aqueous humor by selective diffusion.

▶ **Protection and nerve supply.** The cornea is a vital structure of the eye and as a result extremely sensitive. It receives its *ample sensory supply* from the ophthalmic division of the trigeminal nerve. The slightest tactile sensation causes an eye-closing reflex (see p. 12). Any injury to the cornea (erosion, foreign-body penetration, or ultraviolet keratoconjunctivitis) exposes sensory nerve endings and causes intense pain with reflexive tearing and involuntary eye closing.

Note
The triad of involuntary eye closing (blepharospasm), reflexive tearing (epiphora), and pain always suggests a possible corneal injury (see Chapter 18, p. 322).

5.2 Examination Methods

Nonophthalmologists can evaluate the transparency of the cornea (opacities of the stroma and epithelium suggest scarring or infiltration of the epithelium), its *surface luster* (lack of luster suggests an epithelial defect), and possible *superficial corneal injuries*. A simple ruler can be used to measure the size of the cornea, and *sensitivity* can be tested with a cotton swab (see ▶ Fig. 1.8).

The **ophthalmologist** uses instruments to evaluate corneal morphology and function in greater detail.

5.2.1 Slit Lamp Examination

The slit lamp is the primary instrument used in evaluating the cornea. The ophthalmologist chooses between 8 times and up to 40 times magnification for examining all levels of the cornea with a narrow beam of collimated light (▶ Fig. 5.2).

The slit lamp is the primary instrument for examination of the cornea. It emits slit-shaped bundles of parallel light beams. The slit beam provides direct, indirect, and retrograde illumination of the cornea.

▶ **Direct illumination.** The slit beam is moved over the entire cornea; thus the thickness of the cornea and depth of the anterior chamber can be estimated.

▶ **Indirect illumination.** The light of the slit lamp is directed at the corneal limbus from the side, so

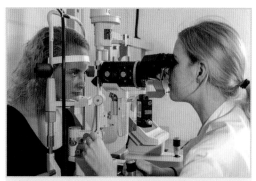

Fig. 5.2 Slit lamp examination of the cornea. The slit lamp (slit aperture) can be used to examine all levels of the cornea with a narrow beam of collimated light.

we have a total reflection by the otherwise completely transparent cornea. Subtle opacities or discrete corneal edema show up with this technique by not totally reflecting the slit lamp light.

▶ **Retrograde illumination.** The cornea is illuminated by light reflected from the iris by a slit lamp beam directed straight into the eye. Subtle epithelial and endothelial findings or small blood vessels become visible.

5.2.2 Dye Examination of the Cornea

Defects in the surface of the cornea can be visualized with fluorescein or rose bengal solution (in either case, administer one drop of 1% solution). Since these dyes are not usually absorbed by the epithelium, they can be used to visualize *loss of epithelium over a wide area* (such as corneal erosion, see p. 322) and *extremely fine defects* (as in superficial punctate keratitis, see p. 81). Illumination with a cobalt blue filter enhances the fluorescent effect.

> **Note**
> These dye methods can reveal corneal epithelial defects (corneal erosion) even without the use of a slit lamp, which is helpful in examining small children.

Wound leakage, that is, a permeable area in the cornea through which intraocular fluid can escape, can be easily diagnosed with the Seidel test (▶ Fig. 5.3). The most frequent causes of wound leakage are perforating injuries, filtration surgery for glaucoma, or cataract operations. To visualize the leaky area, the tear film is dyed with fluorescein (▶ Fig.

5.3a) and the eye is examined under a blue light filter on the slit lamp. The fluorescein shows the intraocular fluid being washed out of the eye (▶ Fig. 5.3b–e).

5.2.3 Corneal Topography

The keratoscope (Placido's disk) permits gross evaluation of the uniformity of the surface of the cornea. This instrument consists of a round disk marked with concentric black and white rings around a central aperture. The examiner holds the disk in his or her hand and looks through the aperture. The *mirror images of the rings on the patient's cornea* indicate the presence of astigmatism (in which case they appear distorted). However, this inexact evaluation method lacks the precision required for modern applications such as refractive surgery. Therefore, the surface of the cornea is now normally evaluated by computerized corneal topography (video keratoscopy). In this examination, the contours of the cornea are measured by a computer in the same manner as by the keratoscope. The refractive values of specific corneal regions are then represented in a color-coded dioptric map. Bright red, for example, represents a steep curvature with a high refractive power. This technique provides a contour map of the distribution of the refractive values over the entire cornea (▶ Fig. 5.4a, b).

5.2.4 Determining Corneal Sensitivity

Nonophthalmologists may perform a simple preliminary examination of corneal sensitivity with a distended cotton swab (see ▶ Fig. 1.8). This examination also helps the ophthalmologist confirm the diagnosis in the presence of a suspected viral infection of the cornea or trigeminal or facial neuropathy as these disorders are associated with reduced corneal sensitivity. Ophthalmologists may use an automatic Dräger esthesiometer **for precise testing of corneal sensitivity** and **for follow-up examinations**. This instrument can incrementally raise the sensitivity stimulus. This makes it possible to determine whether and how rapidly corneal sensitivity increases following corneal transplantation.

5.2.5 Measuring the Density of the Corneal Epithelium

A sufficiently high density of endothelial cells is very important for the transparency of the cornea; for details see Transparency on page 69. **Gross**

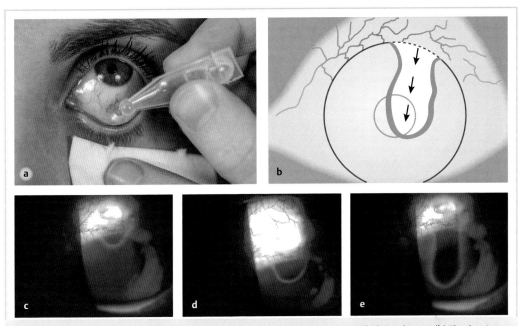

Fig. 5.3 Seidel test for the diagnosis of a corneal leak. (a) Fluorescein drops are instilled into the eye. **(b)** The drawing shows how intraocular fluid runs down over the cornea from the wound leak. The fluorescein makes the escaping fluid visible under a blue light filter **(c–e)**.

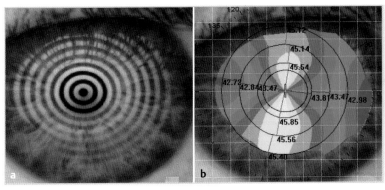

Fig. 5.4 Computerized corneal topography (video keratoscopy). (a) Projection of a Placido's disk onto the cornea. (b) The computer transforms the data from the ring projection into refractive values represented in a color-coded dioptric map.

estimation of the endothelial cell density is possible for a circumscribed area of the cornea using a **slit lamp** and indirect illumination. Both the viewing axis and illumination axis are offset from the visual axis. **Precise quantification** and morphological evaluation of endothelial cells over large areas is only possible by means of **specular microscopy**, a technique designed especially for this purpose (▶ Fig. 5.5). Exact analysis is necessary when the number of cells appears extremely low under slit lamp examination and the patient is a candidate for cataract surgery. If exact analysis then verifies that the number of cells is extremely low (below 300–400 cells/mm²), cataract surgery is

combined with a corneal transplant. This is done to ensure that the patient will be able to see even after cataract surgery, which sacrifices additional endothelial cells.

5.2.6 Measuring the Diameter of the Cornea

An abnormally large or small cornea (megalocornea or microcornea) will be apparent from simple visual inspection. A suspected size anomaly can be easily verified by **measuring** the cornea **with a ruler**. The corneal diameter can be determined more accurately with calipers (usually done under general anesthesia, see ▶ Fig. 10.21) or with the **Wessely keratometer**. This is a type of tube with a condensing lens with millimeter graduations at one end. The examiner places this end on the patient's eye and looks through the other end.

Megalocornea in an infant always requires further diagnostic investigation to determine whether buphthalmos is present (see p. 169). Microcornea may be a sign of congenital defects in other ocular tissues that could result in impaired function (microphthalmos).

5.2.7 Corneal Pachymetry

The thickness of the cornea (about 520 μm centrally) is important for precise measurement of the intraocular pressure. The thicker the cornea, the higher the intraocular pressure; the thinner the cornea, the lower the intraocular pressure. For details, see Chapter 10 on Glaucoma (see p. 144).

Precise measurement of the thickness of the cornea is also crucial in refractive surgery. For details, see Radial keratotomy on page 91 and Astigmatic keratotomy on page 90. Improving refraction often requires making incisions through 90% of the thickness of the cornea while meticulously avoiding full penetration of the cornea. There are two pachymetry techniques for measuring corneal thickness with the high degree of precision that this surgery requires:

- Optical pachymetry with a **slit lamp and measuring attachment** can be carried out with the patient in a seated position, or
- **Ultrasonic** pachymetry; this has the advantage of greater precision and can also be performed with the patient supine.

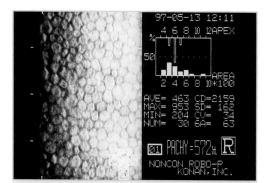

Fig. 5.5 Automatic measurement of endothelial cell density. Specular microscopy allows a precise endothelial cell count (CD=2159 endothelial cells/ mm^2) while simultaneously measuring the thickness of the cornea (pachymetry; pachy = 572 μm).

Recent developments now permit pachymetry by means of specular microscopy. For details see Chapter 5.2.8 and ▶ Fig. 5.5.

5.2.8 Confocal Corneal Microscopy

Confocal corneal microscopy is an examination technique that makes it possible to scan the cornea *over a wide area* from the outer layer to the inner layer. It differs in this regard from slit lamp examination, which tends to be *a focal* examination along a shaft of light perpendicular to the eye. Confocal corneal microscopy visualizes cell structures at maximum magnification that cannot be observed in detail with a slit lamp. These include corneal nerves, amoebas and hyphae.

5.2.9 Ocular Coherence Tomography (OCT)

This high-resolution examination method produces a tissue image that closely resembles a histologic section. Any morphological change is visualized like an optical biopsy (▶ Fig. 5.6).

5.3 Developmental Anomalies

5.3.1 Protrusion Anomalies

Keratoconus

> **Definition**
> Conical, usually bilateral central deformation of the cornea with parenchymal opacification and thinning of the cornea.

▶ **Epidemiology.** Keratoconus is the most *frequently encountered* deformation of the cornea. Occurrence is familial, although women are more likely to be affected than men.

▶ **Etiology.** Keratoconus is probably a genetic disorder. It can occur in families with varying paths of hereditary transmission. Occasionally keratoconus is associated with trisomy 21 syndrome (Down's syndrome) as well as with atopic dermatitis and other connective-tissue disorders such as Marfan's syndrome.

▶ **Symptoms.** The clinical course of the disorder is episodic; the increasing protrusion of the cornea usually produces bilateral irregular myopic astigmatism. Left untreated, in rare cases keratoconus can cause tears of Descemet's membrane due to the

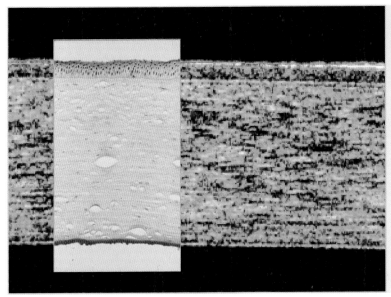

Fig. 5.6 High-resolution corneal OCT. The corneal OCT with superimposed histopathologic corneal section illustrates the detail possible today in representing corneal epithelium, Bowman's membrane, and corneal stroma like an optical biopsy (see also ▶ Fig. 5.1).

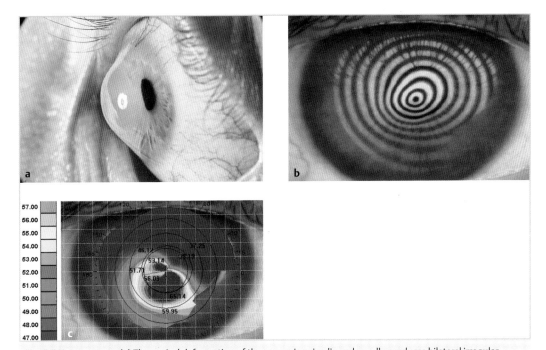

Fig. 5.7 Keratoconus. (a) The conical deformation of the cornea is episodic and usually produces bilateral irregular myopic astigmatism. (b) The Placido's disk image shows distortion and distraction of the ring images. (c) The corresponding color mapping shows decentration of the corneal apex downward and extremely high refractive values (about 65 diopters) in the apex area and a flat cornea (about 37 diopters) in the periphery.

continuous stretching. The entire cornea can then bulge out at this site. This is referred to as acute keratoconus. **Symptoms of acute keratoconus** include sudden loss of visual acuity accompanied by intense pain, photophobia, and increased tearing.

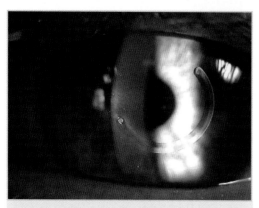

Fig. 5.8 Intracorneal ring segment. Intrastromal implantation of this type of ring segment at the base of the keratoconus serves to stop the progress of the keratoconus and to reduce myopia and astigmatism.

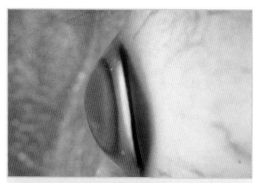

Fig. 5.9 Keratoglobus. The hemispherical protrusion can lead to myopia.

▶ **Diagnostic considerations.** The diagnosis is usually made with a keratoscope or ophthalmometer (reflex images will be irregular). The examiner can also detect keratoconus without diagnostic aids by standing behind the patient and pulling the patient's upper eyelids downward. The conical protrusion of the surface of the cornea (▶ Fig. 5.7) will then be readily apparent due to the deformation of the margin of the eyelid (*Munson's sign*).

▶ **Treatment.** Degeneration of visual acuity can usually be corrected initially with eyeglasses; hard contact lenses will be required as the disorder progresses. However, after a certain point, the patient repeatedly will lose the contact lenses. Recently, crosslinking has become available to patients with verified progressive keratoconus. In this process the cornea is soaked with riboflavin and then irradiated with UV light. This causes linking of collagen fibers and stabilizes the cornea. The cornea can be additionally stabilized by implantation of corneal ring segments (▶ Fig. 5.8). The implantation of such ring segments (see p. 92) is also used for reduction of myopia. Then the only possible treatment is penetrating keratoplasty (transplantation of a corneal graft from a donor into the patient's cornea, see p. 88).

▶ **Prognosis.** The prognosis for penetrating keratoplasty in treating keratoconus is good because the cornea is avascular in keratoconus.

Keratoglobus and Cornea Plana

Very rare disorders include keratoglobus, a congenital deformation resulting in hemispherical protrusion (▶ Fig.5.9) that tends to produce myopia, and flattening of the cornea (cornea plana) that tends to produce hyperopia.

5.3.2 Corneal Size Anomalies (Microcornea and Megalocornea)

Corneal size anomalies are usually congenital and on the whole are rare. An abnormally small cornea (microcornea) has a diameter less than 10.0 mm. It usually causes severe hyperopia that in advanced age often predisposes the patient to angle closure glaucoma (see ▶ Table 10.2). An abnormally large cornea (megalocornea) may be as large as 13 to 15 mm. Corneal enlargement in the newborn and infants may be acquired due to increased intraocular pressure (buphthalmos). Combinations of microcornea and megalocornea together with other ocular deformities may also occur.

5.4 Infectious Keratitis

5.4.1 Protective Mechanisms of the Cornea

As discussed in Chapter 5.1, the cornea has certain defensive mechanisms that are required because of its constant exposure to microbes and environmental influences. The mechanisms include:
- Reflexive eye closing.
- Flushing effect of tear fluid (lysozyme).
- The hydrophobic epithelium forming a diffusion barrier.
- Epithelium being able to regenerate quickly and completely.

5.4.2 Corneal Infections: Predisposing Factors, Pathogens, and Pathogenesis

When certain pathogens succeed in breaching the corneal defenses through superficial injuries or minor epithelial defects, the bradytrophic corneal tissue will respond to the specific pathogen with characteristic keratitis.

▶ **Predisposing factors.** Predisposing factors that promote inflammation are:
- Blepharitis.
- Infection of the ocular appendages (for example, dacryostenosis accompanied by bacterial infestation of the lacrimal sac).
- Changes in the corneal epithelial barrier (bullous keratopathy or dry eyes).
- Contact lenses.
- Lagophthalmos.
- Neuroparalytic disorders.
- Trauma.
- Topical and systemic immunosuppressive agents.

▶ **Pathogens causing corneal infections.** These may include:
- Viruses.
- Bacteria.
- Acanthamoeba.
- Fungi.

▶ **Pathogenesis.** Once these pathogens have invaded the bradytrophic tissue through a superficial corneal lesion, a typical chain of events will ensue:
- Corneal lesion.
- Pathogens invade and colonize the corneal stroma (red eye).
- Antibodies will infiltrate the site.
- As a result, the cornea will opacify and the point of entry will open further, revealing the corneal infiltrate.
- Irritation of the anterior chamber with hypopyon (typically pus will accumulate on the floor of the anterior chamber; see ▶ Fig. 5.10).
- The pathogens will infest the entire cornea.
- As a result the stroma will melt down to Descemet's membrane, which is relatively strong. This is known as a **descemetocele**; only Descemet's membrane is still intact. Descemet's membrane will be seen to protrude anteriorly when examined under a slit lamp.
- As the disorder progresses, perforation of Descemet's membrane occurs and the aqueous humor will be seen to leak. This is referred to as

a **perforated corneal ulcer** and is an indication for immediate surgical intervention (emergency keratoplasty; see Chapter 5.7.1). The patient will notice progressive loss of vision and the eye will be soft.
- **Prolapse of the iris** (the iris will prolapse into the newly created defect) closing the corneal perforation posteriorly. Adhesion of the iris will produce a **white corneal scar**.

This sequence of events can vary in speed and severity. Depending on the voracity of the pathogens and the state of the patient's immune system, an infiltrate can form *within a few hours* or days and quickly progress to a corneal ulcer, melting of the stroma, and even a descemetocele. This rapidly progressing form of infectious corneal ulcer (usually bacterial) is referred to as a **serpiginous corneal ulcer**. It penetrates the cornea particularly rapidly and soon leads to intraocular involvement (the pathogens will be active beyond the visible rim of the ulcer). A serpiginous corneal ulcer is one of the most dangerous clinical syndromes as it can rapidly lead to loss of the eye.

5.4.3 General Notes on Diagnosing Infectious Forms of Keratitis

Prompt diagnosis and treatment of corneal infections are crucial in avoiding permanent impairment of vision. The diagnosis of any type of infectious keratitis essentially includes the following steps:
- Identifying the pathogen and testing its resistance. This is done by taking a smear from the base of the ulcer to obtain sample material and inoculating culture media for bacteria and fungi. Wearers of contact lenses should also have cultures taken from the lenses, and the contact lens container in particular, to ensure that they are not the source of the bacteria or fungus.
- Slides of smears, unstained and treated with Gram and Giemsa stains, are examined to detect bacteria.
- Where a viral infection is suspected, testing corneal sensitivity is indicated as this will be diminished in *viral* keratitis.

5.4.4 Bacterial Keratitis

▶ **Epidemiology.** Over 90% of corneal inflammations are caused by bacteria.

▶ **Etiology.** The pathogens listed in ▶ Table 5.1 are among the most frequent causes of bacterial keratitis in the urban population in temperate climates.

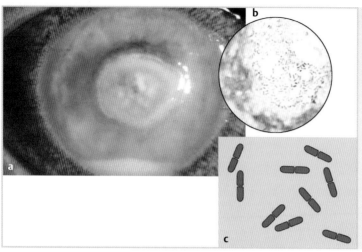

Fig. 5.10 Bacterial corneal ulcer. (a) The clinical findings include a central bacterial corneal ulcer with hypopyon. (b,c) Histologic findings through the microscope: Gram-positive rod bacteria in the corneal stroma.

Table 5.1 The most common bacterial pathogens that cause keratitis

Bacterium	Typical characteristics of infection
Staphylococcus aureus	Infection progresses slowly with little pain
Staphylococcus epidermidis	As in Staphylococcus aureus infection
Streptococcus pneumoniae	Typical serpiginous corneal ulcer: the cornea is rapidly perforated with early intraocular involvement; very painful
Pseudomonas aeruginosa	Bluish-green mucoid exudate, occasionally with a ring-shaped corneal abscess. Progression is rapid with a tendency toward melting of the cornea over a wide area; painful
Moraxella	Painless oval ulcer in the inferior cornea that progresses slowly with slight irritation of the anterior chamber

Note
Most bacteria are unable to penetrate the cornea as long as the epithelium remains intact. Only gonococci and diphtheria bacteria can penetrate an intact corneal epithelium.

▶ **Symptoms.** Patients report moderate to severe pain (except in *Moraxella* infections; see ▶ Table 5.1), photophobia, impaired vision, tearing, and purulent discharge. *Purulent discharge* is typical of *bacterial* forms of keratitis; *viral* forms produce a *watery* discharge.

▶ **Diagnostic considerations.** Positive identification of the pathogens is crucial. **Serpiginous corneal ulcers** (see p. 75) are frequently associated with severe reaction of the anterior chamber including accumulation of cells and pus in the inferior anterior chamber (hypopyon, ▶ Fig. 5.10a) and posterior adhesions of the iris and lens (posterior synechiae).

▶ **Differential diagnosis.** Positive identification of the pathogen is required to exclude a fungal infection.

▶ **Treatment**

Note
Because of the risk of perforation, any type of corneal ulcer is an emergency requiring treatment by an ophthalmologist.

▶ **Conservative treatment.** Treatment is initiated with **topical antibiotics** (such as *aminoglycosides:* kanamycin, gentamicin; *macrolides:* azithromycin, erythromycin; *fluoroquinolones:* levofloxacin, ofloxacin, moxifloxacin; *other antibiotics:* chloramphenicol, colistin, oxytetracycline) with a very broad spectrum of activity against most gram-positive and gram-negative organisms until the results of pathogen and resistance testing are known. Immobilization of the ciliary body and iris by therapeutic mydriasis is indicated in the presence of *intraocular irritation* (manifested by hypopyon). Bacterial keratitis can be treated initially on an outpatient basis with eye drops and ointments.

An *advanced ulcer*—that is, with a protracted clinical course—suggests indolence and poor compliance on the part of the patient. *Hospitalization* is indicated in these cases. Subconjunctival application of antibiotics may be required to increase the effectiveness of the treatment.

▶ **Surgical treatment.** Indications are based on the following situations:

- *Abrasion:* the removal of corneal epithelium and superficial portions of the ulcer (wound débridement) prevents premature epithelialization and facilitates the access of the antibiotics to the infiltrate.
- *Thermocauterization/cryotherapy:* treatment of the base of the ulcer with a hot instrument tip (vapor cautery) cleans and removes necrotic tissue. In infestation with acanthamoebas, cryotherapy is applied.
- *Covering with connective tissue/amniotic membrane transplantation (AMT):* Broad areas of superficial necrosis or insufficient healing may require a membrane (flap preparation from placenta tissue) to accelerate healing under the protecting flap. Corneal scarring may be observed after closure of the defect (▶ Fig. 5.11).
- *Riboflavin UVA crosslinking:* crosslinking is thought to have a bactericidal effect.
- *Keratoplasty à* chaud: in descemetocele or an already perforated ulcer, an emergency keratoplasty is indicated (see Chapter 5.7.1). If the tear ducts are blocked, they should be corrected operatively after the ulcer has healed (see ▶ Fig. 3.10) to rule out a source of infection.

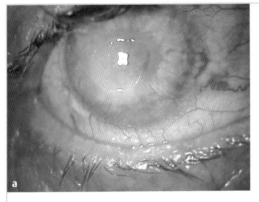
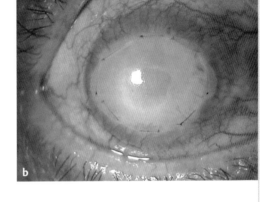
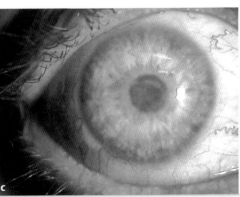

Fig. 5.11 Amniotic membrane transplantation (AMT). (a) Nonhealing, central corneal ulcer with opacification of the cornea and strongly reactive corneal vascularization from the limbus. **(b)** Amniotic membrane, transplanted and anchored with multiple corneal fibers, covers the area of the ulcer completely. The margin of the ulcer is visible through the amniotic membrane. **(c)** Healed cornea with persisting central corneal scars in the area of the ulcer. The corneal vascularization has disappeared and the situation is stable again. Penetrating keratoplasty (PKP) is necessary if the patient does not achieve satisfactory vision because of corneal scarring.

Note
As soon as the results of bacteriologic and resistance testing are available, the physician should verify that the pathogens will respond to current therapy.

Failure of keratitis to respond to treatment may be due to one of the following **causes**, particularly if the pathogen has not been positively identified.
1. The patient is not applying the antibiotic (poor compliance).
2. The pathogen is resistant to the antibiotic.
3. The keratitis is not caused by bacteria but by one of the following pathogens:
   ○ Herpes simplex virus.
   ○ Fungi.
   ○ *Acanthamoeba.*
   ○ Rare specific pathogens such as *Nocardia* or mycobacteria (as these are very rare, they are not discussed in further detail in this chapter).

5.4.5 Viral Keratitis

Viral keratitis is frequently caused by:
• Herpes simplex virus.
• Varicella-zoster virus.
• Adenovirus.

Other *rare* causes include cytomegalovirus, measles virus, or rubella virus.

Herpes Simplex Keratitis

▶ **Epidemiology and pathogenesis.** Herpes simplex keratitis is among the more common causes of corneal ulcer. About 90% of the population are carriers of the herpes simplex virus. A typical feature of the ubiquitous herpes simplex virus is an unnoticed primary infection that often heals spontaneously. Many people then remain carriers of the neurotropic virus, which can lead to recurrent infection at any time proceeding from the trigeminal ganglion. *A corneal infection is always a recurrence.* A primary herpes simplex infection of the eye will present as blepharitis or conjunctivitis. Recurrences may be triggered by external influences (such as exposure to ultraviolet light), stress, menstruation, generalized immunologic deficiency, or febrile infections.

▶ **Symptoms.** Herpes simplex keratitis is usually *very painful* and associated with photophobia, lacrimation, and swelling of the eyelids. Vision may be impaired depending on the location of findings, for example in the presence of central epitheliitis.

▶ **Forms and diagnosis of herpes simplex keratitis.** The following forms of herpes simplex keratitis are differentiated according to the specific layer of the cornea in which the lesion is located. Recurrences are more frequent in the stroma and endothelium.

▶ **Dendritic keratitis.** This is characterized by branching epithelial lesions (necrotic and vesicular swollen epithelial cells, ▶ Fig. 5.12). These findings will be *visible with the unaided eye* after application of fluorescein dye and are characteristic of dendritic keratitis. Corneal sensitivity is usually reduced. Dendritic keratitis may progress to stromal keratitis.

▶ **Stromal keratitis.** Purely stromal involvement without prior dendritic keratitis is characterized by an intact epithelium that will not show any defects after application of fluorescein dye. Slit lamp examination will reveal central *disciform* corneal infiltrates (disciform keratitis) with or without a whitish stromal infiltrate. Depending on the frequency of recurrence, superficial or deep vascularization may be present. Reaction of the anterior chamber will usually be accompanied by endothelial plaques (protein deposits on the posterior surface of the cornea that include phagocytosed giant cells).

▶ **Endotheliitis.** Endotheliitis or endothelial keratitis is caused by the presence of herpes viruses in the aqueous humor. This causes swelling of the endothelial cells and opacification of the adjacent corneal stroma. Involvement of the endothelial cells in the angle of the anterior chamber causes a secondary increase in intraocular pressure (*secondary glaucoma*). Other findings include inflamed cells and pigment cells in the anterior chamber, and endothelial plaques; involvement of the iris with segmental loss of pigmented epithelium is detectable by slit lamp examination.

▶ **Acute retinal necrosis syndrome.** Involvement of the posterior eyeball for all practical purposes is seen only in immunocompromised patients (e.g., recipients of bone marrow transplants and AIDS patients) (see Viral retinitis, Chapter 12.7.4).

▶ **Treatment.** Infections involving the epithelium are treated with trifluridine (3–5 times per day) or ganciclovir (1.5 mg eye gel) as a superficial virostatic agent. **Stromal and intraocular herpes simplex infections** can be treated with acyclovir, which is available for topical use (in ointment form 3–5 times per day) and systemic use.

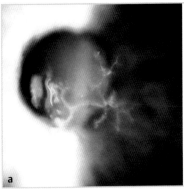
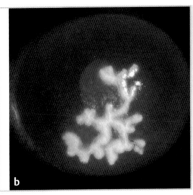

Fig. 5.12 Herpes simplex keratitis: dendritic keratitis. Characteristic findings include branching epithelial lesions. **(a)** Noncontrast, with no dye. **(b)** With fluorescein dye.

Note

Corticosteroids are contraindicated in epithelial herpes simplex infections but can be used to treat stromal keratitis where the epithelium is intact.

Herpes Zoster Keratitis

Definition

Keratitis due to endogenous recurrence of chickenpox (caused by the varicella-zoster virus; see Herpes zoster ophthalmicus, Chapter 2.5.5).

▶ **Etiology.** Proceeding from the trigeminal ganglion, the virus reinfects the region supplied by the trigeminal nerve. The eye is only affected where the ophthalmic division of the trigeminal nerve is involved. In this case, the nasociliary nerve supplying the interior of the eye will also be affected. Hutchinson's sign, vesicular lesions on the tip of the nose, will be present (see ▶ Fig. 2.14).

▶ **Diagnostic considerations.** Herpes zoster ophthalmicus also occurs in superficial and deep forms, which in part are similar to herpes simplex infection of the cornea (red eye with dendritic keratitis, stromal keratitis, and keratouveitis). Corneal sensitivity is usually decreased or absent.

▶ **Treatment.** The eye is treated with acyclovir ointment in consultation with a dermatologist, who will usually treat skin changes with systemic acyclovir (in the form of infusions or tablets). If the corneal epithelium is intact, the irritation of the anterior chamber can be carefully treated with steroids and immobilization of the pupil and ciliary body by therapeutic mydriasis.

5.4.6 Mycotic Keratitis

▶ **Epidemiology.** Mycotic keratitis was once very rare, occurring almost exclusively in farm laborers (see Etiology for contact with possible causative agents). However, this clinical syndrome has become far more prevalent today as a result of the increased and often unwarranted use of antibiotics and steroids.

▶ **Etiology.** The most frequently encountered pathogens are *Aspergillus* and *Candida albicans*. The most frequent causative mechanism is an injury with fungus-infested organic material such as a tree branch.

▶ **Symptoms.** Patients usually have only slight symptoms.

▶ **Diagnostic considerations.** The red eye is apparent upon **inspection** (normally the disorder is unilateral), as is a corneal ulcer with an undermined margin (▶ Fig. 5.10). The ulcer will continue to expand beneath the visible margins (serpiginous corneal ulcer, p. 76). Hypopyon may also be present (as shown in ▶ Fig. 5.13a). **Slit lamp** examination will reveal typical whitish stromal infiltrates, especially with mycotic keratitis due to *Candida albicans*. The infiltrates and ulcer spread very slowly. *Satellite lesions*—several adjacent smaller infiltrates grouped around a larger center—are characteristic but will not necessarily be present.

▶ **Identification of the pathogen.** *Microbiological identification* of fungi is difficult and can be time consuming (for *histologic* identification, see ▶ Fig. 5.13b). It is important to obtain samples from beyond the visible margin of the ulcer. Fungal cultures should always be obtained where bacterial cultures are negative.

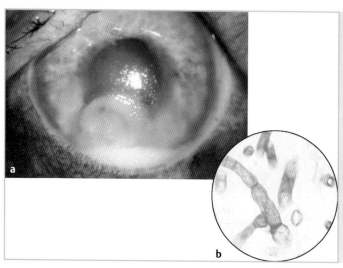

Fig. 5.13 Mycotic keratitis. (a) The clinical findings include a corneal ulcer that extends beyond the visible margin and hypopyon. **(b)** The histologic findings include hyphae in the corneal stroma.

▶ **Treatment**

▶ **Conservative treatment.** Systemic therapy is only indicated in the case of an intraocular involvement. Other cases will respond well to topical treatment with antimycotic agents such as natamycin, nystatin, amphotericin B, and voriconazole. In general, the topical antimycotic agents will have to be specially prepared by the pharmacist. Conservative therapy can be administered to outpatients or to inpatients if necessary. The treatment can be long-term.

▶ **Surgical treatment.** Emergency keratoplasty (see p. 89) is indicated when the disorder fails to respond or responds too slowly to conservative treatment and findings worsen under treatment.

5.4.7 Acanthamoeba Keratitis

▶ **Epidemiology.** This is a rare type of keratitis and one that may have been diagnosed too rarely in the past.

▶ **Etiology.** *Acanthamoeba* is a saprophytic protozoon. Infections usually occur in *wearers of contact lenses*, particularly in conjunction with trauma and moist environments such as saunas.

▶ **Symptoms.** Patients complain of intense pain, photophobia, and lacrimation.

▶ **Diagnostic considerations.** The patient will often have a history of several weeks or months of unsuccessful antibiotic treatment.

Inspection will reveal a unilateral reddening of the eye. Usually there will be no discharge. The infection *can* present as a subepithelial infiltrate, as an intrastromal disciform opacification of the cornea, or as a ring-shaped corneal abscess (▶ Fig. 5.14a).

The disorder is difficult to diagnose, and even immunofluorescence studies in specialized laboratories often fail to provide diagnostic information. Amebic cysts can be readily demonstrated only by histologic and pathologic studies of excised corneal tissue (▶ Fig. 5.14b). Recently it has become possible to demonstrate amebic cysts with the aid of **confocal corneal microscopy** (see Chapter 5.2.8). Patients who wear contact lenses should have them sent in for laboratory examination.

▶ **Treatment**

▶ **Conservative treatment.** Nowadays, the treatment of *Acanthamoeba* keratitis rests on three pillars:

• Membrane disruption (diamidine).
• Inhibition of respiratory enzymes (biguanide).
• Broad-spectrum antibiotics.

A typical combination in current use is: 0.1% propamidine isetionate (Brolene, in some countries only available through international pharmacies) plus polyhexamethylene biguanide (PHMB) as 0.2% eye drops (Lavasept) plus neomycin and pentamidine, which must be prepared by a pharmacist. Cycloplegia (immobilization of the pupil and ciliary body) is usually required as well.

▶ **Surgical treatment.** Emergency keratoplasty is indicated when conservative treatment fails (see p. 89).

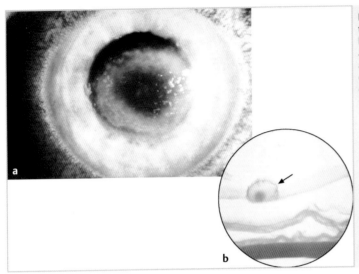

Fig. 5.14 Acanthamoeba keratitis. (a) The clinical findings include keratitis with a ring-shaped corneal abscess. (b) The histologic findings after keratoplasty include typical double-walled amebic cysts in the corneal stroma above Descemet's membrane (arrow).

5.5 Noninfectious Keratitis and Keratopathy

This category encompasses a wide variety of corneal disorders, some of which, such as keratoconjunctivitis sicca (see p. 40), occur very frequently. Causes include:

- Inflammations (blepharitis and conjunctivitis).
- Injuries (rubbing the eyes, foreign bodies beneath the upper eyelid, contact lens incompatibility, exposure to intense ultraviolet irradiation).
- Age-related changes, e.g., senile ectropion with trichiasis (see p. 18), senile entropion (see p. 17), keratoconjunctivitis sicca (see p. 40).
- Surgery (cataract or LASIK [laser-assisted in-situ keratomileusis]).
- Endogenous factors (facial neuropathy).
- Exogenous factors (medications or preservatives).

5.5.1 Superficial Punctate Keratitis

Definition
Superficial punctate corneal lesions due to lacrimal system dysfunction from a number of causes (see Etiology).

▶ **Epidemiology and etiology.** Superficial punctate keratoconjunctivitis is a *very frequent finding* as it can be caused by a wide variety of exogenous factors such as foreign bodies beneath the upper eyelid, contact lenses, smog, etc. It may also appear as a secondary symptom of many other forms of keratitis (see the forms of keratitis discussed in the following sections).

▶ **Symptoms.** Depending on the cause and severity of the superficial corneal lesions, symptoms range from a nearly asymptomatic clinical course (such as in neuroparalytic keratitis, in which the cornea loses its sensitivity; see p. 83) to an intense foreign-body sensation in which the patient has a sensation of sand in the eye with typical signs of epiphora, severe pain, burning, and blepharospasm. Visual acuity is usually only minimally compromised.

▶ **Diagnostic considerations and differential diagnosis.** Fluorescein dye is applied and the eye is examined under a slit lamp. This visualizes fine epithelial defects. The specific dye patterns that emerge give the ophthalmologist information about the etiology of the punctate keratitis (▶ Fig. 5.15).

▶ **Treatment and prognosis.** Depending on the cause, the superficial corneal changes will respond rapidly or less so to *treatment with artificial tears*, whereby every effort should be made to eliminate the causative agents (▶ Fig. 5.15). Depending on the severity of findings, artificial tears of varying viscosity (ranging from eye drops to high-viscosity gels) are prescribed and applied with varying frequency. In exposure keratitis, a high-viscosity gel or ointment is used because of its long retention time; superficial punctate keratitis is treated with eye drops.

Keratoconjunctivitis Sicca

This is one of the most frequent causes of superficial keratitis. The syndrome itself is attributable to dry eyes due to lack of tear fluid and is discussed in Chapter 3.4.1.

5.5.2 Exposure Keratitis

Definition
Keratitis resulting from drying of the cornea in the case of lagophthalmos.

▶ **Epidemiology.** Exposure keratitis is a relatively frequent clinical syndrome. For example, it may occur in association with facial paralysis following a stroke.

▶ **Etiology.** Due to **facial nerve palsy**, there is insufficient closure of the eyelids over the eyeball (lagophthalmos), and the inferior one-third to one-half of the cornea remains exposed and unprotected (exposure keratitis). Superficial punctate keratitis (see p. 81) initially develops in this region and can progress to corneal erosion (see ▶ Fig. 18.5) or ulcer (see p. 75). The upper regions of the cornea are moist and protected longer because of Bell's phenomenon.

Other **causes for exposure keratitis without facial nerve palsy** include
- Uncompensated exophthalmos in Graves's disease.
- Insufficient eyelid closure following eyelid surgery to correct ptosis.
- Insufficient eye care in patients receiving artificial respiration on the intensive care ward.

▶ **Symptoms.** Similar to superficial punctate keratitis (although usually more severe) but *unilateral*.

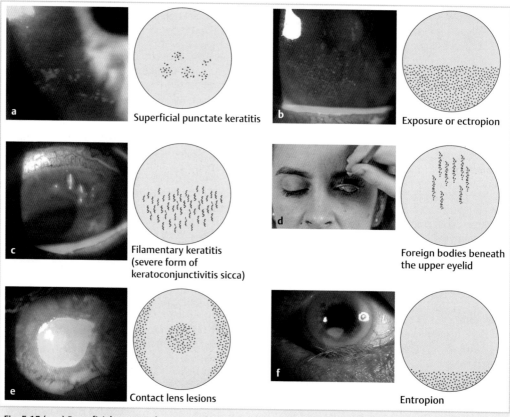

a Superficial punctate keratitis

b Exposure or ectropion

c Filamentary keratitis (severe form of keratoconjunctivitis sicca)

d Foreign bodies beneath the upper eyelid

e Contact lens lesions

f Entropion

Fig. 5.15 (a–e) Superficial punctate keratitis and corneal erosion. Typical staining patterns in the various forms of superficial punctate keratitis and the transition into corneal erosion **(e, f)**. The cause of the disorder can be inferred from the specific pattern of corneal lesions.

▶ **Diagnostic considerations.** Application of fluorescein dye will reveal a typical pattern of epithelial lesions (▶ Fig. 5.15b).

▶ **Treatment.** Application of artificial tears is usually not sufficient where eyelid motor function is impaired. In such cases, *high-viscosity gels, ointment packings* (for antibiotic protection), and a *watch glass bandage* are required. The watch glass bandage must be applied so as to create a moist airtight chamber that prevents further desiccation of the eye (see ▶ Fig. 2.9). In the presence of persistent facial nerve palsy that shows no signs of remission, *lateral tarsorrhaphy* is the treatment of choice. The same applies to treatment of exposure keratitis due to insufficient eyelid closure from other causes (see Etiology).

> **Note**
> Poor corneal care in exposure keratitis can lead to superficial punctate keratitis, erosion, bacterial superinfection with corneal ulcer (see p. 75), and finally to corneal perforation.

5.5.3 Neuropalytic Keratitis

> **Definition**
> Keratitis associated with palsy of the ophthalmic division of the trigeminal nerve.

▶ **Epidemiology.** Palsy of the ophthalmic division of the trigeminal nerve is less frequent than facial nerve palsy.

▶ **Etiology.** The trigeminal nerve is responsible for the cornea's sensitivity to exogenous influences. A conduction disturbance in the trigeminal nerve is usually a *sequela of damage to the trigeminal ganglion* from trauma, radiation therapy of an acoustic neurinoma, or surgery. It will lead to *loss of corneal sensitivity.* As a result of this loss of sensitivity, the patient will not feel any sensation of drying in the eye, and the blinking frequency drops below the level required to ensure that the cornea remains moist. As in exposure keratitis, superficial punctate lesions will form initially, followed by larger epithelial defects that can progress to a corneal ulcer if bacterial superinfection occurs.

▶ **Symptoms.** Because patients with loss of trigeminal function are free of pain, they will experience

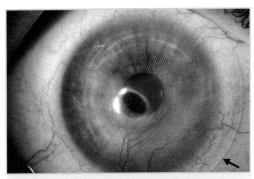

Fig. 5.16 Neuropalytic ulcer. Paracentral, deep corneal ulcer down to Descemet's membrane (descemetocele) with incipient vascularization, provided with a therapeutic contact lens (arrow).

only slight symptoms such as a foreign-body sensation or an eyelid swelling.

▶ **Diagnostic considerations.** Corneal damage, usually central or slightly below the center of the cornea, may range from superficial punctate keratitis (visible after application of fluorescein dye) to a deep corneal ulcer with perforation (▶ Fig. 5.16). The eye will be red and in extreme cases may be leaking aqueous humor.

▶ **Differential diagnosis.** Corneal ulcer due to herpes virus infection (see p. 78).

▶ **Treatment.** This is essentially *identical to treatment of exposure keratitis.* It includes moistening the cornea, antibiotic protection as prophylaxis against infection, and, if conservative methods are unsuccessful, tarsorrhaphy.

Primary and Recurrent Corneal Erosion

These changes are generally the result of a corneal trauma and are dealt with in Chapter 18, page 322.

5.5.4 Problems with Contact Lenses

▶ **Etiology.** These problems occur either with *poorly seated rigid contact lenses* that rub on the surface of the cornea or from *overwearing soft contact lenses.*

If contact lenses are worn for extended periods of time despite symptoms, severe inflammation, corneal ulceration, and vascularization of the corneal periphery may result.

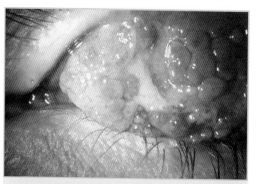

Fig. 5.17 Giant papillae from contact lens incompatibility. Wartlike protrusions of connective tissue on the palpebral conjunctiva due to contact lens or preservative incompatibility (with simple eversion of the upper eyelid).

▶ **Symptoms.** Patients find the contact lenses increasingly uncomfortable and notice worsening of their vision. These symptoms are especially pronounced after removing the contact lenses as the lenses mask the defect in the corneal epithelium.

▶ **Diagnostic considerations.** The ophthalmologist will detect typical corneal changes after applying fluorescein dye (▶ Fig. 5.15e). Keratoconjunctivitis on the superior limbus with formation of giant papillae, wartlike protrusions of connective tissue frequently observed on the superior tarsus (▶ Fig. 5.17), are signs of contact lens or preservative incompatibility.

▶ **Treatment.** The patient should temporarily discontinue wearing the contact lenses, and inflammatory changes should be controlled with steroids until the irritation of the eye has abated.

Note
Protracted therapy with topical steroids should be monitored regularly by an ophthalmologist as superficial epithelial defects heal poorly under steroid therapy. Protracted high-dosage steroid therapy causes a secondary increase in intraocular pressure and cataract in one-third of all patients.

The specific ophthalmologic findings will determine whether the patient should be advised to permanently discontinue wearing contact lenses or whether changing contact lenses and cleaning agents will be sufficient.

5.5.5 Bullous Keratopathy

Definition
Opacification of the cornea with epithelial bullae due to loss of function of the endothelial cells.

▶ **Epidemiology.** Bullous keratopathy is among the most frequent indications for corneal transplants.

▶ **Etiology.** The transparency of the cornea largely depends on a functioning endothelium with a high density of endothelial cells (see p. 69). Where the endothelium has been severely damaged by inflammation, trauma, or major surgery in the anterior eye, the few remaining endothelial cells will be unable to prevent *aqueous humor from entering the cornea*. This results in hydration of the cornea with stromal edema and epithelial bullae (▶ Fig. 5.18a, b). Loss of endothelial cells may also have genetic causes (so-called Fuchs's endothelial dystrophy, see p. 87).

▶ **Symptoms.** The gradual loss of endothelial cells causes *slow deterioration of vision*. The patient typically will have poorer vision in the morning than in the evening, as corneal swelling is greater during the night with the eyelids closed.

▶ **Diagnostic considerations.** Slit lamp examination will reveal thickening of the cornea, epithelial edema, and epithelial bullae.

▶ **Differential diagnosis.** Bullous keratopathy can also occur with glaucoma (see p. 164). However, in these cases the intraocular pressure is typically increased.

▶ **Treatment.** Where the damage to the endothelial cells is not too far advanced and only occasional periods of opacification occur (such as in the morning), *hyperosmolar solutions* such as sodium chloride hypertonic) can improve the patient's eyesight by removing water. However, this is generally only a temporary solution. Beyond a certain stage a *corneal transplant* (for example a penetrating keratoplasty, see p. 88) is indicated.

5.6 Corneal Deposits, Degeneration, and Dystrophies

As bradytrophic avascular tissue, the cornea is particularly susceptible to deposits of foreign material and degeneration (see p. 86).

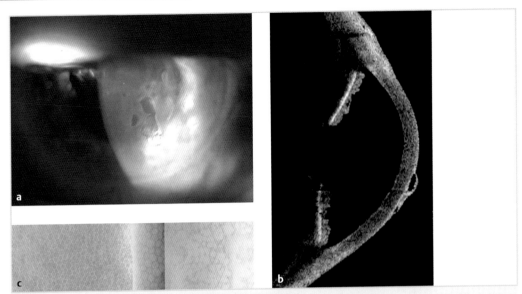

Fig. 5.18 Bullous keratopathy. (a) Corneal edema due to a lack of endothelial cells with clearly recognizable blister-shaped (bullous) elevation of the epithelium. **(b)** Specular image microscopy makes clear the extent and localization of the epithelial elevation. **(c)** Endothelial cell microscopy shows the destroyed endothelial cells (right). In comparison, the left side (a wide-angle view) and the middle (magnified view) of the image show an intact endothelium with a clearly visible honeycomb structure. The actual size of the area shown on the left side of the image is about 0.5 mm².

5.6.1 Corneal Deposits

Arcus Senilis

This is a grayish-white ring-shaped fatty deposit near the limbus that can occur at any age but usually appears in advanced age (▶ Fig. 5.19). Arcus senilis is *usually bilateral* and is a frequently encountered phenomenon. It occurs as a result of lipid deposits from the vessels of the limbus along the entire periphery of the cornea, which normally increase with advanced age. A lipid-free clear zone along the limbus will be discernible. Patients under the age of 50 years who develop arcus senilis should be examined to exclude hypercholesterolemia as a cause. Arcus senilis *requires no treatment* as it does not cause any visual impairments.

The **deposits and pigmentations** discussed in the following section do not generally impair vision.

Corneal Verticillata

Bilateral gray or brownish epithelial deposits that extend in a swirling pattern from a point inferior to the pupil. This corneal change typically occurs with the use of certain *medications*, most frequently with chloroquine and amiodarone. *Fabry's disease*

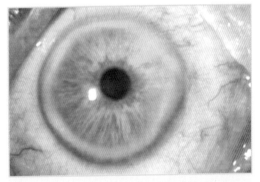

Fig. 5.19 Arcus senilis. Typical grayish-white, ring-shaped fatty deposits near the limbus.

(glycolipid lipidosis) can also exhibit these kinds of corneal changes, which can help to confirm the diagnosis.

Iron Lines

Any irregularity in the surface of the cornea causes the eyelid to distribute the tear film irregularly over the surface of the cornea; a small puddle of tear fluid will be present at the site of the irregularity. *Iron deposits* form in a characteristic manner at this site in the corneal epithelium. The most frequently

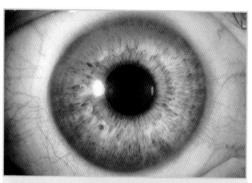

Fig. 5.20 Kayser–Fleischer ring in Wilson's disease. Yellow corneal copper deposits in the peripheral Descemet's membrane. The ring appears as a zone of granular deposition predominantly in the vertical meridian. The ring tends to change its color depending on the illumination.

observed iron lines are the physiologic iron deposits at the site where the eyelids close (the Hudson–Stähli line), Stocker's line with pterygium, Ferry's line with a filtering bleb after glaucoma surgery, and Fleischer's ring with keratoconus. Iron lines have also been described following surgery (radial keratotomy [p. 91]; photorefractive keratectomy [p. 92]; keratoplasty [p. 88]) and in the presence of corneal scars.

Kayser–Fleischer Ring

This golden-brown to yellowish-green corneal ring is caused by copper deposits at the level of Descemet's membrane in Wilson's disease (liver and lens degeneration with decreased serum levels of ceruloplasmin). This ring is so characteristic that the ophthalmologist often is the first to diagnose this rare clinical syndrome (▶ Fig. 5.20).

> **Note**
> In the early stages, a Kayser–Fleischer ring is best detected using gonioscopy.

5.6.2 Corneal Degeneration

Calcific Band Keratopathy

After many years of chronic inflammation of the anterior chamber (chronic uveitis and keratitis) with shrinkage of the eyeball or in patients with juvenile polyarthritis, *calcific deposits occur in Bowman's layer,* causing a transverse zone of opacification in the region of the palpebral fissure. The limbus region will remain clear (▶ Fig. 5.21). This change *significantly* impairs vision. The opacification can be completely removed and vision restored by chelating the calcifications with a sodium EDTA solution.

Peripheral Furrow Keratitis

This includes a *heterogeneous group of disorders in terms of morphology and etiology.* All are noninfectious and lead to **thinning and melting of the peripheral cornea** that may progress to perforation. *Etiologic* factors include:
- Autoimmune processes (collagenosis, marginal keratitis, and sclerokeratitis).
- Trophic dysfunctions (pitting due to lack of tear film).
- Unknown degenerative processes (Terrien's marginal degeneration or Mooren's ulcer).

These corneal changes are most frequently observed in *patients with rheumatoid arthritis.* Treating the underlying disorder is essential in these cases. Otherwise the changes are rare. **Keratomalacia** is a **special** form of the disorder in which *vitamin A deficiency* causes xerosis of the conjunctiva combined with night blindness. This disorder remains one of the most frequent causes of blindness in the developing countries in which malnutrition is prevalent.

5.6.3 Corneal Dystrophies

Definition
This term refers to a group of hereditary corneal metabolic dysfunctions that always lead to bilateral opacification of the various layers of the cornea (see Classification, below).

▶ **Epidemiology.** Corneal dystrophy tends to be *rare.* The most frequent form is Fuchs's endothelial dystrophy, followed by epithelial corneal dystrophy.

▶ **Etiology.** The various corneal dystrophies are *genetic disorders.* They usually manifest themselves in the first or second decade of life except for Fuchs's endothelial dystrophy, which only becomes symptomatic between the ages of 40 and 50 years.

▶ **Classification.** The following forms of dystrophy are differentiated according to the individual layers of the cornea in which they occur:

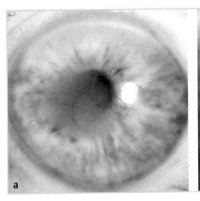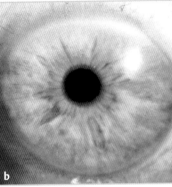

Fig. 5.21 Calcific band keratopathy. (a) Brownish-white calcific deposits occur in Bowman's layer, severely impairing the patient's vision. (b) The findings after chelation of the calcific deposits with an EDTA solution.

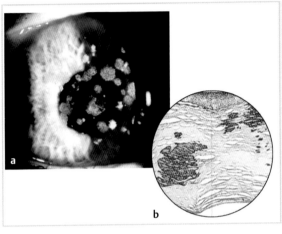

Fig. 5.22 Granular stromal corneal dystrophy. (a) The clinical findings include fragmented opacities surrounded by areas of clear cornea between the deposits. (b) The histologic findings, demonstrating hyaline deposits under Masson's trichrome stain.

- **Epithelial corneal dystrophy.**
- **Stromal corneal dystrophy**. The most prevalent forms include:
  - Granular dystrophy (hyaline deposits, ▶ Fig. 5.22).
  - Lattice dystrophy (amyloid deposits).
  - Macular dystrophy (deposits of acidic mucopolysaccharides, ▶ Fig. 5.23).
- **Endothelial dystrophy,** such as Fuchs's endothelial dystrophy (the most frequently encountered form of corneal dystrophy).

▶ **Morphological classification.** In the last 20 years molecular genetic findings have led to a genotype classification of corneal dystrophies that regroups lattice and granular dystrophy as epithelial dystrophies.

▶ **Symptoms and diagnostic considerations.** All patients suffer from a steadily increasing loss of visual acuity due to the generally gradual opacification of the cornea. This loss of visual acuity may progress to the point where a corneal transplant becomes necessary.

Macular dystrophy is the most rapidly debilitating form of the **stromal dystrophies**, resulting in a severe loss of visual acuity in the second decade of life.

Epithelial and stromal corneal dystrophies are also often accompanied by painful and recurrent corneal erosion. **Fuchs's endothelial dystrophy** involves a gradual loss of endothelial cells that in time leads to *bullous keratopathy* (hydration of the cornea with stromal edema and epithelial bullae) (see p. 84). The patient typically will have poorer vision in the morning than in the evening, as corneal swelling is greater during the night with the eyelids closed.

▶ **Treatment.** Depending on the severity of the loss of visual acuity (see above), a *corneal transplant* may be indicated; see Penetrating Keratoplasty, page 88. Because the cornea remains avascular in these disorders, the prognosis is good.

In **Fuchs's endothelial dystrophy**, a corneal transplant is the treatment of choice. Where the symptoms are not too far advanced, *frequent application of hyperosmolar solutions* can remove water

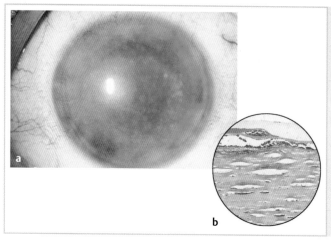

Fig. 5.23 Macular stromal corneal dystrophy. (a) The clinical findings include nodular opacities surrounded by areas of clear cornea between the deposits. **(b)** The histologic findings, showing deposits of acidic mucopolysaccharides on AMP staining.

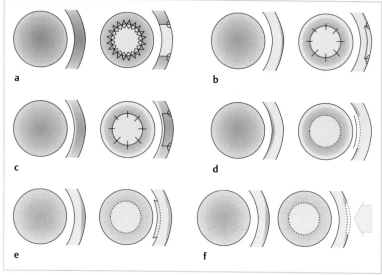

Fig. 5.24 Therapeutic corneal procedures. See text for more detailed explanations. **(a)** Penetrating keratoplasty (PKP). **(b)** Anterior lamellar keratoplasty (ALK). **(c)** Deep anterior lamellar keratoplasty (DALK). **(d)** Descemet membrane endothelial keratoplasty (DMEK). **(e)** Posterior lamellar keratoplasty: Descemet stripping automated endothelial keratoplasty (DSAEK). **(f)** Phototherapeutic keratoplasty (PTK).

from the cornea. However, this is generally only a temporary solution. The corneal transplantation is performed in combination with a cataract extraction; patients with Fuchs's endothelial dystrophy that affects their vision are usually older and also have a cataract. The two procedures are combined because corneal decompensation often results from Fuchs's endothelial dystrophy following the surgical trauma of cataract extraction (see p. 71).

5.7 Corneal Surgery

Corneal surgery includes curative or therapeutic procedures and refractive procedures (▶ Fig. 5.24, ▶ Fig. 5.25).

- **Curative** corneal procedures are intended to improve vision by eliminating *corneal opacification.*
- **Refractive** corneal procedures change the refractive power of a *clear* cornea.

5.7.1 Curative Corneal Procedures

Penetrating Keratoplasty (PKP)

▶ **Principle.** This involves replacement of diseased corneal tissue with a full-thickness donor graft of corneal tissue of varying diameter (▶ Fig. 5.24a). A clear, regularly refracting button of donor cornea is placed in an opacified or irregularly refracting cornea. The corneal button is sutured with a continu-

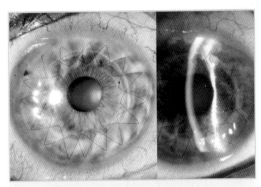

Fig. 5.25 Penetrating keratoplasty (PKP). The donor corneal button is sutured with a continuous double suture.

ous single or double suture (▶ Fig. 5.25) or with interrupted sutures. For special considerations in corneal transplants, see also Morphology and Healing in Chapter 5.1 (p. 68).

Penetrating keratoplasty can be performed as an **elective procedure** to improve visual acuity or as an emergency procedure (**emergency keratoplasty**). Emergency keratoplasty is indicated to treat a perforated or nonhealing corneal ulcer to remove the perforation site and save the eye (*tectonic keratoplasty*).

▶ **Indications.** Corneal diseases that affect the full thickness of the corneal stroma (corneal scars, dystrophy, or degeneration) or protrusion anomalies such as keratoconus or keratoglobus with or without central corneal opacification.

▶ **Allograft rejection (complications).** The body's immune system can respond with a chronic focal allograft rejection (▶ Fig. 5.26a, b) or a diffuse allograft rejection (▶ Fig. 5.26c). The graft will become opacified.

Lamellar Keratoplasty (LKP)

▶ **Principle.** This involves replacement of a particular corneal layer with a partial-thickness donor graft. The following surgical procedures are possible.

▶ **Anterior lamellar keratoplasty**
• Anterior lamellar keratoplasty (ALK, ▶ Fig. 5.24b): replacement of only the superficial stromal opacification with a partial-thickness donor graft of clear corneal tissue.
• Deep anterior lamellar keratoplasty (DALK, ▶ Fig. 5.24c): the corneal stroma is completely excised and replaced by a clear graft. The Descemet

membrane and the endothelial layer stay in place.

The donor corneal button is sutured in place with a continuous or interrupted suture.

▶ **Posterior lamellar keratoplasty**
• DSAEK (Descemet stripping automated endothelial keratoplasty).
• DMEK (Descemet membrane endothelial keratoplasty).

In both procedures, the Descemet's membrane and the diseased endothelium is removed first (descemetorhexis) in patients with endothelial disease, particularly Fuchs's corneal dystrophy.

In DSAEK, a thin graft, consisting of a few stroma layers, Descemet's membrane, and healthy endothelium is implanted in the eye and pressed into place with an air bubble. In the more modern procedure of DMEK, only the Descemet's membrane and the endothelium are implanted.

The advantage of these procedures is stability of the corneal architecture and of astigmatism.

▶ **Indications.** The ALK is a suitable procedure for opacities and scarring of the superficial corneal stroma (posttraumatic, degenerative, dystrophic and postinflammatory).

For ALK an intact Descemet's membrane and a healthy endothelial layer are necessary, as well as for DALK. DALK is a feasible procedure for deep stromal opacities and scarring.

Posterior lamellar keratoplasty (DMEK, DSAEK) is used for the treatment of diseases of the corneal endothelial layer (Fuchs's corneal dystrophy, pseudophakic bulbous keratopathy). This fascinating, relatively new procedure leaves most of the outer corneal aspects intact.

▶ **Allograft rejection (complications).** Allograft rejection is less frequent than in the case of penetrating keratoplasty. There is also less danger of infection as lamellar keratoplasty does not involve opening the globe. Graft rejection rarely occurs in posterior lamellar keratoplasty.

Phototherapeutic Keratectomy

▶ **Principle.** Superficial corneal scars can be ablated with an excimer laser (wavelength of 193 nm). The lesion is excised parallel to the surface of the cornea to avoid refractive effects (▶ Fig. 5.24f). The edges of the ablated area are merged smoothly with the rest of the corneal surface, eliminating any irregularities.

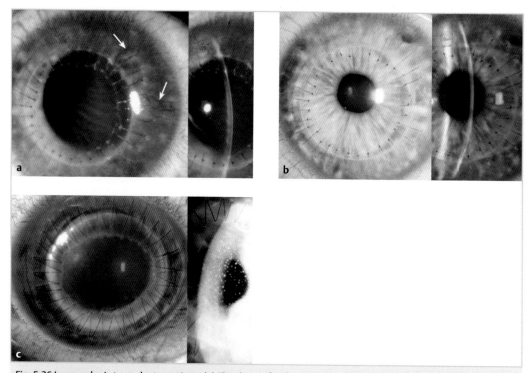

Fig. 5.26 Immunologic transplant reactions. (a) The chronic focal reaction proceeds from vascular branches extending to the graft (arrows). The graft shows focal opacification (left image) and is thickened (right image) with a progressive frontal line (Khodadoust's line). **(b)** The same eye after two weeks of topical and systemic steroid therapy. The graft is clear again and has a normal thickness. **(c)** Acute diffuse transplantation reaction. The graft is opacified and thickened. The slit lamp image shows precipitates posterior to the cornea.

▶ **Indications.** Indications are identical to those for lamellar keratoplasty. However, this method is only suitable for ablation of relatively superficial corneal opacifications—i.e., in the upper 20% of the corneal stroma.

▶ **Disadvantage.** Despite attempting ablation parallel to the surface of the cornea, phototherapeutic keratectomy often creates a hyperopic effect.

5.7.2 Refractive Corneal Procedures

Refractive corneal surgery—i.e., the surgical treatment of refractive errors—has developed into a separate field in recent years. Refractive errors are common in the population. In Germany, about 60% of people over the age of 16 years wear spectacles, and another 3% have contact lenses. The percentage of refractive errors increases with age: in those between 20 and 30 years of age about one-third have refractive errors; in those between 30 and 44 the figure is 40%; in those between 45 and 59 it is

76%; and in those over the age of 60 it is 94%. Refractive errors occurring in patients over the age of 45 is classified as presbyopia. Different surgical procedures cover the whole field of correction of refractive errors (▶ Fig. 5.27).

Astigmatic Keratotomy (AK)

▶ **Principle.** Limbus-parallel incisions of the cornea in the steep meridian make the cornea flatter and reduce the dioptric power in this meridian (▶ Fig.5.27: preoperatively 46 and 42.5 diopter; postoperatively: 43.5 and 43.0 diopter). The longer the incision and the closer to the center of the cornea, the greater the flattening effect. *Every corneal incision is a relaxing incision.*

▶ **Indications.** Higher-degree, regular astigmatism, e.g., status post penetrating keratoplasty. A maximum of 5 diopters can be corrected.

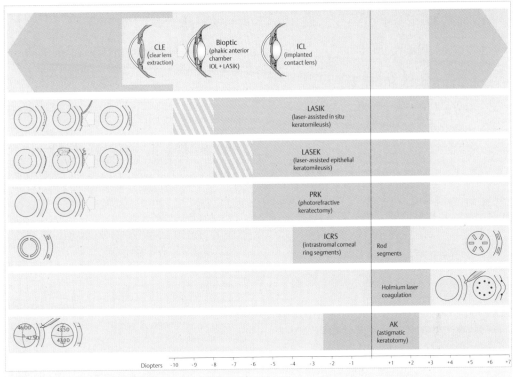

Fig. 5.27 Refractive corneal procedures. See text for explanation.

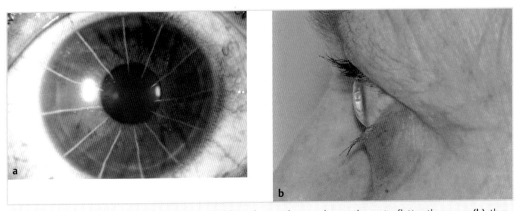

Fig. 5.28 Radial keratotomy. The radial incisions **(a)** from the periphery to close to the center flatten the cornea **(b)**, thus reducing the refractory power of the eye.

▶ **Advantage.** A well-established procedure with incisions outside the optical axis.

▶ **Disadvantage.** An effect is only observable in very deep incisions (90–95% of corneal depth). In general, the refractive outcome of the procedure is hard to calculate.

Radial Keratotomy (RK)

Radial keratotomy was the first refractive operation that was developed, and it opened up the field of refractive surgery. Due to numerous disadvantages, RK is a procedure of limited importance today (see below).

▶ **Principle.** Correction of myopia by flattening the central dome of the cornea with 4 to 16 radial incisions extending through as much as 90% of the thickness of the cornea (▶ Fig. 5.28). This increases the steepness of the corneal periphery and lowers the center of the cornea, reducing its refractive power. This method does not influence the optical center of the cornea.

▶ **Indications.** Moderate myopia (less than 6 diopters).

▶ **Advantage.** Incisions are outside the optical axis.

▶ **Disadvantage.** The outcome of the operation is influenced by the initial refraction, intraocular pressure, corneal thickness, and patient's age and sex. Refractive fluctuations of up to 1.5 diopters during the course of a day can also have a negative influence on surgical results. Refraction becomes unstable within a year in one-fifth of all cases.

Conductive Keratoplasty (Holmium Laser Coagulation, High-Frequency Coagulation)

▶ **Principle.** The holmium laser or high-frequency device is focused on the corneal stroma to create shrinkage effects by heat generation. Placing the areas symmetrically steepens the central cornea, which can correct hyperopia to some degree (▶ Fig.5.27).

▶ **Indications.** Hyperopia correction up to 3.0 diopters.

▶ **Advantage.** Established procedure with surgical effects outside the optical axis.

▶ **Disadvantage.** Remaining stromal scars can lead to glare.

Intacs: Intrastromal Corneal Ring Segments (ICRS) and Rod Segments

▶ **Principle.** Via two small corneal incisions, semicircular intrastromal tunnels are created and two clear polymethylmethacrylate (PMMA) ring segments are implanted. Between these ring segments the central cornea flattens and myopia is corrected. Hyperopia is corrected by making six small peripheral incisions in the corneal stroma, into which six straight rod segments are placed to produce a steeper corneal center. The refractive power depends on the thickness of the implanted ring or rod segment.

▶ **Indications.** Myopia correction up to −4.0 diopters; hyperopia correction up to +2.0 diopters.

▶ **Advantage.** The center of the cornea (optical axis) remains untouched. Intacs can be removed easily, if necessary.

▶ **Disadvantage.** Occasional glare problems can occur due to accumulation of fat around the segments. In addition, vascularization of the cornea adjacent to the segments or erosion of the corneal stroma over the segments is reported.

Photorefractive Keratectomy (PRK)

▶ **Principle.** Tissue is ablated to change the corneal curvature and to achieve a refractive correction. Flattening the corneal curvature corrects myopia, whereas steepening the curvature corrects hyperopia. The amount of tissue removed at different sites can be varied with layer-by-layer excimer laser ablation and the use of apertures. This makes it possible to correct for myopia, by removing more tissue from the center of the cornea, or for hyperopia, by removing more tissue from the periphery (▶ Fig. 5.27).

▶ **Indications.** Correction of myopia up to −6.0 diopters; hyperopia correction up to +3.0 diopters; astigmatism up to 3.0 diopters.

▶ **Advantage.** Established procedure, with a 95% success rate and good long-term results.

▶ **Disadvantage.** Occasionally painful during the phase in which the previously removed corneal epithelium grows back over the ablation area. Vision may be unstable in the immediate postoperative period. A persistent sensitivity to glare due to central corneal opacification (haze) is possible.

Excimer Laser Epithelial Keratomileusis (LASEK)

▶ **Principle.** The superficial corneal layer (epithelium) is loosened with alcohol and set aside, or removed with a specially designed microtome. Then the refractive procedure is performed with the excimer laser (PRK). Finally, the epithelial layer is brought back to recover the cornea again and held in place with a soft contact lens (▶ Fig. 5.27).

▶ **Indications.** Myopia correction up to −6.0 diopters, occasionally up to −8.0 diopters; hyperopia up to +3.0 diopters; astigmatism up to 3.0 diopters.

▶ **Advantage.** Procedure is suitable even in thinner corneas, and for larger ablation areas. Fewer glare problems than in PRK.

▶ **Disadvantage.** Occasionally pain due to an incomplete epithelial layer. Vision is not immediately stable. Myopic corrections of more than −6.0 diopters are the limit of this surgical procedure.

Excimer Laser In Situ Keratomileusis (LASIK)

▶ **Principle.** Myopia is corrected with preservation of Bowman's layer. A superficial corneal flap (approximately 150 μm) is created with a microkeratome. The keratome is withdrawn, the flap is reflected, and the exposed underlying corneal stroma is ablated with an excimer laser to correct the myopia. Then the flap is repositioned on the corneal bed and fixed in place by force of its own adhesion (▶ Fig. 5.27).

▶ **Indications.** Myopia correction up to −8.0 diopters, occasionally −10.0 diopters; hyperopia correction up to +3.0 diopters; astigmatism up to +3.0 diopters.

▶ **Advantage.** Fast visual recovery, stable results, no pain. A secondary enhancement can be achieved by relifting of the flap and additional laser treatment.

▶ **Disadvantage.** Postoperative dry eye syndrome (80% of corneal nerves are cut by the microkeratome). Glare problems occur occasionally.
  Flap complications are rare but severe (free cap, lost flap, "buttonhole" folds). Biomechanical properties of the cornea need to be respected. If too much stromal tissue is ablated, corneal ectasia may result.

Wavefront Correction (Aberrometry)

In addition to spherical and cylindrical refractive errors, there are so-called higher-order aberrations. (These involve a complex, nonhomogeneous distribution of the refraction. The power is not given in diopters but as the intensity of the wavefront aberration.) These deficiencies of the optical system can be corrected with special excimer laser programs (wavefront guided ablation) during PRK, LASIK, or LASEK procedures.

Implanted Contact Lens (ICL)

▶ **Principle.** Over a 3-mm limbal tunnel incision, a foldable intraocular lens is implanted and positioned in the posterior chamber between iris and crystalline lens (▶ Fig. 5.27).

▶ **Indications.** Myopic corrections from −10.0 to −20.0 diopters; hyperopic corrections from +3.0 to +8.0 diopters; astigmatism up to 2.0 diopters.

▶ **Advantage.** Cornea remains intact. The ICL can be removed or exchanged.

▶ **Disadvantage.** This is an intraocular procedure with the associated basic risk profile (hemorrhage, infection). Development of cataract and glaucoma is possible.

Phakic Anterior Chamber Lens

▶ **Principle.** An anterior chamber lens supported by the iridocorneal angle or an iris-fixated "iris-claw" lens is implanted through a 3-mm incision at the limbus (▶ Fig. 5.29).

▶ **Indication.** Defective vision from +6 to −10 diopters.

▶ **Advantages and disadvantages.** As discussed under Implanted Contact Lens above.

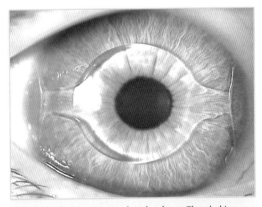

Fig. 5.29 Phakic anterior chamber lens. The phakic anterior chamber lens is supported by small elastic side struts in the iridocorneal angle and corrects the patient's defective vision to emmetropia. Take care to avoid contact between the artificial lens and the anterior surface of the iris and the posterior surface of the cornea.

Bioptic (Intraocular Lens Implantation and LASIK)

▶ **Principle.** This is a two-step procedure. The first step is the flap preparation of the LASIK. The flap is replaced. Then a phakic intraocular lens (phakic IOL) is placed in the anterior or posterior chamber or iris-fixated. After about 8 to 12 weeks the "fine tuning" of the procedure can be performed by relifting the flap and targeting the desired refractive result by excimer laser ablation (▶ Fig. 5.27).

▶ **Indications.** Myopic corrections from −10.0 diopters up to −28.0 diopters; hyperopic corrections up to +7.0 diopters; astigmatism up to 3.0 diopters.

▶ **Advantage.** Combination of two established procedures. The precise refractive goal can be achieved by the second-step enhancement. The phakic IOL can be explanted.

▶ **Disadvantage.** Intraocular procedure, glare, development of glaucoma and cataract, dry eye syndrome.

Clear Lens Extraction (CLE)

▶ **Principle.** This is the removal of a clear crystalline lens, using the same procedure as for regular cataract extraction (phacoemulsification via a 3-mm tunnel incision). The implantation of an IOL with the patient's target refraction completes the procedure (▶ Fig. 5.27).

▶ **Indications.** Myopic corrections up to −28.0 diopters; hyperopia corrections up to +8.0 diopters; astigmatism up to 3.0 diopters.

▶ **Advantage.** Established procedure of IOL implantation. Implantation of multifocal IOLs possible as pseudoaccommodative procedure.

▶ **Disadvantage.** Intraocular procedure. In highly myopic patients, a higher risk of postoperative retinal detachment is encountered.

Chapter 6

Sclera

6 Sclera

Gerhard K. Lang

6.1 Basic Knowledge

▶ **Function.** The sclera and the cornea form the rigid outer covering of the eye. All six ocular muscles insert into the sclera.

▶ **Morphology.** The sclera is fibrous, whitish-opaque, and consists of nearly acellular connective tissue with a higher water content than the cornea. The sclera is thickest (1 mm) anteriorly at the limbus of the cornea, where it joins the corneal stroma, and at its posterior pole. It is thinnest (0.3 mm) at the equator and beneath the insertions of the rectus muscles. The site where the fibers of the optic nerve enter the sclera is known as the lamina cribrosa. In the angle of the anterior chamber, the sclera forms the trabecular meshwork and the canal of Schlemm. The aqueous humor drains from there into the intrascleral and episcleral venous plexus through about 20 canaliculi.

▶ **Neurovascular supply.** Vortex veins and the short anterior and posterior ciliary arteries penetrate the sclera. The ciliary nerves pass through the sclera from posterior to anterior.

6.2 Examination Methods

The anterior sclera can be examined directly, approximately to the equator, with the help of a slit lamp and the patient's eye movements. Evaluation of the sclera posterior to the equator requires indirect methods such as **ultrasound**.

Transillumination can provide evidence of possible abnormal changes in the posterior sclera. However, this method is not as precise as an ultrasound examination.

6.3 Color Changes

The sclera is normally a dull white, like porcelain. Altered color suggests one of the following changes:
- **Conjunctival** and/or **ciliary injection** and inflammation will give the sclera a red appearance.
- A sclera that is **very thin** will appear **blue** because of the underlying choroid (this occurs in the newborn, in osteogenesis imperfecta, and following inflammation; see ▶ Fig. 6.4).
- In **jaundice,** the sclera turns **yellow**.
- In **ochronosis** (alkaptonuria) (see p. 66), the sclera will take on **brownish** color. This should be distinguished from pigmented changes in the conjunctiva.

6.4 Staphyloma and Ectasia

Staphyloma refers to a bulging of the sclera in which the underlying uveal tissue in the bulge is also thinned or degenerated. By far the most common form is *posterior staphyloma in severe myopia,* a bulging of the entire posterior pole of the eyeball (▶ Fig. 6.1). Staphyloma can also occur secondary to scleritis (see ▶ Fig. 6.4).

Ectasia is a thinning and bulging of the sclera without uveal involvement, as can occur secondary to inflammation.

Both staphyloma and ectasia are secondary or incidental findings. No treatment is available.

6.5 Trauma

The sclera is frequently involved in penetrating trauma (see p. 326). Deep injuries that extend far posteriorly usually also involve the choroid and retina. Surgery to treat larger injuries extending 8 mm past the limbus should also include a retinal repair

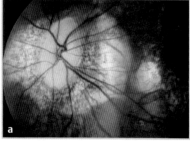 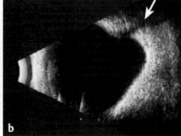

Fig. 6.1 Posterior staphyloma in a highly myopic eye. (a) Ophthalmologic image of posterior staphyloma of the sclera. (b) Ultrasound image, showing the posterior scleral bulge and oblique course of the optic nerve through the sclera (arrow).

(retinal cryopexy or retinal tamponade) (see ▶ Fig. 12.27).

6.6 Inflammations

Inflammations are the most clinically significant scleral changes encountered in ophthalmologic practice. They more often involve the anterior sclera (episcleritis and anterior scleritis) than the posterior sclera (posterior scleritis).

▶ **Classification.** Forms of scleral inflammation are differentiated as follows:
- **Location.** Anterior or posterior—i.e., anterior or posterior to the equator of the globe.
- **Depth**
  - Superficial (episcleritis).
  - Deep (scleritis).
- **Nature**
  - Diffuse (usually scleritis).
  - Circumscribed or segmental (episcleritis).
  - Nodular, with formation of small mobile nodules (scleritis and episcleritis).
  - Necrotizing (scleritis only).
  - Nonnecrotizing (scleritis only).

6.6.1 Episcleritis

Definition
Circumscribed, usually segmental, and generally *nodular* inflammation of the episclera (connective tissue between sclera and conjunctiva).

▶ **Epidemiology.** Episcleritis is the most common form of scleral inflammation.

▶ **Etiology.** Episcleritis is rarely attributable to one of the systemic underlying disorders listed in ▶ Table 6.1, and is only occasionally due to bacterial or viral inflammation. Often episcleritis will have no readily discernible cause.

▶ **Symptoms.** Episcleritis can be unilateral or bilateral. It is usually associated with segmental reddening and slight tenderness to palpation.

▶ **Findings.** The episcleral vessels lie within the fascial sheath of the eyeball (Tenon's capsule) and are arranged radially. In episcleritis, these vessels and the conjunctival vessels above them become hyperemic (▶ Fig. 6.2). Tenon's capsule and the episclera are infiltrated with inflammatory cells, but the sclera itself is not swollen. The presence of small *mobile* nodules is typical of nodular episcleritis.

Table 6.1 Systemic diseases that can cause scleritis

Frequent causes	Rare causes
• Rheumatoid arthritis	• Tuberculosis
• Polymyositis	• Lues
• Dermatomyositis	• Borreliosis
• Ankylosing spondylitis	• Reiter's syndrome
• Spondyloarthritis	
• Vasculitis	
• Wegener's granulomatosis	
• Herpes zoster ophthalmicus	
• Syphilis	
• Gout	

▶ **Differential diagnosis.** The disorder should be distinguished from conjunctivitis (see Note box) and scleritis, (see below).

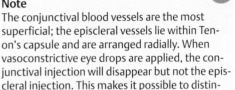

Note
The conjunctival blood vessels are the most superficial; the episcleral vessels lie within Tenon's capsule and are arranged radially. When vasoconstrictive eye drops are applied, the conjunctival injection will disappear but not the episcleral injection. This makes it possible to distinguish conjunctivitis from episcleritis.

▶ **Treatment and prognosis.** Episcleritis usually resolves spontaneously within 1 to 2 weeks, although the nodular form can persist for extended periods of time. Severe symptoms are treated with topical steroids (eye drops) or with a nonsteroidal anti-inflammatory agent.

6.6.2 Scleritis

Definition
Diffuse or localized inflammation of the sclera. Scleritis is classified according to location:
- Anterior (inflammation anterior to the equator of the globe).
- Posterior (inflammation posterior to the equator of the globe).
- Anterior scleritis is further classified according to its nature:
  - Nonnecrotizing anterior scleritis (nodular or diffuse).
  - Necrotizing anterior scleritis (with or without inflammation).

▶ **Epidemiology.** Scleritis is far less frequent than episcleritis. Patients are generally older, and women are affected more often than men.

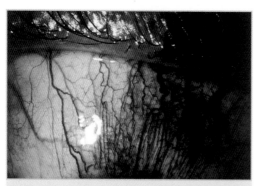

Fig. 6.2 Segmental episcleritis. Typical hyperemia and inflammation of the radial episcleral blood vessels.

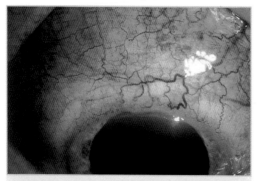

Fig. 6.3 Diffuse nonnecrotizing scleritis. Typical signs include thickening and edema of the sclera and deep, diffuse reddening.

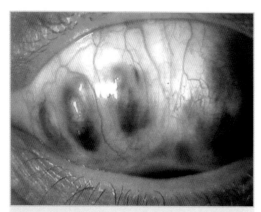

Fig. 6.4 Circumscribed scleral staphyloma secondary to scleritis. The underlying choroid shows through at the bulge where the sclera is thinned, giving it a bluish tinge.

▶ **Etiology.** Approximately 50% of scleritis cases (which tend to have severe clinical courses) are attributable to systemic autoimmune or rheumatic disease (▶ Table 6.1), or are the result of immunologic processes associated with infection. This applies especially to anterior scleritis. Posterior scleritis is not usually associated with any specific disorder. As with episcleritis, scleritis is only occasionally due to bacterial or viral inflammation.

▶ **Symptoms and findings.** All forms except for scleromalacia perforans are associated with *severe pain* and general reddening of the eye.

▶ **Anterior nonnecrotizing scleritis (nodular form).** The nodules consist of edematous swollen sclera and are *not mobile* (in contrast to episcleritis).

▶ **Anterior necrotizing scleritis (diffuse form).** The inflammation is more severe than in the nodular form. It can be limited to a certain segment or may include the entire anterior sclera (▶ Fig. 6.3).

▶ **Anterior necrotizing scleritis with inflammation.** Circumscribed reddening of the eyes is a typical sign. There may be deviation or injection of the blood vessels of the affected region, accompanied by vascular patches in the episcleral tissue. As the disorder progresses, the sclera thins as the scleral lamellae of collagen fibrils melt, so that the underlying choroid shows through (▶ Fig. 6.4). The inflammation gradually spreads from its primary focus. Usually it is associated with uveitis.

▶ **Anterior necrotizing scleritis without inflammation (scleromalacia perforans).** This form of scleritis typically occurs in *female patients* with a long history of seropositive rheumatoid arthritis. The clinical course of the disorder is usually asymptomatic and begins with a yellow necrotic patch on the sclera. As the disorder progresses, the sclera also thins so that the underlying choroid shows through. This is the *only* form of scleritis that *may be painless.*

▶ **Posterior scleritis.** Sometimes there will be no abnormal findings in the anterior eye, and pain will be the only symptom. Associated inflammation of the orbit may result in proptosis (exophthalmos) and impaired ocular motility due to myositis of the ocular muscles. Intraocular findings may include exudative retinal detachment and/or choroidal detachment. Macular and optic disc edema are frequently present (▶ Fig. 6.5).

Note

The reddening in scleritis is due to injection of the deeper vascular plexus on the sclera and to injection of the episclera. Inspecting the eye in daylight will best reveal the layer of maximum injection.

▶ **Differential diagnosis.** Conjunctivitis and episcleritis (see Chapter 6.6.1).

▶ **Treatment**
▶ **Anterior nonnecrotizing scleritis.** Topical or systemic *nonsteroidal* anti-inflammatory therapy.

▶ **Anterior necrotizing scleritis with inflammation.** Systemic *steroid* therapy is usually required to control pain. If corticosteroids do not help or are not tolerated, immunosuppressive agents may be used.

▶ **Anterior necrotizing scleritis without inflammation (scleromalacia perforans).** As no effective treatment is available, grafts of preserved sclera, lyophilized dura, or an amnion membrane patch may be required to preserve the globe if the course of the disorder is fulminant.

▶ **Posterior scleritis.** Treatment is the same as for anterior necrotizing scleritis with inflammation.

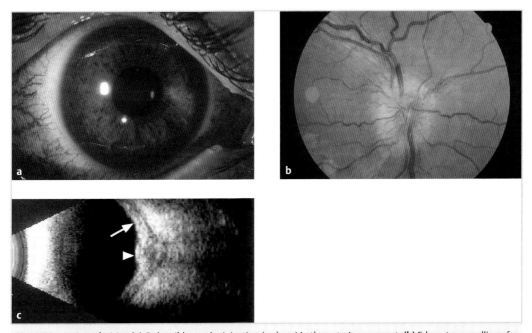

Fig. 6.5 Posterior scleritis. (a) Only mild vascular injection (red eye) in the anterior segment. **(b)** Edematous swelling of the optic nerve head. **(c)** In the ultrasound image, significant swelling of the choroid (arrow) and prominence of the optic disc (arrowhead) are seen.

Chapter 7

Lens

7

7 Lens

Gerhard K. Lang

7.1 Basic Knowledge

▶ **Function of the lens.** The lens is one of the essential refractive media of the eye and focuses incident rays of light on the retina. It adds a variable element to the eye's total refractive power (10–20 diopters, depending on individual accommodation) to the fixed refractive power of the cornea (approximately 43 diopters).

▶ **Shape.** The fully developed lens is a **biconvex, transparent structure**. The curvature of the posterior surface, which has a radius of 6 mm, is greater than that of the anterior surface, which has a radius of 10 mm.

▶ **Weight.** The lens is approximately 4 mm thick, and its weight increases with age to five times its weight at birth. The lens of an adult weighs about 220 mg.

▶ **Position and suspension.** The lens lies in the posterior chamber of the eye between the posterior surface of the iris and the vitreous body in a **saucer-shaped depression of the vitreous body** known as the hyaloid fossa. Together with the iris it forms an optical diaphragm that separates the anterior and posterior chambers of the eye. Radially arranged **zonule fibers** that insert into the lens around its equator connect the lens to the ciliary body. These fibers hold the lens in position (▶ Fig. 7.1) and transfer the **tensile** force of the ciliary muscle (see Chapter 16.1.3, Accommodation).

▶ **Embryology and growth.** The lens is a **purely epithelial structure** without any nerves or blood vessels. It moves into its intraocular position in the first month of fetal development as surface ectoderm invaginates into the primitive optic vesicle, which consists of neuroectoderm. *A purely ectodermal structure*, the lens differentiates during gestation into central geometric lens fibers, an anterior layer of epithelial cells, and an acellular hyaline capsule (▶ Fig. 7.2). The normal **direction of growth** of epithelial structures is centrifugal; fully developed epithelial cells migrate to the surface and are peeled off. However, the lens grows in the *opposite* direction. The youngest cells are always on the surface and the oldest cells in the center of the lens. The growth of primary lens fibers forms the **embryonic nucleus**. At the **equator**, the epithelial cells further differentiate into lens fiber cells (▶ Fig. 7.2). These new secondary fibers displace the primary fibers toward the center of the lens. Formation of a **fetal nucleus** that encloses the embryonic nucleus is complete at birth. Fiber formation at the equator, which continues throughout life, produces the **infantile nucleus** during the first and second decades of life, and the **adult nucleus** during the third decade. Completely enclosed by the lens capsule, the lens never loses any cells so that its tissue is continuously compressed throughout life (▶ Fig. 7.3). The various density zones created as the lens develops are readily discernible as discontinuity zones (▶ Fig. 7.4).

▶ **Metabolism and aging of the lens.** The lens is nourished by **diffusion from the aqueous humor**. In this respect it resembles a tissue culture, with the aqueous humor as its substrate and the eyeball as the container that provides a constant temperature.

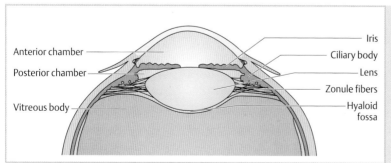

Fig. 7.1 Shape of the lens and its position in the eye. The lens is a biconvex structure suspended on the zonule fibers. It lies in the hyaloid fossa and separates the anterior and posterior chambers of the eye.

Anterior chamber
Posterior chamber
Vitreous body
Iris
Ciliary body
Lens
Zonule fibers
Hyaloid fossa

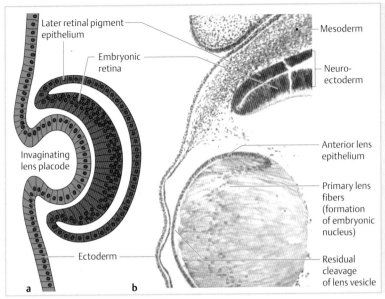

Fig. 7.2 Embryology of the lens. (a) First month of fetal development. The ectoderm invaginates and is isolated in what becomes the optic cup. **(b)** The lens vesicle is completely invaginated. The primary lens fibers grow and begin to form the embryonic nucleus.

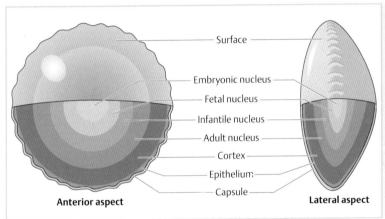

Fig. 7.3 Anatomy of the lens.

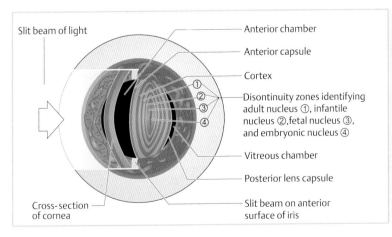

Fig. 7.4 Slit lamp examination of the lens. The various density zones (1 to 4) created as the lens develops are visible as discontinuity zones.

Note

The metabolism and detailed biochemical processes involved in aging are complex and not completely understood. Because of this, it has not been possible to influence cataract (see p. 105) development with medications.

The metabolism and growth of the lens cells are self-regulating. Metabolic activity is essential for the preservation of the integrity, transparency, and optical function of the lens. The epithelium of the lens helps to maintain the ion equilibrium and permit **transportation of nutrients, minerals, and water into the lens**. This type of transportation, referred to as a "pump-leak system," permits active transfer of sodium, potassium, calcium, and amino acids from the aqueous humor into the lens as well as passive diffusion through the posterior lens capsule. Maintaining this equilibrium (homeostasis) is essential for the transparency of the lens and is closely related to the water balance. The **water content of the lens** is normally stable and in equilibrium with the surrounding aqueous humor. The water content of the lens decreases with age, whereas the content of insoluble lens proteins (albuminoid) increases. The lens becomes harder, less elastic (i.e., it undergoes loss of accommodation, see p. 372), and less transparent. A **decrease in the transparency of the lens with age** is as unavoidable as wrinkles in the skin or gray hair. Manifestly reduced transparency is present in 95%

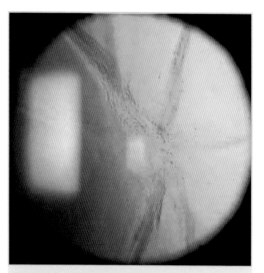

Fig. 7.5 Retroillumination of the lens (Brückner's test). Opacities appear black in the red pupil.

of persons over the age of 65, although individual exceptions are not uncommon. The central portion or nucleus of the lens becomes sclerosed and slightly yellowish with age.

7.2 Examination Methods

▶ **Cataracts.** Retroillumination of the lens (Brückner's test) is the *quickest preliminary examination method* for lens opacities (see Cataracts, Chapter 7.4). Under a light source or ophthalmoscope (set to 10 diopters), opacities will appear black in the red pupil (▶ Fig. 7.5). The lens can be examined *in greater detail and in three dimensions* under focal illumination with a slit lamp with the pupil maximally dilated. The extent, type, location, and density of opacities and their relation to the visual axis can be evaluated. Mature lens opacities can be diagnosed with the unaided eye by the presence of a white pupil (leukocoria).

Note

Where the fundus is not visible in the presence of a mature lens opacity, ultrasound studies (one-dimensional A-scan and two-dimensional B-scan studies) are indicated to exclude involvement of the deeper structures of the eye.

▶ **Iridodonesis and phacodonesis.** Tremulous motion of the iris and lens observed during slit lamp examination suggests subluxation of the lens; see Chapter 7.5).

7.3 Developmental Anomalies of the Lens

Anomalies of lens shape are very rare. Lenticonus is a circumscribed conical protrusion of the anterior pole (anterior lenticonus) or posterior pole (posterior lenticonus). A hemispherical protrusion is referred to as lentiglobus. Symptoms include myopia and reduced visual acuity. Some patients with Alport's syndrome (kidney disease accompanied by sensorineural hearing loss and anomalies of lens shape) have *anterior* lenticonus. *Posterior lenticonus* may be associated with a lens opacity (▶ Fig. 7.6). Treatment is the same as for congenital or juvenile cataract.

Microphakia refers to a lens of abnormally small diameter. Any interruption of the development of the eye generally leads to microphakia. This can occur for example in Weill–Marchesani syndrome (see ▶ Table 7.5).

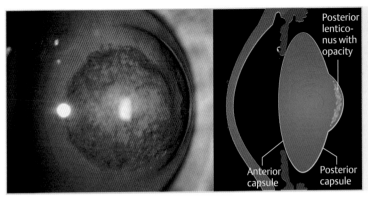

Fig. 7.6 Posterior lenticonus. Conical protrusion of the posterior pole, here associated with a posterior subcapsular opacity.

(labels on figure: Posterior lenticonus with opacity; Anterior capsule; Posterior capsule)

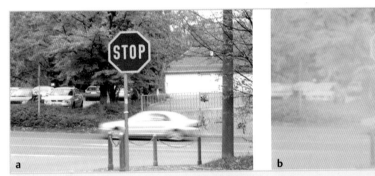

Fig. 7.7 Symptoms of cataract. **(a)** Visual image without a cataract. **(b)** Visual image with a cataract: there are gray areas and partial loss of image perception with alterations in color perception.

7.4 Cataract

Definition

A cataract is present when the transparency of the lens is reduced to the point that the patient's vision is impaired. The term cataract comes from the Greek word *katarraktes* (down-rushing; waterfall), because earlier it was thought that the cataract was a congealed fluid from the brain that had flowed in front of the lens.

▶ **General symptoms.** Development of the cataract and its symptoms is generally an *occult process*. Patients experience the various symptoms such as seeing only shades of gray, visual impairment, blurred vision, distorted vision, glare or star bursts, monocular diplopia, altered color perception, etc. to varying degrees, and these symptoms will vary with the specific type of cataract (see ▶ Table 7.3 and ▶ Fig. 7.7).

Note
Diagnosis of a cataract is generally very unsettling for patients, who immediately associate it with surgery. One should therefore refer only to a cataract when it has been established that surgery is indicated. If the cataract has not progressed to an advanced stage or the patient can cope well with the visual impairment, one should refer instead to a "lens opacity."

▶ **Classification.** Cataracts can be classified according to several different criteria:
• Time of occurrence (acquired or congenital cataracts).
• Maturity.
• Morphology.

No one classification system is completely satisfactory. We prefer the system shown in ▶ Table 7.1.

Table 7.1 Classification of cataracts according to time of occurrence

Acquired cataracts (over 99% of cataracts)	Congenital cataracts (fewer than 1% of cataracts)

• Senile cataract (over 90% of cataracts)
• Cataract with systemic disease
  ○ Diabetes mellitus (most frequent)
  ○ Galactosemia
  ○ Renal insufficiency
  ○ Mannosidosis
  ○ Fabry's disease
  ○ Lowe's syndrome
  ○ Wilson's disease
  ○ Myotonic dystrophy
  ○ Tetany
  ○ Skin disorders
• Secondary and complicated cataracts
  ○ Cataract with heterochromia (most frequent)
  ○ Cataract with chronic iridocyclitis
  ○ Cataract with retinal vasculitis
  ○ Cataract with retinitis pigmentosa
• Postoperative cataracts
  ○ Most frequently following vitrectomy and silicone oil retinal tamponade
  ○ Following filtering operations
• Traumatic cataracts
  ○ Contusion or perforation rosette (most frequent)
  ○ Infrared radiation (glassblower's cataract)
  ○ Electrical injury
  ○ Ionizing radiation
• Toxic cataract
  ○ Corticosteroid-induced cataract (most frequent)
  ○ Less frequently from chlorpromazine, miotic agents, or busulfan
	• Hereditary cataracts
	  ○ Autosomal-dominant
	  ○ Autosomal-recessive
	  ○ Sporadic
	  ○ X-linked
	• Cataracts due to early embryonic (transplacental) damage
	  ○ Rubella (40–60%)
	  ○ Mumps (10–22%)
	  ○ Hepatitis (16%)
	  ○ Toxoplasmosis (5%)

7.4.1 Acquired Cataract

Senile Cataract

▶ **Epidemiology.** Senile cataract is by far the most frequent form of cataract, accounting for 90% of cataracts. About 5% of 70-year-olds and 10% of 80-year-olds suffer from a cataract requiring surgery.

> **Note**
> Ninety percent of cataracts are senile cataracts.

▶ **Etiology.** The precise causes of senile cataract have not been identified. As occurrence is often familial, it is important to obtain a detailed family history.

▶ **Classification and forms of senile cataracts.** The classification according to **maturity** (▶ Table 7.2) follows the degree of visual impairment and the maturity, which earlier was important to determine the time of surgery. We follow a **morphological classification** as morphological aspects such as the hardness and thickness of the nucleus now influence the surgical procedure (▶ Table 7.3):

▶ **Nuclear cataract.** In the fourth decade of life, the pressure of peripheral lens fiber production causes hardening of the entire lens, especially the nucleus. The nucleus takes on a *yellowish-brown color (brunescent nuclear cataract)*. This may range from reddish-brown to nearly black discoloration of the entire lens (black cataract). Because they increase the refractive power of the lens, nuclear cataracts lead to lenticular myopia and occasionally produce a second focal point in the lens with resulting monocular diplopia (▶ Fig. 7.8).

> **Note**
> Nuclear cataracts develop very slowly. Due to the lenticular myopia, near vision (even without eyeglasses) remains good for a long time.

▶ **Cortical cataract.** Nuclear cataracts are often associated with changes in the lens cortex. It is interesting to note that patients with cortical cataracts tend to have acquired hyperopia in contrast to

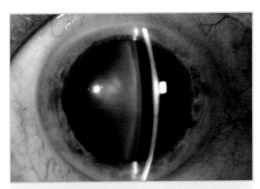

Fig. 7.8 Nuclear cataract. The nucleus of the lens has a yellowish-brown color resulting from constant inward densification of peripheral lens fiber production.

Table 7.2 Classification of cataracts in relation to maturity

Cataract form	Visual acuity
Developing cataract	Still full (0.8–1.0)
Immature cataract	Reduced (0.4–0.5)
Developed cataract	Severely reduced (1/50–0.1)
Mature cataract, hypermature cataract	Light and dark perception, perception of hand movements in front of the eye

patients with nuclear cataracts, who tend to be myopic (see above).

Whereas changes in *nuclear* cataracts are due to hardening, *cortical* changes are characterized by *increased water content*. Several morphological changes will be apparent upon slit lamp examination with maximum mydriasis:

- *Vacuoles.* Fluid accumulations will be present in the form of small narrow cortical vesicles. The vacuoles remain small and increase in number.
- *Water fissures.* Radial patterns of fluid-filled fissures will be seen between the fibers.
- *Separation of the lamellae.* Not as frequent as water fissures, these consist of a zone of fluid between the lamellae (often between the clear lamellae and the cortical fibers).
- *Cuneiform cataract.* This is a frequent finding in which the opacities radiate from the periphery of the lens like spokes of a wheel.

Note ❗

Cortical cataracts progress more rapidly than nuclear cataracts. Visual acuity may temporarily improve during the course of the disease. This is due to a stenopeic effect as light passes through a clear area between two radial opacities.

▶ **Posterior subcapsular cataract.** This is a *special form of cortical cataract* that begins in the visual axis. Beginning as a small cluster of granular opacities, this form of cataract expands peripherally in a disklike pattern. As opacity increases, the rest of the cortex and the nucleus become involved (the usual spectrum of senile cataract).

Note ❗

Posterior subcapsular cataract leads to early, rapid, and severe loss of visual acuity. Near vision is usually significantly worse than distance vision (near-field miosis). Dilating eye drops can improve visual acuity in this form of cataract. Patients are severely hampered by intense glare.

▶ **Mature cataract.** The lens is diffusely white due to *complete opacification of the cortex.* A brownish lens nucleus is often faintly discernible (▶ Fig. 7.9). Where water content is increased, a lens with a mature cataract can swell and acquire a silky luster (intumescent cataract in which the capsule is under pressure). The increasing thickness of the lens increases the resistance of the pupil and with it the risk of angle closure glaucoma (see p. 164).

Note ❗

Vision is reduced to perception of light and dark, and the interior of the eye is no longer visible. The cataract operation leads to restoration of both the patient's visual acuity and the ophthalmologist's access to a diagnostic view into the eye.

▶ **Hypermature cataract.** If a mature cataract progresses to the point of complete liquefaction of the cortex, the dense brown nucleus will subside within the capsule. Its superior margin will then be visible in the pupil as a dark brown silhouette against the surrounding grayish-white cortex. The pressure in the lens capsule decreases. The contents of the limp and wrinkled capsular bag gravitate within the capsule. This condition, referred to as *Morgagni's cataract,* is the final stage in a cataract that has usually developed over the course of two decades. The approximate onset of the cataract can usually be inferred from such findings (▶ Fig. 7.10).

Note ❗

Prompt cataract extraction not only restores visual acuity but also prevents development of phacolytic glaucoma.

Table 7.3 Overview of forms of senile cataract

Cataract form	Morphology	Incidence	Symptoms	Visual acuity	Progression	Peculiarities, glare, eyesight in twilight	Diagnosis and prognosis for vision
Nuclear cataract		About 30%, particularly in more severe myopia	• Shades of gray (like looking through frosted glass) • Blurred vision • Distorted vision • Double or triple vision • Intense glare in bright light • Diminished contrast • Changes in color perception (rare)	• Impairment is relatively late • Increasingly poor *distance vision* • *Good near vision* remains unchanged due to myopic effect of cataract	Slow	• Eyesight in twilight is often better than in daylight because the mydriasis in darkness allows light past the opacity • Glare less pronounced • Monocular diplopia due to two focal points in the lens	• Morphology by transillumination (Brückner's test) • Detailed diagnosis in slit lamp examination • Prediction of expected postoperative visual acuity: *laser interference visual acuity testing*
Cortical cataract		About 50%		• *Early loss of visual acuity!* • Hyperopic effect of cataract compromises distance vision less than near vision	Rapid (temporary improvement in visual acuity due to stenopeic effect)	• Patient is severely hampered by glare (sun, snow, headlights). Patients typically prefer dark glasses and wide-brimmed hats • Marked improvement of vision in twilight and at *night (nyctalopia)*	
Posterior subcapsular cataract		About 20%		• *Early loss of visual acuity* • *Near vision* particularly affected, *distance vision better*	Rapid		
Mature cataract		Final stage	• Objects no longer discernible • Patients with bilateral cataracts are practically blind and dependent on others in everyday life	Visual acuity reduced to perception of light and dark; perception of hand movements in front of the eye	All cataract forms will progress to a mature/hypermature form given enough time	In intense light, patient will perceive gross movements and persons as silhouettes	• Leukocoria (white pupil) detectable with unaided eye • Slit lamp permits differentiation • Retinoscopy to determine visual acuity is often ineffective with dense opacities
Hypermature cataract							

When the lens capsule becomes permeable for liquefied lens substances, it will lose volume due to leakage. The capsule will become wrinkled. The escaping lens proteins will cause intraocular irritation and attract macrophages that then cause congestion of the trabecular meshwork (*phacolytic glaucoma*: see Chapter 10.5.1).

Note
Emergency extraction of the hypermature cataract is indicated in phacolytic glaucoma to save the eye.

7.4.2 Cataract in Systemic Disease

▶ **Epidemiology.** Lens opacities can occasionally occur as a sign of systemic disease.

▶ **Types of cataract in systemic disease**
▶ **Diabetic cataract.** The typical diabetic cataract is rare in young diabetic patients. Transient metabolic decompensation promotes the occurrence of a typical radial snowflake pattern of cortical opacities (snowflake cataract). Transient hyperopia and myopia can occur.

Note
Diabetic cataract progresses rapidly. Senile cataracts are observed about five times as often in older diabetics as in patients the same age with normal metabolism. These cataracts usually also occur 2–3 years earlier.

▶ **Galactosemic cataract.** This *deep posterior cortical opacity* begins after birth. Galactosemia is a rare cause of early cataract in children lacking an enzyme required to metabolize galactose. The newborn receives ample amounts of galactose in the mother's milk. Due to a lack of uridylyl transferase, or less frequently galactokinase, galactose cannot be metabolized to glucose, and the body becomes inundated with galactose or with galactose 1-phosphate. If the disorder is diagnosed promptly and the child is maintained on a galactose-free diet, the opacities of the first few weeks of life will be reversible.

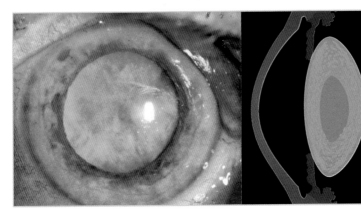

Fig. 7.9 Mature cataract.
- There is diffuse, complete opacification of the lens. A brownish nucleus is faintly visible posterior to the cortical layer.
- The interior of the eye is no longer visible.
- Visual acuity is reduced to perception of light and dark.

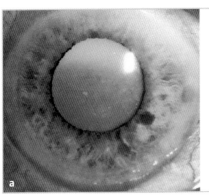
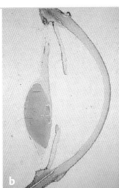

Fig. 7.10 Hypermature cataract. (a) The brown nucleus has subsided in the liquefied cortex. **(b)** The histologic image obtained at autopsy shows the position of the subsided nucleus and the shrunken capsular bag.

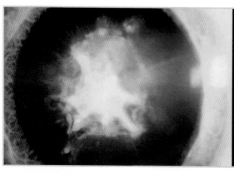
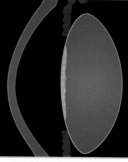

Fig. 7.11 Dermatogenous cataract. Typical symptoms include a crest-shaped whitish opacity beneath the anterior lens capsule along the visual axis.

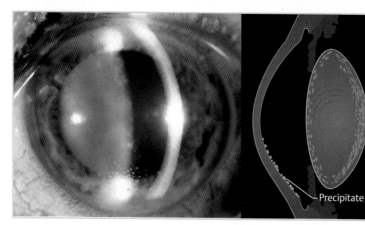
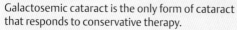

Precipitate

Fig. 7.12 Complicated cataract in chronic iridocyclitis. This diffuse opacity originates from the posterior subcapsular cataract. Inflammatory precipitates indicative of chronic uveitis are also visible on the posterior surface of the cornea.

Note

Galactosemic cataract is the only form of cataract that responds to conservative therapy.

▶ **Dialysis cataract.** Hemodialysis to eliminate metabolic acidosis in renal insufficiency can disturb the osmotic equilibrium of lens metabolism and cause swelling of the cortex of the lens.

Other *rare metabolic diseases* that can cause cataract include mannosidosis, Fabry's disease, Lowe's syndrome (oculocerebrorenal syndrome), and Wilson's disease (hepatolenticular degeneration).

▶ **Cataract with myotonic dystrophy.** Opacities first occur between the ages of 30 and 50 years, initially in a thin layer of the anterior cortex and later also in the subcapsular posterior cortex in the form of rosettes. Detecting these opacities is important for *differential diagnosis* as cataracts do not occur in Thomsen's disease (myotonia congenita) or Erb's progressive muscular dystrophy.

Symptoms that *confirm the diagnosis* include cataract, active signs of myotonia (delayed opening of

the fist), and passive signs of myotonia (decreased relaxation of muscles in the extremities following direct percussion of the muscle and absence of reflexes).

▶ **Tetany cataract.** The opacity lies within a broad zone inferior to the anterior lens capsule and consists of a series of gray punctate lesions. Symptoms that *confirm the diagnosis* include low blood calcium levels, a positive hyperventilation test, and signs of tetany: positive Chvostek, Trousseau and Erb signs.

▶ **Dermatogenous cataract.** This may occur with chronic neurodermatitis and less frequently with other skin disorders such as scleroderma, poikiloderma, and chronic eczema. Characteristic signs include an anterior crest-shaped thickening of the protruding center of the capsule (▶ Fig. 7.11).

7.4.3 Complicated Cataracts

This form of cataract can occur as a complication of any protracted intraocular inflammation, especially heterochromia, chronic iridocyclitis, retinal vasculitis, and retinitis pigmentosa. The result is a

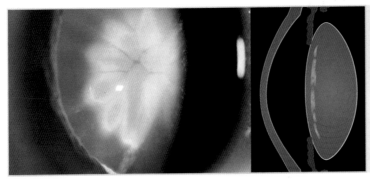

Fig. 7.13 Contusion cataract. A contusion rosette posterior to the anterior lens capsule has developed after severe blunt trauma to the eyeball.

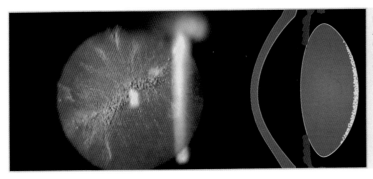

Fig. 7.14 Cortisone cataract. A dense pumicelike opacity has developed in the posterior capsule after prolonged systemic steroid therapy for bronchial asthma.

pumicelike posterior subcapsular cataract that progresses axially toward the nucleus. This form of cataract produces extreme light scattering (▶ Fig. 7.12).

7.4.4 Cataract after Intraocular Surgery

Cataracts usually develop earlier in the operated eye as compared to the opposite, unoperated eye after intraocular surgery. This applies especially to filtering operations. A secondary cataract (usually a nuclear cataract) will generally occur following vitrectomy and silicone oil tamponade. In contrast, posterior subcapsular cataract after vitrectomy with gas tamponade (gas cataract) resolves after resorption of the gas.

7.4.5 Traumatic Cataract

The incidence of these lens opacities is higher in men than in women due to occupational and sports injuries. The following types of traumatic cataracts are differentiated.

▶ **Frequent traumatic cataracts**
• **Contusion cataract.** Contusion of the eyeball will produce a rosette-shaped subcapsular opacity on the anterior surface of the lens. It will nor-

mally remain unchanged but will migrate into the deeper cortex over time due to the apposition of new fibers (▶ Fig. 7.13). This can be significant for expert medical assessment.

▶ **Rarer traumatic cataracts**
• **Infrared radiation cataract** (glassblower's cataract): This type of cataract occurs after decades of prolonged exposure to the infrared radiation of fire without eye protection. Characteristic findings include splitting of the anterior lens capsule, whose edges will be observed to curl up and float in the anterior chamber. Occupational safety regulations have drastically reduced the incidence of this type of cataract.
• **Electrical injury.** This dense subcapsular cataract can be caused by lightning or high-voltage electrical shock.
• **Cataract from ionizing radiation.** See Chapter 18.6.3.

7.4.6 Toxic Cataract

▶ **Steroid cataract.** Prolonged topical or systemic therapy with corticosteroids can result in a posterior subcapsular opacity. The exact dose–response relationship is not known (▶ Fig. 7.14).

Other toxic cataracts can result from chlorpromazine, miotic agents (especially cholinester-

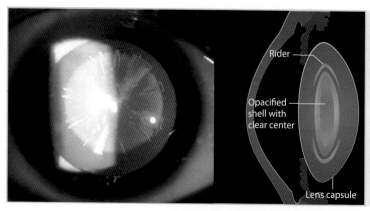

Fig. 7.15 Lamellar cataract. The lens opacities ("riders") are located in only one layer of lens fibers—often only in the equatorial region, as shown here.

Rider

Opacified shell with clear center

Lens capsule

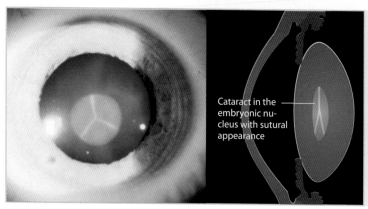

Fig. 7.16 Nuclear cataract. This variant of the lamellar cataract affects only the outer layer of the embryonic nucleus, seen here as a sutural cataract.

Cataract in the embryonic nucleus with sutural appearance

ase inhibitors), and busulfan (Myleran, GlaxoSmith-Kline) used in the treatment of chronic myelocytic leukemia.

7.4.7 Congenital Cataract

There are many congenital cataracts. They are either hereditary or acquired through the placenta.

Hereditary Congenital Cataracts

Familial forms of congenital cataracts may be autosomal-dominant, autosomal-recessive, sporadic, or X-linked. They are easily diagnosed on the basis of their characteristic symmetric morphology.

▶ **Forms of hereditary congenital cataract**
▶ **Lamellar or zonular cataract.** Opacities are located in one layer of lens fibers, often as "riders" only in the equatorial region (▶ Fig. 7.15).

▶ **Nuclear cataract.** This is a variant of the lamellar cataract in which initially only the outer layer of the embryonic nucleus is affected (▶ Fig. 7.16).

▶ **Coronary cataract.** This is characterized by fine radial opacities in the equatorial region.

▶ **Cerulean cataract.** This is characterized by fine round or club-shaped blue peripheral lens opacities.

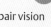
Note
Most familial lens opacities do not impair vision and are not progressive.

This also applies to rare lens opacities involving the capsule such as anterior and posterior polar cataracts, anterior pyramidal cataract, and Mittendorf's dot (remnant of the embryonic hyaloid artery on the posterior capsule of the lens) (see p. 177).

Cataract from Transplacental Infection in the First Trimester of Pregnancy

A statistical study in 1986 by Pau cites the following incidences of congenital cataract with respect to systemic disease contracted by the mother during the first trimester of pregnancy:

- Rubella 40–60%.
- Mumps 10–22%.
- Hepatitis 16%.
- Toxoplasmosis 5%.

Most of these cases involved *total cataracts* due to virus infection contracted by the mother during early pregnancy. This infection occurred during the fifth to eighth week of pregnancy, the phase in which the lens develops. Because the protective lens capsule has not yet been formed at this time, viruses can invade and opacify the lens tissue.

The most frequent cause of cataract is a rubella infection contracted by the mother, which also produces other developmental anomalies (Gregg's syndrome involving lens opacity, an open ductus arteriosus, and sensorineural hearing loss). The cataract is bilateral and total and can be diagnosed by the presence of leukocoria (white pupil) and chorioretinal scarring secondary to choroiditis.

7.4.8 Treatment of Cataracts

Medication

In spite of theoretical approaches in animal research, the effectiveness of conservative cataract treatment in humans has not been demonstrated.

> **Note**
> At present, no conservative methods are available to prevent, delay, or reverse the development of a cataract. Galactosemic cataracts are the only exception to this rule (see p. 109).

Surgical Treatment

Cataract surgery is the most frequently performed procedure in ophthalmology.

When Is Surgery Indicated?

Earlier surgical techniques were dependent upon the maturity of the cataract. This is no longer the case in modern cataract surgery.

▶ **Optical indications.** Restoration of visual acuity is by far the most frequent indication for cataract surgery.

- In the presence of **bilateral cataracts,** the eye with the worse visual acuity should undergo surgery when the patient feels visually handicapped. However, this threshold will vary depending on the patient's occupational requirements.
- In the presence of a **unilateral cataract,** the patient is often inclined to postpone surgery as long as vision in the healthy eye is sufficient.

▶ **Medical indications.** These are situations in which the health of the eye is endangered.

- In the presence of a **mature cataract,** it is important to advise the patient to undergo surgery as soon as possible to prevent a phacolytic glaucoma.
- In the case of **retinal disease** (e.g., diabetic retinopathy) a cataract extraction may be necessary to clear the optical axis for retinal diagnosis and laser treatment.

Will the Operation Be Successful?

The prospect of a successful outcome is important for the patient. Most patients define a successful outcome in terms of a significant improvement in vision. Therefore, it is important that the patient undergoes a thorough preoperative eye examination to exclude any ocular disorders—aside from the cataract—that may worsen visual acuity and compromise the success of the cataract operation. Such disorders include uncontrolled glaucoma, uveitis, macular degeneration, retinal detachment, atrophy of the optic nerve, and amblyopia.

> **Note**
> A detailed history of the patient's other ocular disorders and vision prior to development of the cataract should be obtained before surgery.

Several methods are helpful for assessing the **prognosis with respect to expected visual acuity** (retinal resolution) following cataract surgery. These include:

- *Macular optical coherence tomography* (OCT).
- *Laser interference visual acuity testing (see p. 277).*
- *Evaluation of the choroid figure* (in severe opacifications such as a mature cataract, see p. 107).

Reliability of Cataract Surgery

Cataract surgery is now performed as a microsurgical technique under an operating microscope. Modern standardized techniques such as extracapsular cataract extraction (ECCE), phacoemulsification, and microincision cataract surgery (MICS), microsurgical instruments, atraumatic suture material (30-µm thin nylon suture thread), and specially trained surgeons performing many cataract operations (high-volume surgeons) have made it possible to successfully perform cataract surgery *without serious complications in 99% of patients.* The procedure lasts a total of about 30 minutes and, like the postoperative phase, is painless.

The risk of losing vision or the entire eye during a cataract extraction, with hemorrhage during surgery or endophthalmitis after surgery, is about 0.05%. It is mandatory, however, to discuss the risks of the cataract surgery with the patient before the operation.

Due to the great safety of cataract surgery, the operation can now be performed earlier.

Inpatient or Outpatient Surgery?

Usually cataract surgery is carried out on an outpatient basis. The patient can be *hospitalized for about three days,* depending on the adequacy of postoperative care at home. Older patients who live alone may be unable to care for themselves adequately and maintain the regimen of prescribed medications for the operated eye in the immediate postoperative phase. The operation *can be performed as an outpatient procedure* if the ophthalmologist's practice is able to ensure adequate care.

Possible Types of Anesthesia

Cataract extraction can be performed under *local anesthesia* or *general anesthesia.* Today, most operations are performed under local anesthesia. Aside from the patient's wishes, there are medical reasons for preferring one form of anesthesia over another.

▶ **General anesthesia (intubation anesthesia or laryngeal mask; LMA).** This is recommended for patients who are extremely apprehensive and nervous, are deaf, or have mental disabilities; it is also indicated for patients with Parkinson's disease or rheumatism, who are unable to lie still without pain.

▶ **Local anesthesia (retrobulbar, peribulbar, or topical anesthesia).** This is recommended for patients with increased anesthesia risks, and is the preferred approach in outpatient surgery.

Preoperative Consultation on Options for Refractive Correction

See ▶ Table 7.4 for more details.

▶ **Intraocular lens.** In almost all cataract extractions, an intraocular lens (IOL) is implanted, preferably in the place of the natural lens *(posterior chamber lens, PC-IOL).* If it is impossible to anchor a posterior chamber lens for technical reasons because of a lacking capsule sac, an intraocular lens is implanted in the anterior chamber. The anterior chamber lens (ACL), is supported in the iridocorneal angle or is fixated onto the iris ("iris-claw lens"). An eye with an artificial lens is referred to as a *pseudophakia.* The different kinds of IOLs are discussed in the section on IOL technology.

▶ **Biometry.** The refractive power of the lens required is determined preoperatively by biometry to reach the targeted refractive result. In a simplified fashion, IOL refractive power is determined by the refractive power of the cornea, IOL refraction constants, and the axial length, determined by ultrasonic measurement. More recent devices (e.g., the Zeiss IOL-Master) perform automated biometry with the measurement of countless additional parameters and the appropriate software.

▶ **Postoperative refractive status.** The usual recommendation is to target emmetropia or mild myopia (−0.25 to −0.5 diopters). The patient will then only need glasses for reading. Postoperative hyperopia (need for glasses at far and near distances) is not satisfactory for the patient. If the patient's fellow eye does not need cataract extraction within a short period of time, the refractive difference between the two eyes should be not more than 2 to 2.5 diopters, to avoid anisometric problems in binocular vision.

Artificial Lens Technology

▶ **Intraocular Lens (IOL).** Every IOL (▶ Fig. 7.17) consists of a central optical part (refractive element) and two haptics, to stabilize the IOL in the capsular bag, ciliary sulcus, or chamber angle:
- **Monofocal IOLs,** with only one specific focus (far or near).
- **Multifocal IOLs,** with a focus for far and near objects. Multifocal IOLs do not yet match the optical quality standards of monofocal IOLs and may create problems due to reduced contrast

Table 7.4 Comparison of a normal eye ① and correction of cataract with a posterior chamber intraocular lens ②, anterior chamber lens ③, contact lens ④, and cataract eyeglasses ⑤

Correction	Monocular image size	Binocular vision: combination	Advantages/ disadvantages
① Normal eye	Normal	① can be combined with ②, ③ and ④ Difference in image size is small enough for the brain to fuse the images	Visual field: full Normal vision
② Posterior chamber lens	2% larger than ①	② can be combined with ①, ②, ③ and ④	Visual field: full IOL: no care necessary Vision (even without glasses): good vision, good orientation
③ Anterior chamber lens	3% larger than ①	③ can be combined with ①, ②, ③ and ④	Visual field: full IOL: no care needed Vision: (even without glasses) good vision, good orientation
④ Contact lens	8–10% larger than ①	④ can be combined with ①, ②, ③, and ④	Visual field: full Older patients often find it difficult to look after and manage lenses Vision: good with contact lenses, poor orientation without contact lenses Injury due to wearing of contact lenses possible Contact lenses not possible with dry eyes
⑤ Cataract eyeglasses	25% larger than ①	⑤ can only be combined with ⑤	Visual Field: limited (peripheral scotoma) Cataract eyeglasses: simple to use, heavy unsatisfactory cosmetic appearance Vision: good with eyeglasses, poor orientation without eyeglasses

vision, glare, and halos at night. Patient selection is crucial, and about 5% of multifocal IOLs need to be explanted due to patient dissatisfaction.

- **Toric IOLs** correct not only spherical ametropia but also up to 3 diopters of astigmatism. Orientation of the IOL (orientation marks), as exactly as possible to the nearest degree, is crucial.
- **Multifocal toric IOLs** combine multifocal optical quality and ametropia correction.

Note
Today, the surgeon is obliged to inform the patient before the cataract operation of all possible artificial lens options.

▶ **IOL design.** The geometrical configuration of IOLs has been subject to constant development. The sharp posterior edge of the optical part (▶ Fig. 7.18) serves as a barrier to lens epithelial cells migrating from the equator of the capsule toward the center, preventing secondary cataract. The sloping side part and the rounded anterior edge of the optic minimize glare and internal light reflections. Additional enhancements of the optical quality include multifocal steps and an aberration-optimized anterior IOL surface.

▶ **IOL materials.** Basically, IOLS can be divided into **nonflexible** and **flexible types**, as well as **one-piece IOLs** (in which the haptics and optic are made of a single material with no connecting points) and **three-piece IOLs** (in which the optic and haptics are made of different materials such as polymethylmethacrylate, polypropylene, and polyamide and connected to each other).

▶ **Nonflexible IOLs.** These are mostly made of polymethylmethacrylate (PMMA). To implant a non-flexible IOL, the incision needs to be larger than the diameter of the IOL (5.5–6.5 mm). Modern nonflexible IOLs are one-piece IOLs.

▶ **Flexible IOLs.** These are folded with a forceps or an injector system and are therefore implantable through 2.0- to 3.0-mm incisions with the same optic size as nonflexible IOLs (▶ Fig. 7.19). Flexible IOLs today are made chiefly of silicone or acrylic.

The development and modification of modern IOLs is a constantly ongoing process.

Alternative Methods of Correcting Refractive Errors

▶ **Cataract eyeglasses.** The development of the intraocular lens (see above) has largely replaced

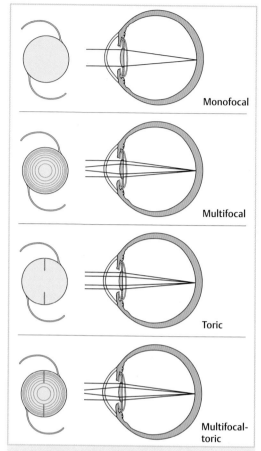

Fig. 7.17 Intraocular lens (IOL) technology. Monofocal, multifocal, and toric IOLs.

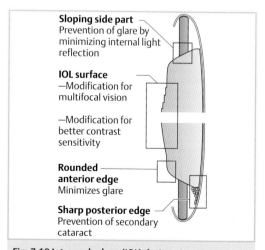

Sloping side part
Prevention of glare by minimizing internal light reflection

IOL surface
—Modification for multifocal vision

—Modification for better contrast sensitivity

Rounded anterior edge
Minimizes glare

Sharp posterior edge
Prevention of secondary cataract

Fig. 7.18 Intraocular lens (IOL) design. Important features of modern IOLs designed to optimize optical quality.

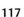

the correction of postoperative aphakia with cataract lenses. Long the standard, this method is *now only necessary in exceptional cases*. Cataract eyeglasses cannot be used to correct *unilateral aphakia*, because the difference in the size of the retinal images is too great (aniseikonia). Thus cataract eyeglasses are only suitable for correcting *bilateral aphakia*. Cataract eyeglasses have the disadvantage of limiting the field of vision (*peripheral* and *ring scotoma*).

▸ **Contact lenses (soft, rigid, and oxygen-permeable).** These lenses provide a near-normal field of vision and are *suitable for postoperative correction of unilateral cataracts*, as the difference in image size is negligible. However, many older patients have difficulty in learning how to cope with contact lenses.

Surgical Techniques

The operation is performed on only one eye at a time. The procedure on the fellow eye is performed after about a week once the first eye has stabilized.

▸ **Historical milestones**
• **Couching** (reclination). Up until the 19th century, a pointed instrument was used to displace the lens into the vitreous body out of the visual axis.
• **1746.** J. Daviel carried out the **first extracapsular cataract extraction** by removing the contents of the lens through an inferior approach.
• **1866.** A. von Graefe carried out the first removal of a cataract through a **superior limbal incision with capsulotomy**.

▸ **Intracapsular cataract extraction (ICCE).** *Until the mid-1980s, this was the method of choice.* Today, intracapsular cataract extraction is used only with subluxation or dislocation of the lens (see p. 120). Using a cryoextractor, the whole lens inside its capsule is frozen and removed (intracapsularly) through a large superior corneal incision (180°).

▸ **Extracapsular cataract extraction (ECCE).** The anterior capsule is opened (capsulorrhexis). Then only the cortex and nucleus of the lens are removed (extracapsular extraction); the posterior capsule and zonule suspension remain intact. This provides a stable base for implantation of the posterior chamber intraocular lens. The necessary incision length is 10 to 12 mm.

Note
Extracapsular cataract extraction with implantation of a posterior chamber intraocular lens is now the method of choice.

Today, *phacoemulsification* (emulsifying and aspirating the nucleus of the lens with a high-frequency ultrasonic needle) is the preferred technique for removing the nucleus. Where the nucleus is very hard, the entire nucleus is expressed or aspirated. Then the softer portions of the cortex are removed by suction with an aspirator/irrigator attachment in an aspiration/irrigation maneuver. The posterior capsule is then polished, and an intraocular lens (IOL) is implanted in the empty capsular bag (▸ Fig. 7.20). Phacoemulsification and IOL implantation require an incision only 2.5 to 3.0 mm in length. Where a tunnel technique is used to make this incision, no suture will be necessary as the wound will close itself.

▸ **Advantages of ECCE.** Extracapsular cataract extraction usually does not achieve the same broad exposure of the retina that intracapsular cataract extraction does, particularly when a secondary cataract is present. However, the extracapsular cataract extraction maintains the integrity of the anterior and posterior chambers of the eye, and the vitreous body cannot prolapse anteriorly as it does after intracapsular cataract extraction. At 0.1 to 0.2%, the incidence of retinal detachment after extracapsular cataract extraction is about ten times less than after intracapsular cataract extraction, which has an incidence of 2 to 3%.

Secondary Cataract

▸ **Epidemiology.** Approximately 30% of cataract patients develop a secondary cataract after extracapsular cataract extraction.

▸ **Etiology.** Extracapsular cataract extraction removes only the anterior central portion of the capsule and leaves epithelial cells of the lens intact along with remnants of the capsule. These epithelial cells are capable of reproducing and can produce a secondary cataract of fibrous or regenerative tissue in the posterior capsule that diminishes visual acuity (▸ Fig. 7.21a).

▸ **Treatment.** A neodymium:yttrium aluminum garnet (Nd:YAG) laser can incise the posterior capsule in the visual axis without requiring invasive eye surgery. This immediately improves vision (▸ Fig. 7.21b).

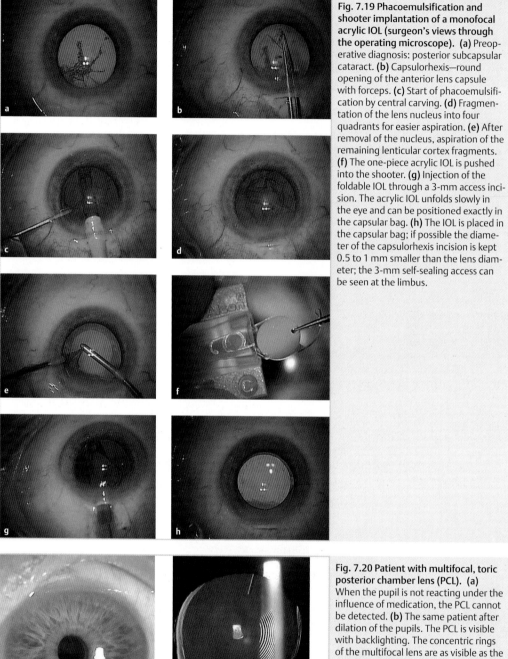

Fig. 7.19 Phacoemulsification and shooter implantation of a monofocal acrylic IOL (surgeon's views through the operating microscope). (a) Preoperative diagnosis: posterior subcapsular cataract. (b) Capsulorhexis—round opening of the anterior lens capsule with forceps. (c) Start of phacoemulsification by central carving. (d) Fragmentation of the lens nucleus into four quadrants for easier aspiration. (e) After removal of the nucleus, aspiration of the remaining lenticular cortex fragments. (f) The one-piece acrylic IOL is pushed into the shooter. (g) Injection of the foldable IOL through a 3-mm access incision. The acrylic IOL unfolds slowly in the eye and can be positioned exactly in the capsular bag. (h) The IOL is placed in the capsular bag; if possible the diameter of the capsulorhexis incision is kept 0.5 to 1 mm smaller than the lens diameter; the 3-mm self-sealing access can be seen at the limbus.

Fig. 7.20 Patient with multifocal, toric posterior chamber lens (PCL). (a) When the pupil is not reacting under the influence of medication, the PCL cannot be detected. (b) The same patient after dilation of the pupils. The PCL is visible with backlighting. The concentric rings of the multifocal lens are as visible as the axis of the toric astigmatism correction (see also ▶ Fig. 7.17).

Special Considerations in Cataract Surgery in Children

▶ **Observe changes in the child's behavior.** Children with congenital, traumatic, or metabolic cataract will not necessarily communicate their visual impairment verbally. However, it can be diagnosed from these **symptoms:**

- Leukocoria.
- Oculodigital phenomenon. The child presses his or her finger against the eye or eyes, because this can produce light patterns the child finds interesting.
- Strabismus. The first sign of visual impairment (▶ Fig. 7.22).
- The child cries when the normal eye is covered.
- The child has difficulty walking or grasping.
- Erratic eye movement is present.
- Nystagmus (see p. 316).

▶ **Operate as early as possible.** Retinal fixation and cortical visual responses develop within the first 6 months of life. This means that children who undergo surgery after the age of 1 year have *significantly poorer chances* of developing normal vision.

Note
Children with congenital cataract should undergo surgery as early as possible to avoid amblyopia.

The prognosis for successful surgery is less favorable for *unilateral cataracts* than for bilateral cataracts. This is because the amblyopia of the cataract eye puts it at an irreversible disadvantage in comparison with the fellow eye as the child learns how to see.

▶ **Plan for the future when performing surgery.** After opening the extremely elastic anterior lens capsule, one can aspirate the soft infantile cortex and nucleus. *Secondary cataracts are frequent complications in infants.* The procedure should therefore include a *posterior capsulotomy with anterior vitrectomy* to ensure an unobstructed visual axis. The operation *preserves the equatorial portions of the capsule* to permit subsequent implantation of a posterior chamber intraocular lens in later years.

▶ **Refraction changes constantly.** The refractive power of the eye changes dramatically within a

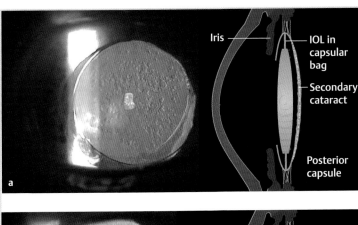

Iris — IOL in capsular bag

— Secondary cataract

Posterior capsule

a

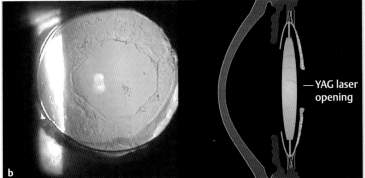

— YAG laser opening

b

Fig. 7.21 Secondary cataract. (a) Regenerative secondary cataracts lead to diminished visual acuity and increased glare. (b) Nd:YAG laser capsulotomy. The posterior capsulotomy removes the obstruction of the visual axis and immediately improves vision.

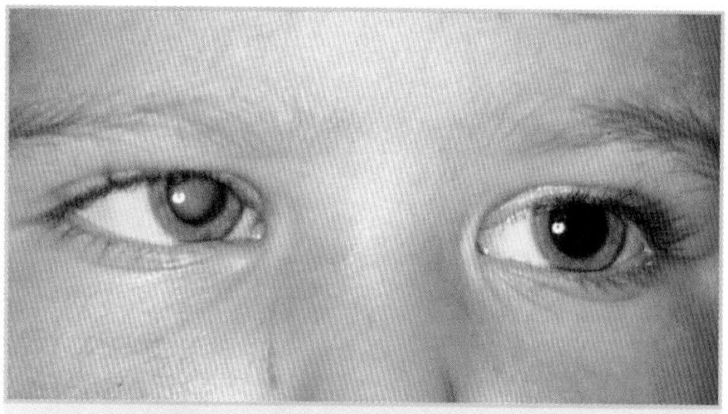

Fig. 7.22 Congenital cataract. A 6-month-old child with a congenital cataract (leukocoria) and esotropia in the right eye.

short period of time as the eye grows. The refraction in the eye of a newborn is 30 to 35 diopters and drops to 15 to 25 diopters within the first year of life (myopic shift).

Refractive Compensation

Two main points need to be noted for optical correction of aphakia in a child: age and whether the cataracts are unilateral or bilateral. Possible methods of correction include the following:

- **Glasses** can be fitted in older children with bilateral, but not unilateral aphakia (▶ Table 7.4). It should be noted that thick cataract glasses may be inappropriate due to their weight, for cosmetic reasons, or due to prismatic distortion and ring scotoma.
- **Contact lenses** are a good option for unilateral and bilateral aphakia. The use of soft contact lenses in infants is difficult and requires intensive cooperation from parents. Usually they are well tolerated up to the age of 2 years.
- **IOL implantation** is nowadays a routine procedure in children over the age of 2 years. The problem in newborns is the myopic shift in the growing eye. An IOL power is therefore calculated by biometry that results in a certain amount of hyperopia, which is then corrected with glasses. During the child's subsequent growth, the hyperopia ideally moves back toward emmetropia.
- **Orthoptic postoperative therapy is required.** *Unilateral cataracts* in particular require orthoptic postoperative therapy in the operated eye to close the gap in relation to the normal fellow eye. For details of occlusion treatment, see Treatment and Avoidance of Strabismic Amblyopia in Chapter 17.2.3.

Note
Refraction should be evaluated by retinoscopy (see Chapter 16) every 2 months during the first year of life and every 3 to 4 months during the second year, and contact lenses and eyeglasses should be changed accordingly.

7.5 Lens Dislocation

Definition
Subluxation (partial dislocation): the suspension of the lens (the zonule fibers) is slackened, and the lens is only partially within the hyaloid fossa (▶ Fig. 7.23).
Luxation (complete dislocation): the lens is torn completely free and has migrated into the vitreous body or, less frequently, into the anterior chamber.

▶ **Etiology.** There are several causes of lens dislocation (▶ Table 7.5). Most frequently it is due to **trauma** (e.g., bulbar contusion, see p. 325). Later in life, **pseudoexfoliation** may also lead to subluxation or luxation of the lens. **Hereditary causes** and **metabolic disease** produce lens displacement *early,* but on the whole are *rare. Additional rare causes* include **hyperlysinemia** (characterized by retarded mental development and seizures) and **sulfite oxidase deficiency** (which leads to mental retardation and excretion of cysteine in the urine).

Note
The most frequent atraumatic causes of lens dislocation are Marfan's syndrome, homocystinuria, and Weill–Marchesani syndrome.

▶ **Symptoms.** Slight displacement may be of no functional significance to the patient. More pronounced displacement produces severe optical distortion with loss of visual acuity.

▶ **Diagnostic considerations.** The cardinal symptoms include tremulous motion of the iris and lens when the eye moves (iridodonesis and phacodonesis). These symptoms are detectable in examination using a slit lamp.

▶ **Treatment.** Optical considerations (see Symptoms) and the risk of secondary angle closure glaucoma due to protrusion of the iris and dislocation of the lens into the anterior chamber are indications for removal of the lens.

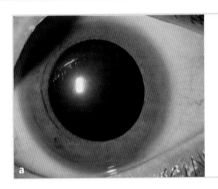 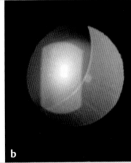

Fig. 7.23 Subluxation of the lens in Marfan's syndrome. (a) The lens is displaced superiorly and medially. As the zonule fibers are intact, a certain amount of accommodation is still possible. **(b)** Same eye: in back light, the subluxation is clearly visible.

Table 7.5 Etiology of lens displacement

Cause	Lens displacement
Hereditary causes (rare)	
• Ectopia lentis: isolated and monosymptomatic	Complete or partial displacement of the lens (for example, into the anterior chamber)
• Marfan's syndrome: characterized by arachnodactyly, long limbs, and laxness of joints	Lens is abnormally round; lens displacement is usually superior and temporal; zonule fibers are elongated but frequently intact
• Weill–Marchesani syndrome: symptoms include short stature and brachydactyly	Lens is abnormally round and often too small; lens is usually eccentric and displaced inferiorly
• Homocystinuria (metabolic disease): characterized by oligophrenia, osteoporosis, and skeletal deformities	Lens displacement is usually medial and inferior; torn zonule fibers appear as a "permanent wave" on the lens
Acquired causes	
• Trauma (probably the most frequent cause)	Zonule defects due to deformation can cause subluxation or luxation of the lens
• Pseudoexfoliation (in advanced age)	Zonule weakness due to loosening of the insertion of the fibers on the lens can cause lens displacement
• Ciliary body tumor (rare)	Lens is displaced by tumor
• Large eyes with severe myopia and buphthalmos (rare)	Zonule defects due to excessive longitudinal growth can cause lens displacement

Chapter 8

Uveal Tract (Vascular Layer)

8 Uveal Tract (Vascular Layer)

Gabriele E. Lang and Gerhard K. Lang

8.1 Basic Knowledge

▶ **Structure.** The uveal tract (also known as the vascular layer, vascular tunic, and uvea) takes its name from the Latin *uva* (grape) because the dark pigmentation and shape of the structure are reminiscent of a grape. The uveal tract consists of the following structures:
- Iris.
- Ciliary body.
- Choroid.

▶ **Position.** The uveal tract lies between the sclera and retina.

▶ **Neurovascular supply. Arterial supply** to the uveal tract is provided by the *ophthalmic artery*.
- The *short posterior ciliary arteries* enter the eyeball with the optic nerve and supply the *choroid*.
- The *long posterior ciliary arteries* pass along the interior surface of the sclera to the *ciliary body* and the *iris*. They form the major arterial circle at the root of the iris and the minor arterial circle in the collarette of the iris.
- The *anterior ciliary arteries* originate from the vessels of the rectus muscles and communicate with the *posterior ciliary vessels*.

Venous blood drains through four to eight *vorticose or vortex veins* that penetrate the sclera posterior to the equator and join the superior and inferior ophthalmic veins (▶ Fig. 8.1). **Sensory supply** is provided by the *long and short ciliary nerves*.

8.1.1 Iris

▶ **Structure and function.** The iris consists of two layers:
- The anterior mesodermal stromal layer.
- The posterior ectodermal pigmented epithelial layer.

The **posterior layer** is opaque and protects the eye against excessive incident light. The **anterior surface** of the lens and the **pigmented layer** are so

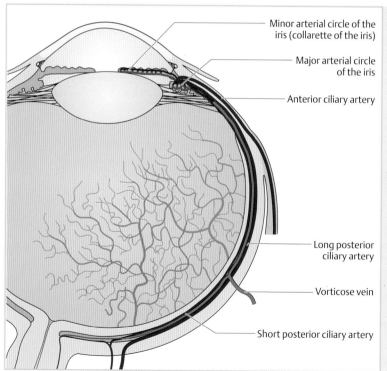

Minor arterial circle of the iris (collarette of the iris)

Major arterial circle of the iris

Anterior ciliary artery

Long posterior ciliary artery

Vorticose vein

Short posterior ciliary artery

Fig. 8.1 Vascular supply to the uveal tract. See discussion in the text.

close together near the pupil that they can easily form adhesions in inflammation.

The **collarette of the iris** covering the minor arterial circle of the iris divides the stroma into *pupillary* and *ciliary* portions. The pupillary portion contains the **sphincter muscle**, which is supplied by parasympathetic nerve fibers, and the **dilator pupillae muscle**, supplied by sympathetic nerve fibers. These muscles regulate the contraction and dilation of the pupil, so that the iris can be regarded as the **aperture** of the optical system of the eye.

Note

Pupil dilation is sometimes sluggish in preterm infants and the newborn because the dilator pupillae muscle develops relatively late.

▶ **Surface.** The normal iris has a richly textured surface structure with **crypts** (tissue gaps) and interlinked **trabeculae**. A faded surface structure *can* be a sign of inflammation, so-called iritis (see p. 128.)

▶ **Color.** The color of the iris varies in the individual according to the **melanin content of the melanocytes (pigment cells)** in the *stroma* and *epithelial layer*. Eyes with a high melanin content are dark brown, whereas eyes with less melanin are grayish-blue. **Caucasians at birth** always have a grayish-blue iris as the *pigmented layer* only develops gradually during the first year of life. Even in **albinos** (see p. 128), i.e., in impaired melanin synthesis, the eyes have a grayish-blue iris because of the melanin deficiency. Under slit lamp retroillumination they appear reddish due to the fundus reflex.

8.1.2 Ciliary Body

▶ **Position and structure.** The **ciliary body** extends from the root of the iris to the ora serrata, where it joins the choroid. It consists of *anterior pars plicata* and the *posterior pars plana,* which lies 3.5 mm posterior to the limbus. Numerous **ciliary processes** extend into the posterior chamber of the eye. The suspensory ligament of the lens, the zonule of Zinn, extends from the pars plana and the intervals between the ciliary processes to the lens capsule.

▶ **Function.** The *ciliary muscle* is responsible for **accommodation.** The double-layered *epithelium covering the ciliary body* **produces** the **aqueous humor**.

8.1.3 Choroid

▶ **Position and structure.** The choroid is the **middle tunic of the eyeball**. It is bounded on the interior by *Bruch's membrane.* The choroid is highly vascularized, containing a vessel layer with large blood vessels and a capillary layer. The blood flow through the choroid is the *highest in the entire body.*

▶ **Function.** The choroid **regulates temperature** and supplies **nourishment to the outer layers of the retina**.

8.2 Examination Methods

The *slit lamp* is used to examine the **surface of the iris** under a focused beam of light. *Normally no vessels will be visible.*

Note

Iris vessels are only visible in atrophy of the iris, in inflammation, or as neovascularization in rubeosis iridi on page 132 (see ▶ Fig. 8.12).

The normal and pathologic vessels can be visualized by *iris angiography* after intravenous injection of fluorescein sodium dye: neovascularizations "leak."

Defects in the pigmented layer of the iris appear red under retroillumination with a slit lamp (church window phenomenon, see ▶ Fig. 8.6). *Slit lamp biomicroscopy* visualizes individual cells such as melanin cells at 40-power magnification.

The *anterior chamber* is *normally transparent.* Inflammation can increase the permeability of the **vessels of the iris** and compromise the barrier between blood and aqueous humor. *Opacification of the aqueous humor* by proteins can be observed with the aid of a *slit lamp* when the eye is illuminated with a lateral focal beam of light (Tyndall effect). This method can also be used to diagnose *cells in the anterior chamber* in the presence of inflammation.

Direct inspection of the **root of the iris** is not possible because it does not lie within the line of sight. However, it can be indirectly visualized by *gonioscopy* (see p. 147). Inspection of the **posterior portion of the pars plana** requires a *three-mirror lens.* The globe is also indented with a metal rod to permit visualization of this part of the ciliary body (for example, in the presence of a suspected malignant melanoma of the ciliary body).

The pigmented epithelium of the retina permits only limited evaluation of the **choroid** by *ophthalmoscopy* and *fluorescein angiography* or indocyanine green angiography. Changes in the choroid such as tumors or hemangiomas can be visualized by ultrasound examination. Where a **tumor is suspected,** transillumination of the eye is indicated. After administration of topical anesthesia, a fiberoptic light source is placed on the eyeball to *visualize the shadow of the tumor on the red of the fundus.*

8.3 Developmental Anomalies

8.3.1 Aniridia

Aniridia is the **absence of the iris.** This **generally bilateral** condition is *transmitted as an autosomal-dominant trait* or occurs *sporadically.* However, peripheral remnants of the iris are usually still present so that ciliary villi and zonule fibers will be visualized under slit lamp examination (▶ Fig. 8.2). Aniridia may also be traumatic (e.g., as the result of penetrating injuries) in which the iris can be completely avulsed from its attachment to the ciliary body, so that no ciliary villi or zonule fibers can be seen.

Note

In sporadic aniridia, a Wilms's tumor of the kidney should be excluded.

Vision is severely compromised as a result of the foveal hypoplasia. The disorder is frequently associated with nystagmus, amblyopia, buphthalmos, and cataract.

Note

Visual acuity will generally be reduced in the presence of nystagmus.

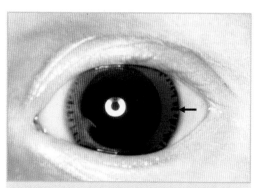

Fig. 8.2 Aniridia. The ciliary villi (arrow) and the lens are visible with slit lamp retroillumination.

8.3.2 Coloboma

Another congenital anomaly results from **incomplete fusion of the embryonic optic cup,** which normally occurs in about the sixth week of pregnancy. These anomalies are known as **colobomas.** They are directed medially and inferiorly and can involve the iris (▶ Fig. 8.3), ciliary body, zonule

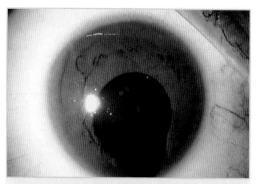

Fig. 8.3 Congenital iris coloboma. The congenital iris coloboma is located medially and inferiorly. The pupil merges with the coloboma without any sharp demarcation.

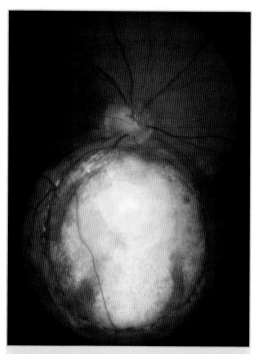

Fig. 8.4 Coloboma of the retina and choroid. This coloboma of the retina, choroid, and optic nerve exposes the underlying white sclera.

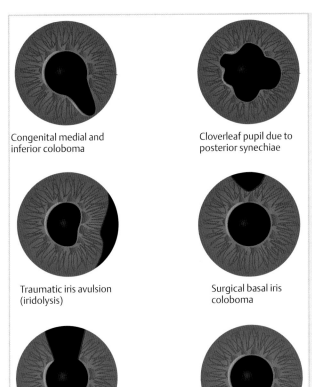

Fig. 8.5 Various iris changes. Ando's surgical iridectomy at the 6 o'clock position prevents a pupillary block glaucoma in eyes filled with oil or gas. Cloverleaf pupil see p.130.

Congenital medial and inferior coloboma

Cloverleaf pupil due to posterior synechiae

Traumatic iris avulsion (iridolysis)

Surgical basal iris coloboma

Surgical segmental iris coloboma

Ando's surgical iridectomy

fibers, and choroid (▶ Fig. 8.4). **Bridge colobomas** exhibit remnants of the iris or choroid. Involvement of the choroid and optic nerve frequently leads to *reduced visual acuity.*

Surgical iris colobomas (▶ Fig. 8.5) in cataract and glaucoma surgery are usually opened superiorly. In this way, they are covered by the upper lid so that the patient is not dazzled and does not see double images.

In contrast to traumatic aniridia (see p. 126), in which the iris is completely torn away, **traumatic colobomas** arise when there is localized separation of the iris from its attachment to the ciliary body (iridodialysis). The separation of the base of the iris can often be recognized by the unrounding of the pupil (▶ Fig. 8.5). If the iridodialysis is in the lower part of the iris, the patient may experience double vision, since the "second pupil" caused by the separation of the iris is not covered by the upper lid (in smaller and very peripheral defects, no double vision occurs). In this case, the iris should be surgically reattached to its base. This operation

is obligatory if an additional cyclodialysis (separation of the ciliary body) causes hypotonia in the eye, since this leads to atrophia bulbi and thus to blindness. In this case, the ciliary body must be reattached.

8.4 Pigmentation Anomalies

8.4.1 Heterochromia

Impaired development of the pigmentation of the iris can lead to a congenital **difference in coloration between the left and right iris (heterochromia).** One iris containing varying pigmentation is referred to as **iris bicolor**. Isolated heterochromia is not necessarily clinically significant (simple heterochromia), yet it can be a sign of abnormal changes. The following types are differentiated:

- **Fuchs's heterochromic cyclitis** (etiology unclear). This refers to *recurrent iridocyclitis* (simultaneous inflammation of several portions of the uveal tract) in adults, with *precipitates on* the posterior surface of the cornea without formation of posterior synechiae (adhesions between the iris and lens). The eye is *free of external irritation*. This disorder is often associated with complicated cataract and increased intraocular pressure (glaucoma).

- **Sympathetic heterochromia.** In *unilateral impairment of the sympathetic nerve supply*, the affected iris is significantly lighter. Heterochromia with unilaterally lighter pigmentation of the iris also occurs in iridocyclitis, acute glaucoma, and anterior chamber hemorrhage (hyphema).
- **Melanosis of the iris.** This refers to *dark pigmentation* of one iris.

Aside from the difference in coloration between the two irises, neither sympathetic heterochromia nor melanosis leads to further symptoms. The only form of heterochromia that leads to abnormal changes is Fuchs's heterochromic cyclitis. The possible complications involved require specific treatment.

8.4.2 Albinism

Albinism (from the Latin *albus,* white) is a congenital **metabolic disease that leads to hypopigmentation of the eye**. The following types are differentiated:
- **Ocular albinism** (involving only the eyes).
- **Oculocutaneous albinism** (involving the eyes, skin, and hair).

In albinism, the iris is light blue because of the melanin deficiency resulting from impaired melanin synthesis. Under slit lamp retroillumination, the *iris appears reddish* due to fundus reflex (▶ Fig. 8.6). Ophthalmoscopy will detect *choroidal vessels* (▶ Fig. 8.7). Associated foveal aplasia results in significant *reduction in visual acuity* and *nystagmus*. Most patients are also *photophobic* because of the missing filter function of the pigmented layer of the iris.

8.5 Inflammation

Inflammations of the uveal tract are classified according to the various portions of the globe:
- Anterior uveitis (**iritis**).
- Intermediate uveitis (**cyclitis**).
- Posterior uveitis (**choroiditis**).

However, some inflammations involve the middle portions of the uveal tract such as **iridocyclitis** (inflammation of the iris and ciliary body) or **panuveitis** (inflammation involving all segments).

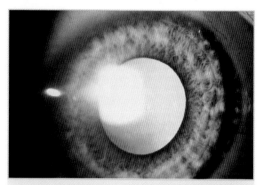

Fig. 8.6 Ocular albinism. The peripheral iris appears red with retroillumination.

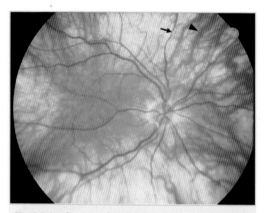

Fig. 8.7 Fundus in ocular albinism. Typical features include the choroidal vessels, which are visualized by ophthalmoscopy (arrowhead: choroidal vessel; arrow: retinal vessel).

8.5.1 Acute Iritis and Iridocyclitis

▶ **Epidemiology. Iritis** is the most frequent form of uveitis. It usually occurs in combination with cyclitis. About three-quarters of all **iridocyclitis** cases have an acute clinical course.

▶ **Etiology.** Iridocyclitis is frequently attributable to **immunologic causes** such as allergic or hyperergic reaction to bacterial toxins. In some rheumatic disorders it is known to be frequently associated with the expression of specific human leukocyte antigens (HLA) such as HLA-B27. Iridocyclitis can also be a **symptom of systemic disease** such as ankylosing spondylitis, Reiter's syndrome, sarcoidosis, etc. (▶ Table 8.1). **Infections** are less frequent and occur secondary to penetrating trauma or sepsis (bacteria, viruses, mycosis, or parasites). *Phaco-*

Table 8.1 Causes of uveitis according to location

Form of uveitis	Possible causes
HLA-B27-associated iridocyclitis	• Idiopathic • Ankylosing spondylitis • Reiter's syndrome • Regional enteritis (Crohn's disease) • Ulcerative colitis • Psoriasis
Non-HLA-B27-associated iridocyclitis	• Idiopathic • Viral • Tuberculosis • Sarcoidosis • Syphilis • Leprosy • Rheumatoid arthritis (Still–Chauffard syndrome) • Heterochromic cyclitis • Phacogenic uveitis • Trauma
Iridocyclitis and choroiditis	• Toxoplasmosis • Sarcoidosis (Boeck's disease) • Tuberculosis • Syphilis • Behçet's disease • Sympathetic ophthalmia • Borreliosis • Brucellosis • Yersiniosis • Listeriosis • Weil's disease • Malignant tumors
Choroiditis	• Toxoplasmosis • Sarcoidosis (Boeck's disease) • Syphilis • Behçet's disease • Histoplasmosis • Toxocara

genic inflammation, possibly with glaucoma, can result when the lens becomes involved.

▶ **Symptoms.** Patients report dull pain in the eye or forehead accompanied by impaired vision, photophobia, and excessive tearing (epiphora).

Note
In contrast to choroiditis (see p. 131), acute iritis or iridocyclitis is painful because of the involvement of the ciliary nerves.

▶ **Diagnostic considerations.** Typical signs include:
• **Ciliary injection.** The episcleral and perilimbal vessels may appear blue and red.
• **Combined injection.** The conjunctiva is also affected.

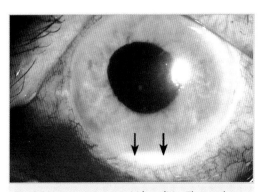

Fig. 8.8 Hypopyon in acute iridocyclitis. The purulent exudate accumulates as a pool (arrows) on the floor of the anterior chamber.

The **iris** is **hyperemic** (the iris vessels will be visible in a light-colored iris). The **structure** appears **diffuse** and **reactive miosis** is present.

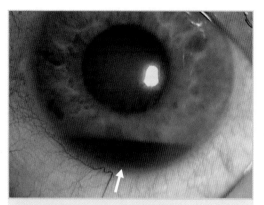

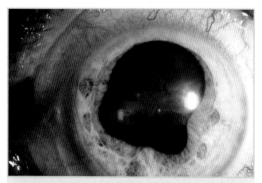

Fig. 8.9 Hyphema. Bleeding into the anterior chamber (arrow) can occur in rubeosis iridis, trauma, or, in rare cases, iridocyclitis.

Fig. 8.10 Posterior synechiae secondary to iridocyclitis (cloverleaf pupil). Acute iridocyclitis produces adhesions between the iris and lens (see also ▶ Fig. 8.5).

Vision is impaired because of cellular infiltration of the anterior chamber and protein or fibrin accumulation (visible as a **Tyndall effect**). The precipitates accumulate on the posterior surface of the cornea in a triangular configuration known as Arlt's triangle. Exudate accumulation on the floor of the anterior chamber is referred to as **hypopyon** (▶ Fig. 8.8). Viral infections may be accompanied by bleeding into the anterior chamber (**hyphema**) (▶ Fig. 8.9). Corneal edema can also develop in rare cases.

> **Note**
> Corneal edema and Tyndall effect (accumulations of protein in the anterior chamber) can be diagnosed when the eye is illuminated with a lateral beam of light from a focused light or slit lamp.

▶ **Differential diagnosis.** See ▶ Table 8.2.

> **Note**
> In acute iritis, the depth of the anterior chamber is normal and reactive miosis is present. In contrast, in acute glaucoma the anterior chamber is shallow and the pupil is dilated (▶ Table 8.2).

▶ **Complications.** Complications include:
- Secondary open angle glaucoma with an increase in intraocular pressure.
- Adhesions between the iris and posterior surface of the cornea (anterior synechiae).
- Adhesions between the iris and lens (posterior synechiae) (▶ Fig. 8.10).

▶ **Treatment.** Topical and, in appropriate cases, systemic antibiotics or antiviral therapy are indicated for iridocyclitis due to a pathogen (with a corneal ulcer, penetrating trauma, or sepsis).

> **Note**
> A conjunctival smear, or a blood culture in septic cases, is obtained to identify the pathogen. Antibiotic therapy should begin immediately as microbiological identification of the pathogen is not always successful.

Therapeutic mydriasis in combination with steroid therapy is indicated to **minimize the risk of synechiae** and ease pain. Where no pathogen can be identified, high-dose topical steroid therapy (prednisolone eye drops every hour in combination with subconjunctival injections of soluble dexamethasone) and nonsteroid antiphlogistic eye drops (4 × daily.) are administered. To minimize the risk of *posterior synechiae,* the pupil must be maximally dilated (atropine, scopolamine, cyclopentolate, and possibly epinephrine eye drops).

> **Note**
> The mydriatic effect of dilating eye drops may be reduced in iritis. This may necessitate the use of longer-acting medications such as atropine, which may have to be applied several times daily.

Occasionally it is possible to break off existing synechiae in this manner, and patches of iris tissue will remain on the anterior surface of the lens. **Secondary open angle glaucoma** is treated by administering beta blockers in eye drop form and carbonic anhydrase inhibitors (local with eye drops or systemic) (see ▶ Table 10.3).

Table 8.2 Differential diagnosis of acute iritis and acute glaucoma

Differential criteria	Acute iritis	Acute glaucoma
Symptoms	Dull pain and photophobia	Intense pain and vomiting
Conjunctiva	Combined injection	Combined injection
Cornea	Clear	Opacified, edematous
Anterior chamber	Normal depth; cells and fibrin are present	Shallow
Pupil	Narrowed (reactive miosis)	Dilated, not round
Globe	Normal pressure	"Rock hard"

▶ **Prognosis.** Symptoms usually improve within a few days when proper therapy is initiated. The disorder can progress to a chronic stage.

8.5.2 Chronic Iritis and Iridocyclitis

▶ **Epidemiology.** About a quarter of all **iridocyclitis** cases have a chronic clinical course.

▶ **Etiology.** See ▶ Table 8.1.

▶ **Symptoms.** See Acute Iritis and Iridocyclitis, Chapter 8.5.1. Chronic iridocyclitis may exhibit only minimal symptoms.

▶ **Diagnostic considerations.** See Chapter 8.5.1.

▶ **Differential diagnosis.** The disorder should be distinguished from acute glaucoma (see p. 164), conjunctivitis (see p. 54), and keratitis (see p. 74).

▶ **Complications.** Total obliteration of the pupil by posterior synechiae is referred to a **pupillary block**. Because the aqueous humor can no longer circulate, **secondary angle closure glaucoma with iris bombé** occurs. **Occlusion of the pupil** also results in fibrous scarring in the pupil. This can lead to the development of posterior subcapsular opacities in the lens (**secondary cataract**). Recurrent iridocyclitis can also lead to calcific band keratopathy (see p. 86).

▶ **Treatment.** In **pupillary block** with a secondary angle closure glaucoma, *Nd:YAG laser iridotomy* can be performed to create a shunt to allow the aqueous humor from the posterior chamber to circulate into the anterior chamber. In the presence of a **secondary cataract**, a cataract *extraction* can be performed when the inflammation has abated.

▶ **Prognosis.** Because of the chronic recurrent course of the disorder, it frequently involves complications such as synechiae or cataract that may progress to blindness from shrinkage of the eyeball.

8.5.3 Choroiditis

▶ **Epidemiology.** There are few epidemiologic studies of choroiditis. The annual incidence is assumed to be four cases per 100,000 people.

▶ **Etiology.** See ▶ Table 8.1.

▶ **Symptoms.** Patients are free of pain, although they report blurred vision and floaters.

Note
Choroiditis is painless, as the choroid is devoid of sensory nerve fibers.

▶ **Diagnostic considerations.** Ophthalmoscopy reveals isolated or multiple choroiditis foci. In *acute disease* they appear as ill-defined white dots (▶ Fig. 8.11). *Once scarring has occurred* the foci are sharply demarcated with a yellowish-brown color. Occasionally the major choroidal vessels will be visible through the atrophic scars.

No cells will be found in the vitreous body in a **primary choroidal process**. However, inflammation proceeding from the retina (**retinochoroiditis**) will exhibit *cellular infiltration of the vitreous body*.

▶ **Differential diagnosis.** This disorder should be distinguished from retinal inflammations, which are accompanied by cellular infiltration of the vitreous body and are most frequently caused by viruses or *Toxoplasma gondii*.

▶ **Treatment.** Choroiditis is treated either with antibiotics or steroids, depending on its etiology.

▶ **Prognosis.** The inflammatory foci will heal within 2 to 6 weeks and form chorioretinal scars.

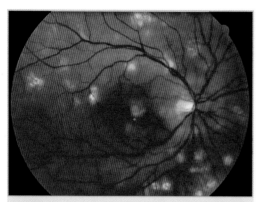

Fig. 8.11 Multifocal choroiditis. The foci of acute inflammation are yellowish and ill-defined; older lesions are yellowish-brown and sharply demarcated.

The scars will result in localized scotomas that will reduce visual acuity if the macula is affected.

8.5.4 Sympathetic Ophthalmia

Definition
Specific bilateral inflammation of the uveal tract due to chronic irritation of one eye, caused by a perforating wound to the eye or intraocular surgery, produces transferred uveitis in the fellow eye.

▶ **Epidemiology.** Sympathetic ophthalmia is very rare.

▶ **Etiology.** Sympathetic uveitis can occur in an *otherwise unaffected eye* even years after penetrating injuries or intraocular surgery in the fellow eye, especially where there was chronic irritation. Tissues in the injured eye (uveal tract, lens, and retina) act as antigens and provoke an autoimmune disorder in the unaffected eye.

▶ **Symptoms.** The earliest symptoms include limited range of accommodation and photophobia. Later there is diminished visual acuity and pain.

▶ **Diagnostic considerations.** Clinical symptoms include combined injections, cells and protein in the anterior chamber and vitreous body, papillary and retinal edema, and granulomatous inflammation of the choroid.

▶ **Differential diagnosis.** The disorder should be distinguished from iridocyclitis and choroiditis from other causes (see ▶ Table 8.1).

▶ **Treatment.** The injured eye, which is usually blind, must be enucleated to eliminate the antigen. High-dose topical and systemic steroid therapy is indicated. Concurrent treatment with immunosuppressives (cyclophosphamide and azathioprine) may be necessary.

▶ **Clinical course and complications.** The disorder has a chronic clinical course and may involve severe complications of uveitis such as secondary glaucoma, secondary cataract, retinal detachment, and shrinkage of the eyeball. Sympathetic ophthalmia can lead to blindness in particularly severe cases.

Note
When the injured eye is blind, prophylactic enucleation is indicated before the onset of sympathetic ophthalmia in the fellow eye. An early sign of sympathetic ophthalmia is a limited range of accommodation with photophobia.

8.6 Neovascularization in the Iris: Rubeosis Iridis

Definition
Rubeosis iridis is neovascularization in the iris that occurs in various retinal disorders.

▶ **Etiology.** Rubeosis iridis is a consequence of ischemic retinal disease. The related hypoxia leads to release of growth factors, such as "vascular endothelial growth factor" (VEGF), that travel to the

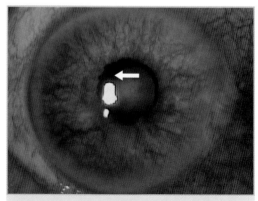

Fig. 8.12 Neovascularization in the iris: rubeosis iridis. Protrusion of the pigmented layer (ectropium uveae, arrow) indicates that the rubeosis iridis has been present for at least several weeks.

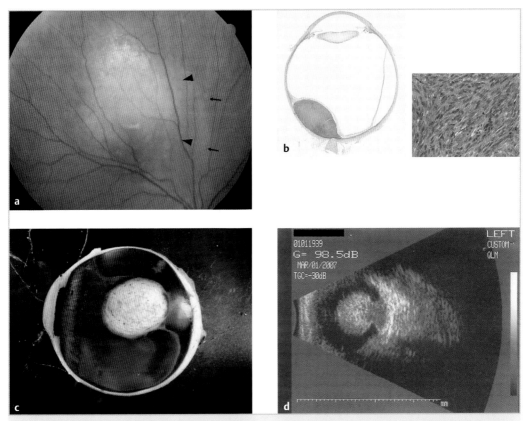

Fig. 8.13 Choroidal melanoma. **(a)** A prominent yellowish-brown choroidal tumor (arrowheads) accompanied by serous retinal detachment (arrows). Compare the ultrasound findings shown in **(d)**. **(b)** This histological image (from another eye, but with identical findings) shows tumor growth into the eye in the direction of the retina, causing visual problems at an advanced stage. **(c)** Eye after enucleation and fixation. The incision of the eye ran through the tumor. **(d)** Echogram of the same eye with base of tumor at the choroid and tumor eruption through Bruch's membrane (= so-called collar button lesion).

anterior chamber and trigger neovascularization of the iris. The newly formed vessels are fragile and this can result in bleeding in the anterior chamber (hyphema). The most frequent causes of rubeosis iridis (▶ Fig. 8.12) are *proliferative diabetic retinopathy* and *retinal vein occlusion*. Retinal periphlebitis is a less frequent cause of neovascularization in the iris.

▶ **Symptoms and diagnostic considerations.** **Neovascularization in the stroma of the iris** is *asymptomatic* for the patient. **Neovascularization in the angle of the anterior chamber** is irreversible and produces secondary angle closure glaucoma with the typical *symptoms of acute glaucoma*: loss of visual acuity, intense pain, conjunctival and ciliary injection, and a "rock hard" eyeball upon palpation (see ▶ Fig. 10.17).

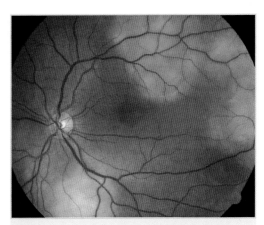

Fig. 8.14 Choroidal metastases. Flat, grayish-brown choroidal tumors.

133

▶ **Differential diagnosis.** Acute glaucoma due to other causes such as acute angle closure glaucoma should be excluded.

▶ **Treatment, prognosis, and prophylaxis.** Rubeosis iridis is tantamount to the *loss of an eye.* Usually it leads to *irreversible blindness.* Prompt laser treatment of retinal disorders is crucial to prevent rubeosis iridis. Secondary angle closure glaucoma is treated by trans-scleral freezing of the ciliary body (cyclocryotherapy) or laser treatment (cyclophotocoagulation) to reduce intraocular pressure. Where this fails or the eye shrinks (phthisis bulbi) and the patient experiences intense pain, enucleation of the eye is indicated.

> **Note**
> Prompt laser treatment is important in high-risk proliferative diabetic retinopathy to prevent rubeosis iridis.

8.7 Tumors

8.7.1 Malignant Tumors (Uveal Melanoma)

With an incidence of 1 in 10,000, malignant uveal melanoma is the most common primary intraocular tumor. It usually occurs as a choroidal melanoma, and is almost always unilateral. *Tumors in the iris* are detected earlier than tumors located in the *ciliary body* and *choroid* (▶ Fig. 8.13a, b).

- **Iris melanomas.** These tumors are *often initially asymptomatic.* However, metastatic melanoma cells in the angle of the anterior chamber can lead to *secondary glaucoma.* Circumscribed iris melanomas are removed by *segmental iridectomy.*
- **Ciliary body melanomas.** Symptoms include changes in accommodation and refraction resulting from displacement of the lens. Ciliary body melanomas are resected en bloc.

- **Choroidal melanomas.** These tumors become clinically symptomatic when involvement of the macula *reduces visual acuity* or the patient notices a shadow in his or her field of vision as a result of the tumor and the accompanying *retinal detachment.* The diagnosis is confirmed with the aid of transillumination, ultrasound, and fluorescein angiography. Choroidal tumors are treated with radioactive isotopes delivered by plaques of radioactive material (*brachytherapy*). *Enucleation* is indicated for tumors whose diameter exceeds 8 mm and whose prominence exceeds 5 mm.
- **Uveal metastases** most frequently develop from carcinomas of the breast or lung. They are usually flat, with little pigmentation. (▶ Fig. 8.14).

8.7.2 Benign Choroidal Tumors

Choroidal nevi (▶ Fig. 8.15) occur in 11% of the population. They can lead to secondary neovascularization with retinal edema. In very rare cases in which the macula is involved, choroidal nevi can lead to impaired vision. However, benign choroidal tumors are normally asymptomatic.

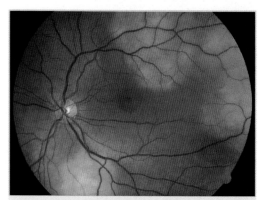

Fig. 8.15 Benign choroidal tumor (nevus). In contrast to uveal melanoma (▶ Fig. 8.13), the nevus is flat, has more pigment, is sharply demarcated, and does not change in size. As it is located underneath the retina, it does not cause any visual problems.

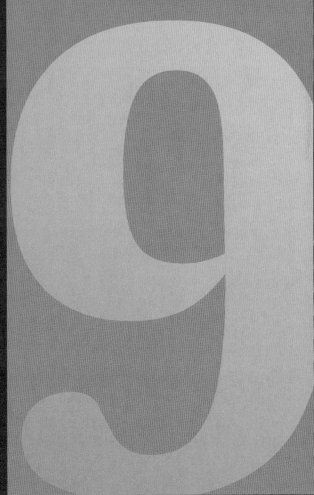

Chapter 9

Pupil

9 Pupil

Oskar Gareis and Gerhard K. Lang

9.1 Basic Knowledge

▶ **Relevance and function.** The pupil refers to the central opening in the iris. It acts as an aperture to improve the quality of the resulting image by controlling the amount of light that enters the eye.

▶ **Pupillary light reflex.** This reflex arc consists of:
- An afferent path that detects and transmits the light stimulus.
- An efferent path that supplies the muscles of the iris (▶ Fig. 9.1).

▶ **Afferent path.** This path begins at the light receptors of the retina (▶ Fig. 9.1, A), and continues along the optic nerve (B), and the optic chiasm (C) where some of the fibers cross to the opposite side. The path continues along the optical tracts (D) until shortly before the lateral geniculate body (E). There the *afferent reflex path* separates from the visual pathway and continues to the pretectal nuclei (F) and from there to *both* Edinger–Westphal nuclei (G). Each of the two pretectal nuclei conducts impulses to *both Edinger–Westphal nuclei.* This bilateral connection has several consequences:

- Both pupils will normally be the same size (*isocoria*) even when one eye is blind. Deviations of up to 1 mm are normal.
- Both pupils will narrow even when only one eye is illuminated (*consensual light reflex*).

▶ **Efferent parasympathetic path.** This path begins in the *Edinger–Westphal nucleus* (G). Its nerve fibers form the parasympathetic part of the oculomotor nerve (H) and travel to the ciliary ganglion (I) in the orbit. Postganglionic nerve fibers pass through the short ciliary nerves to the effector organ, the *sphincter pupillae muscle* (J).

Perlia's nucleus and the Edinger–Westphal nuclei are also responsible for the **near reflex**, which consists of accommodation, convergence, and miosis.

▶ **Efferent sympathetic nerve supply to the pupil.** Three neurons connected by synapses supply the pupil (▶ Fig. 9.2):
- The *central first neuron* begins in the posterior hypothalamus (A), passes the brain stem and the medulla oblongata to the ciliospinal center (Budge's center; B) in the cervical spinal cord (C8 T2).
- The *preganglionic second neuron* extends from the ciliospinal center through the white rami

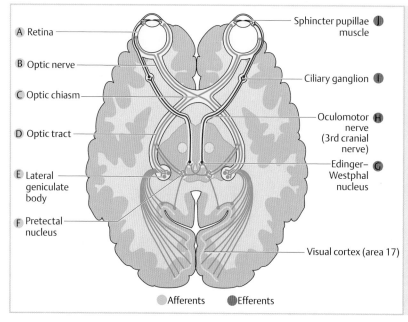

A Retina
B Optic nerve
C Optic chiasm
D Optic tract
E Lateral geniculate body
F Pretectal nucleus

Sphincter pupillae muscle (J)
Ciliary ganglion (I)
Oculomotor nerve (3rd cranial nerve) (H)
Edinger–Westphal nucleus (G)
Visual cortex (area 17)

Afferents Efferents

Fig. 9.1 Parasympathetic pupillary reflex pathway. See discussion in text.

communicantes and sympathetic trunk (C) to the superior cervical ganglion (D). It is vulnerable to certain lesions such as Pancoast tumors because it is immediately adjacent to the tip of the lung.

- The *postganglionic third neuron* extends from the superior cervical ganglion as a neural plexus along the internal carotid artery, ophthalmic artery, and long ciliary nerves to the effector organ, the *dilator pupillae muscle* (E).

▶ **Normal pupil size.** Pupil size ranges from approximately 1 mm (**miosis**) to approximately 8 mm (**mydriasis**).

- Pupils tend to be wider in teenagers and in darkness. They are also wider with joy, fear, or surprise due to increased sympathetic tone, and when the person inhales deeply.
- Pupils tend to be narrower in the newborn due to parasympathetic tone, in the elderly due to decreased mesencephalic inhibition and sympathetic diencephalic activity, in light, during sleep, and when the person is fatigued (due to decreased sympathetic activity).

9.2 Examination Methods

Complete examination of pupillary disorders (see p. 125) includes testing direct and indirect light reflexes, the swinging flashlight test, testing the near reflex, and morphological evaluation of the iris. A synopsis of all findings is required to determine whether a disorder is due to ocular or cerebral causes (see Chapter 9.4).

9.2.1 Testing the Light Reflex

The light reflex is tested in subdued daylight where the pupil is slightly dilated (▶ Table 9.1). The patient gazes into the distance to neutralize near-field miosis.

▶ **Direct light reflex.** The examiner first covers both of the patient's eyes then uncovers one eye. Normally the pupil will constrict after a latency period of about 0.2 seconds. The other eye is tested in the same manner.

▶ **Indirect or consensual light reflex.** The examiner separates the patient's eyes by placing his or her hand on the bridge of the patient's nose. This prevents incident light from *directly striking* the eye being examined, which would elicit a *direct light reflex.* The examiner then illuminates the other eye while observing the reaction of the covered, unilluminated eye. *Normally both pupils will constrict,* even in the unilluminated eye.

▶ **Swinging flashlight test.** This test is used to diagnose a *discrete unilateral or unilaterally more pronounced sensory deficit* in the eye (optic nerve and/or retina). Often damage to the optic nerve or

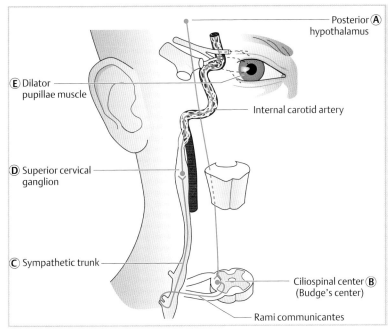

Fig. 9.2 **Sympathetic supply to the eye.** See discussion in text.

Posterior (A) hypothalamus

(E) Dilator pupillae muscle

Internal carotid artery

(D) Superior cervical ganglion

Ciliospinal center (B) (Budge's center)

(C) Sympathetic trunk

Rami communicantes

retina is only partial, such as in partial atrophy of the optic nerve, maculopathy, or peripheral retinal detachment. In these cases, the remaining healthy portions of the afferent pathway are sufficient to trigger constriction of the pupil during testing of the direct light reflex. This constriction will be less than in the healthy eye but may be difficult to diagnose from discrete pupillary reflex findings alone. Therefore, the *reflexive behavior of both eyes should be evaluated in a direct comparison* to detect differences in the rapidity of constriction and subsequent dilation. This is done by moving a light source alternately from one eye to the other in what is known as a swinging flashlight test.

Reproducible results can only obtained if the examiner strictly adheres to this **test protocol**:
- The patient focuses on a remote object in a room with subdued light. This neutralizes convergence miosis, and the pupils are slightly dilated, making the pupillary reflex more easily discernible.
- The examiner alternately illuminates both eyes with a relatively bright light, taking care to maintain a *constant distance, duration of illumination, and light intensity* so that both eyes must adapt to the same conditions.
- The examiner evaluates the *initial constriction* upon illumination and the *subsequent dilation* of the pupil.

Where the pupil constricts more slowly and dilates more rapidly than in the fellow eye, one refers to a *relative afferent pupillary defect*. The defect is "relative" because the difference in pupillary reflex only occurs when there is a difference in the sensory defect to the left and right eye.

9.2.2 Evaluating the Near Reflex

The **near reflex triad** consists of
1. Convergence of the visual axes.
2. Accommodation.
3. Constriction of the pupils (miosis).

The near reflex is tested by having the patient focus on a distant object and then on an object in the near field. Usually this is the patient's finger, which is brought to within 10 cm of the eyes. *The near reflex is intact* if both eyes continuously converge with accommodation and miosis appropriate for the patient's age as the object is moved to within 10 cm of the eyes. The examiner should take care to avoid illuminating the pupil, which will produce a light reflex with miosis.

9.3 Influence of Pharmacologic Agents on the Pupil

For details see ▶ Table 9.2.

> **Note**
> Drug-induced mydriasis is contraindicated in patients with a shallow anterior chamber, due to the risk of acute angle closure.

9.4 Pupillary Motor Dysfunction

Pupillary motor dysfunction must be distinguished from a number of differential diagnoses that include not only ocular disorders but neurologic and internal disorders. Diagnosis is difficult,

Table 9.1 Characteristic pupil findings in unilateral lesions of the pupillary reflex pathway

Localization of the lesion (unilateral)		Direct light reflex	Indirect light reflex		Swinging-flashlight test	Findings
			Ipsilateral	Contralateral		
Afferent pupillary pathway (optic nerve, retina)	Slight lesion	+	++	+	Slight constrictions Faster dilation	Isocoria
	Severe lesion	–	++	–	Dilation	
Efferent pupillary pathway	Oculomotor lesion	–	–	–	No response	Anisocoria
	Ciliary ganglion lesion	+	+	++	Delayed constriction Delayed dilation	

Note: – = response absent; + = weak response; ++ = strong response.

Table 9.2 Influence of pharmacologic agents on the pupil

Substance group and individual active agents	Mechanism and duration of action	Indication and special considerations
Miotics		
Parasympathomimetics		
• Direct parasympatho-mimetics	Act on acetylcholine receptors of the sphincter pupillae muscle (miosis) and the ciliary muscle (increased accommodation)	
• Acetylcholine	Extremely short duration of action (several minutes)	Intraocular application only, e.g., keratoplasty; ineffective as eye drops (rapid breakdown)
• Pilocarpine	Effective for 5–7 h	Alternative medication in glaucoma treatment
• Carbachol	Effective for 7–9 h	Currently very rarely used medication in glaucoma therapy
Mydriatics		
Parasympatholytics		
	Act by blocking acetylcholine receptors of the sphincter pupillae muscle (mydriasis) and the ciliary muscle (accommodation paralysis)	
• Tropicamide	Effective for approximately 4–6 h (shortest-acting mydriatic)	Used for diagnostic purposes
• Cyclopentolate	Effective for approximately 12–24 h More cycloplegic than mydriatic	Used **diagnostically** for objective measurement of refraction; used **therapeutically** to relax the ciliary body (e.g., in iritis)
• Scopolamine	Effective for approximately 1 week	Used therapeutically for protracted mydriasis, for example following surgical repair of retinal detachment or in iridocyclitis
• Atropine	Effective for more than 1 week (longest-acting mydriatic)	In all long-term therapeutic mydriasis, e.g., after surgical repair of detached retina and iridocyclitis
Sympathomimetics		
○ Direct sympathomimetics	Act on the epinephrine receptors of the dilator pupillae muscle	
• Epinephrine	Only slightly effective; rapidly broken down by amino-oxidases	Used in the diagnosis of Horner's syndrome and in intraocular application for better mydriasis during surgery
• Phenylephrine	Effective for approximately 6 h Advantage: does not cause accommodation paralysis	Used chiefly for diagnostic purposes due to its short duration of action
○ Indirect sympathomimetics	Inhibit reabsorption of norepinephrine	
• Cocaine 4%	Effective for approximately 6 h	Today used as eye drops only for diagnostic purposes and in Horner's syndrome (see p. 141)

because *isocoria or anisocoria are nonspecific clinical symptoms.* Therefore, functional tests are indicated to confirm the diagnosis. The following section uses diagrams of the initially presenting clinical symptoms to illustrate the various types of pupillary dysfunction. The text presents the differential diagnoses with the functional studies used to confirm the respective diagnosis.

Isocoria with constricted or dilated pupils is primarily of interest to the neurologist and less so to the ophthalmologist. These disorders are therefore discussed at the end of the section.

9.4.1 Isocoria with Normal Pupil Size

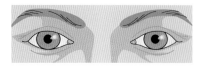

Relative Afferent Pupillary Defect

▶ **Causes.** Unilateral sensory disorder such as retinal detachment, neuritis of the optic nerve, atrophy of the optic nerve, or retinal vascular occlusion.

▶ **Diagnostic considerations.** Direct light reflex is decreased or absent (relative afferent pupillary defect) in the affected eye.
• The consensual light reflex in the affected eye is weak or absent but normal in the unaffected eye.
• The swinging flashlight test reveals dilatation in the affected eye when illuminated (*Marcus Gunn pupil*) or reduced constriction and earlier dilatation in the presence of lesser lesions (afferent pupillary defect).
• Near reflex is normal.
• Unilaterally reduced visual acuity and/or field of vision.

Note
Unilateral blindness (afferent defect) does not produce anisocoria.

Bilateral Afferent Pupillary Defect

▶ **Causes.** Bilateral sensory disorder such as maculopathy or atrophy of the optic nerve.

▶ **Diagnostic considerations**
• Delayed direct and consensual light reflexes.
• The swinging flashlight test produces identical results in both eyes (where disorder affects both sides equally).
• Near reflex is normal.
• Bilaterally reduced visual acuity and/or field of vision.

9.4.2 Anisocoria with a Dilated Pupil in the Affected Eye

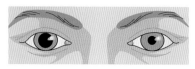

Complete Oculomotor Palsy

▶ **Causes.** Processes in the base of the skull such as tumors, aneurysms, inflammation, or bleeding.
• Processes in the area of the superior orbital fissure or apex of the orbit.

▶ **Diagnostic considerations**
• Direct and consensual light reflexes without constriction in the affected eye (fixed pupil).
• Near reflex miosis is absent.
• Impaired motility and double vision.

Note
Sudden complete oculomotor palsy (loss of motor and parasympathetic function) is a sign of a potentially life-threatening disorder. In unconscious patients, unilateral mydriasis is often the only clinical sign of this.

Tonic Pupil

▶ **Causes.** Postganglionic damage to the parasympathetic pathway, presumably in the ciliary ganglion, that frequently occurs with diabetes mellitus, alcoholism, viral infection, and trauma.

▶ **Diagnostic considerations**
• Direct and consensual light reflexes show absent or delayed reaction, possibly with wormlike segmental muscular contractions.
• Dilation is also significantly delayed.
• Near reflex is slow but clearly present; accommodation with delayed relaxation is present.
• Motility is unimpaired.
• Pharmacologic testing with 0.1 % pilocarpine:
  ○ Significant miosis in the affected eye (denervation hypersensitivity).
  ○ No change in the pupil of the unaffected eye (too weak).
• Adie's tonic pupil syndrome: the tonic pupil is accompanied by absence of the Achilles and patellar tendon reflexes.

Note
Tonic pupil is a relatively frequent and completely harmless cause of unilateral mydriasis.

Iris Defects

▶ **Causes**
- Trauma (aniridia or sphincter tears).
- Secondary to acute angle closure glaucoma.
- Synechiae (postiritis or postoperative).

▶ **Diagnostic considerations.** Patient history and slit lamp examination.

Following Eye Drop Application (Unilateral Administration of a Mydriatic)

Simple Anisocoria

▶ **Causes.** Presumably due to asymmetrical supranuclear inhibition of the Edinger–Westphal nucleus.

▶ **Diagnostic considerations**
- Direct and consensual light reflexes and swinging flashlight test show constant difference in pupil size.
- Near reflex is normal.
- Pharmacologic testing: cocaine test (4% cocaine eye drops are applied to both eyes and pupil size is measured after 1 hour): bilateral pupil dilation indicates an intact neuron chain.

9.4.3 Anisocoria with a Constricted Pupil in the Affected Eye

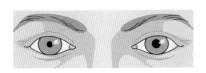

Horner's Syndrome

▶ **Causes.** Damage to the sympathetic pathway.
- Central (first neuron):
  - Tumors.
  - Encephalitis.
  - Diffuse encephalitis.
- Peripheral (second neuron):
  - Syringomyelia.
  - Diffuse encephalitis.

- Trauma.
- Rhinopharyngeal tumors.
- Goiter.
- Aneurysm.
- Processes in the tip of the lung.
- Peripheral in the strict sense (third neuron):
  - Vascular processes.
  - Internal carotid aneurysm.

▶ **Clinical picture**
- Miosis (approximately 1–2 mm difference) due to failure of the dilator pupillae muscle.
- Ptosis (approximately 1–2 mm difference) due to failure of the muscle of Müller.
- Enophthalmos due to failure of the rudimentary lower eyelid retractors. This makes the lower eyelid project so that the eye appears smaller. This condition only represents a type of pseudoenophthalmos.
- Decreased sweat gland secretion (only present in preganglionic disorders as the sweat glands receive their neural supply via the external carotid).

▶ **Diagnostic considerations**
- Direct and consensual light reflexes are intact, which distinguishes this disorder from a parasympathetic lesion; the pupil dilates more slowly (dilation deficit).
- Near reflex is intact.
- Pharmacologic testing with cocaine eye drops.
  - **Peripheral Horner's syndrome.** *On the affected side, there is slight mydriasis (decrease in norepinephrine due to nerve lesion). On the unaffected side, there is significant mydriasis.*
  - **Central Horner's syndrome.** *On the affected side, the pupil is dilated. On the unaffected side, the pupil is also dilated (the norepinephrine in the synapses is not inhibited).*

Following Eye Drop Application

Unilateral administration of a miotic as in glaucoma therapy.

9.4.4 Isocoria with Constricted Pupils

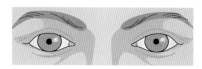

Argyll Robertson Pupil

▶ **Causes.** The precise location of the lesion is not known; presumably the disorder is due to a lesion in the pretectal region and the Edinger–Westphal nucleus such as tabes dorsalis (Argyll Robertson phenomenon), encephalitis, diffuse encephalitis, syringomyelia, trauma, bleeding, tumors, and alcoholism.

▶ **Diagnostic considerations**
- Direct and consensual light reflexes are absent.
- Near reflex is intact or there is overcompensation (the Edinger–Westphal nucleus is being controlled via the convergence center).
- The pupil is not round, and constriction is not always symmetrical.
- There is no reaction to darkness or pharmacologic stimuli.

Bilateral Pupillary Constriction due to Pharmacologic Agents

▶ **Causes**
- Morphine.
- Deep general anesthesia.
- Pilocarpine eye drops.

Toxic Bilateral Pupillary Constriction

▶ **Causes.** For example, mushroom poisoning.

Inflammatory Bilateral Pupillary Constriction

▶ **Causes**
- Encephalitis.
- Meningitis.

9.4.5 Isocoria with Dilated Pupils

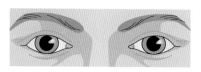

Parinaud's Syndrome

▶ **Causes.** Tumors such as pineal gland tumors that selectively damage fibers between the pretectal nuclei and the Edinger–Westphal nucleus.

▶ **Diagnostic considerations**
- Fixed dilated pupils that do not respond to light.
- Normal near reflex.
- Limited upward gaze (due to damage to the vertical gaze center) and retraction nystagmus.

Intoxication

▶ **Causes.** Atropine, spasmolytic agents, anti-Parkinsonian agents, antidepressants, botulism (very rare but important), carbon monoxide, cocaine.

Disorders

- Migraine.
- Schizophrenia.
- Hyperthyreosis.
- Hysteria.
- Epileptic seizure.
- Increased sympathetic tone (Bumke's anxiety pupils).
- Coma.
- Death agony.

Chapter 10

Glaucoma

10 Glaucoma

Gerhard K. Lang

10.1 General Introductory Remarks

Glaucoma has been recognized as a clinical disease for 150 years. Until recently, intraocular pressure (IOP) was considered to be the only pathogenetic factor, but its significance has now been qualified to some extent. Three elements in the development of glaucoma need to be taken into account: risk factors, the pathogenetic mechanism, and injury.

Three risk factors need to be taken into account:

- Intraocular pressure.
- Vascular dysregulation.
- Systemic blood pressure.

In many other diseases there is also another aspect: *cure*. However, as is well known, glaucoma is not curable.

10.2 Basic Knowledge

Definition

The term "glaucoma" covers several diseases with differing etiologies that share the common finding of optic neuropathy with characteristic pathologic findings in the optic nerve head and a specific pattern of visual field defects. The disease is often, but not always, associated with increased intraocular pressure. The final stage of glaucoma is blindness.

Primary glaucoma refers to glaucoma that is not caused by other ocular disorders.

Secondary glaucoma may occur as the result of another ocular disorder or as an undesired side effect of medication or other treatment.

▶ **Epidemiology.** Throughout the world there are about 70 million people suffering from glaucoma and 7 million who have been blinded by the disease. Glaucoma is the *second most frequent cause of blindness* in developing countries after diabetes mellitus. Some 15–20% of blind persons have lost their eyesight as a result of glaucoma. In Germany, for example, approximately 10% of the population over the age of 40 years suffers from increased intraocular pressure. Approximately 10% of patients seen by ophthalmologists have glaucomas. Of the German population, 8 million persons are at risk of developing glaucoma, 800,000 have already developed the disease (i.e., have glaucoma that has been diagnosed by an ophthalmologist), and 80,000 face the risk of goinvthe glaucoma is not promptly diagnosed and treated.

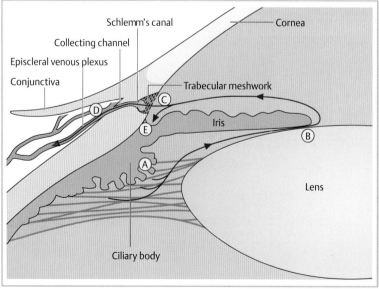

Fig. 10.1 Physiology of aqueous humor circulation. On its way from the nonpigmented cells of the ciliary epithelia (**A**) to underneath the conjunctiva (**D**), the aqueous humor overcomes physiologic resistance from two sources—resistance from the pupil (**B**) and resistance from the trabecular meshwork (**C**). **E**, uveoscleral outflow.

Schlemm's canal — Cornea
Collecting channel
Episcleral venous plexus
Conjunctiva
Trabecular meshwork
Iris
Lens
Ciliary body

▶ **Physiology and pathophysiology of aqueous humor circulation** (▶ Fig. 10.1). The average *normal intraocular pressure of 15 mm Hg* in adults is significantly higher than the average tissue pressure in almost every other organ in the body. This high pressure is important for optical imaging and helps to ensure:

- Uniformly smooth curvature of the surface of the cornea.
- Constant distance between the cornea, lens, and retina.
- Uniform alignment of the photoreceptors of the retina and the pigmented epithelium on Bruch's membrane, which is normally taut and smooth.

The aqueous humor is formed by the ciliary processes and secreted into the posterior chamber of the eye (▶ Fig. 10.1, A). At a rate of about 2 to 6 µL/min and a total anterior and posterior chamber volume of about 0.2 to 0.4 mL, about 1–2% of the aqueous humor is replaced each minute.

The aqueous humor passes through the pupil into the anterior chamber. As the iris lies flat along the anterior surface of the lens, the aqueous humor cannot overcome the pupillary resistance (**first physiologic resistance**; ▶ Fig. 10.1, B) until sufficient pressure has built up to lift the iris off the surface of the lens. The flow of the aqueous humor from the posterior chamber into the anterior chamber is therefore not continuous but pulsatile.

Any *increase in the resistance to pupillary outflow (pupillary block)* leads to an increase in the pressure in the posterior chamber; the iris inflates anteriorly on its root like a sail and presses against the trabecular meshwork (see ▶ Table 10.2). This is the *pathogenesis of angle closure glaucoma.*

Various factors can increase the resistance to pupillary outflow (▶ Table 10.1). The aqueous humor flows out of the angle of the anterior chamber through two channels:

- The trabecular meshwork (▶ Fig. 10.1, C) receives about 85% of the outflow, which then drains into the canal of Schlemm. From here it is conducted by 20 to 30 radial collecting channels into the episcleral venous plexus (▶ Fig. 10.1, D).
- A uveoscleral vascular system receives about 15% of the outflow, which joins the venous blood (▶ Fig. 10.1, E).

Table 10.1 Factors that increase resistance to pupillary outflow and predispose to angle closure glaucoma

Increased contact between the margin of the pupil and lens with	Increased viscosity of the aqueous humor with

• Small eyes
• Large lens (increased lens volume) due to:
  ○ Age (lens volume increases with age by a factor of 6)
  ○ Diabetes mellitus (osmotic swelling of the lens)
• Miosis
  ○ Age (atrophy of the sphincter and dilator muscles)
  ○ Medications (miotic agents in glaucoma therapy)
  ○ Iritis (reactive miosis)
  ○ Diabetic iridopathy (thickening of the iris)
• Posterior synechiae (adhesions between lens and iris)
	• Inflammation (protein, cells, or fibrin in the aqueous humor)
	• Bleeding (erythrocytes in the aqueous humor)

The trabecular meshwork (▶ Fig. 10.1, C) is the **second source of physiologic resistance**. The trabecular meshwork is a body of loose spongelike avascular tissue between the scleral spur and Schwalbe's line. Increased resistance is present in *open angle glaucoma.*

▶ **Classification.** Glaucoma can be classified according to the specific pathophysiology (▶ Table 10.2).

10.3 Examination Methods

10.3.1 Oblique Illumination of the Anterior Chamber

The anterior chamber is illuminated by a beam of light tangential to the plane of the iris. In eyes with an anterior chamber of *normal depth,* the iris is uniformly illuminated. This is a sign of a deep anterior chamber with an open angle (see ▶ Fig. 1.9).

Table 10.2 Classification of glaucoma

Form of glaucoma		Incidence	Angle (anatomic)	Angle (gonioscopy)	Outflow impediment
Open angle glaucoma	Primary	Over 90% of glaucomas	Open	Completely open. Structures appear normal.	In the trabecular meshwork
	Secondary	2–4% of glaucomas	Open	Completely open. Trabecular meshworks and secondary occluding cells visible	Erythrocytes, pigment, inflammatory cells, pseudo-exfoliation material occlude the trabecular meshwork
Angle closure glaucoma	Primary (pupillary block glaucoma)	About 5% of glaucomas	Blocked	Occluded. No angle structures visible	Iris tissue occludes the trabecular meshwork
	Secondary	2–4% of glaucomas	Blocked	Occluded. No angle structures visible. Occluding structures visible	Displacement of the trabecular meshwork produces anterior synechiae, scarring, and neovascularization (rubeosis iridis)
Juvenile glaucoma		1% of glaucomas	Undifferentiated	Open. Occluding embryonic tissue and lack of differentiation visible	In the trabecular meshwork (which is not fully differentiated and/or is occluded by embryonic tissue)
Absolute glaucoma	This is not a separate form of glaucoma, rather it describes an eye blinded by glaucoma that is often painful				

In eyes with a *shallow anterior chamber* and an angle that is partially or completely closed, the iris protrudes anteriorly and is not uniformly illuminated (see ▶ Fig. 1.9).

10.3.2 Slit Lamp Examination

The *central and peripheral depth of the anterior chamber* should be evaluated on the basis of the thickness of the cornea. An anterior chamber that is less than three times as deep as the thickness of the cornea in the center with a peripheral depth less than the thickness of the cornea suggests a narrow angle (▶ Fig. 10.2a). Gonioscopy or an anterior segment OCT is essential for further evaluation.

> **Note**
> To evaluate the depth of the anterior chamber, set the slit for a narrow light beam and let the light strike the eye at a slight angle (as in ▶ Fig. 10.2).

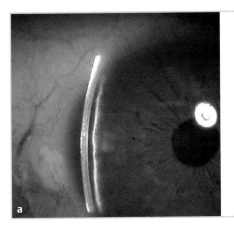
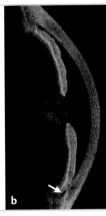

Fig. 10.2 Slit lamp examination to evaluate the depth of the anterior chamber. (a) The depth of the anterior chamber is less than the thickness of the cornea on its periphery: a shallow anterior chamber. Gonioscopy is indicated. **(b)** OCT imaging clearly shows that the iridocorneal angle is narrowed down to a slit (arrow).

10.3.3 Gonioscopy

The iridocorneal angle (▶ Fig. 10.3b) is determined at the slit lamp with a gonioscope that is positioned directly on the cornea (▶ Fig. 10.3a).

Gonioscopy can differentiate the following conditions:

- Open angle: open angle glaucoma.
- Occluded angle: angle closure glaucoma.
- Angle access is narrowed: configuration with imminent risk angle of an acute closure glaucoma.
- Angle is occluded: secondary angle closure glaucoma, for example due to neovascularization in rubeosis iridis.
- Angle open but with inflammatory cellular deposits, erythrocytes, or pigment in the trabecular meshwork: secondary open angle glaucoma.

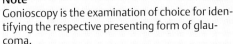

Note
Gonioscopy is the examination of choice for identifying the respective presenting form of glaucoma.

10.3.4 Measuring Intraocular Pressure

▶ **Palpation (see ▶ Fig. 1.12).** Comparative palpation of both eyeballs is a preliminary examination that can detect increased intraocular pressure (IOP).

- If the examiner can indent the eyeball, which fluctuates under palpation, pressure is less than 20 mm Hg.

- An eyeball that is not resilient but rock hard is a sign of about 60 to 70 mm Hg of pressure (acute angle closure glaucoma).

▶ **Schiøtz indentation tonometry.** This examination *measures the degree to which the cornea can be indented* in the supine patient. The lower the intraocular pressure, the deeper the tonometer pin sinks and the greater distance the needle moves.

Indentation tonometry (▶ Fig. 10.4a) often provides inexact results. For example, the rigidity of the sclera is reduced in myopic eyes, which will cause the tonometer pin to sink more deeply for that reason alone. Because of this, indentation tonometry has been largely supplanted by applanation tonometry but it is still an option for bedfast patients. Local anesthesia is required for the measurement.

▶ **Applanation tonometry.** This method is the *most common method of measuring intraocular pressure* (▶ Fig. 10.4b). It permits the examiner to obtain a measurement on a sitting patient within a few seconds (Goldmann's method) or on a supine patient (Draeger's method). A flat tonometer tip has a diameter of 3.06 mm for applanation of the cornea over a corresponding area (7.35 mm^2). Staining with fluorescein is necessary for measurement of surface anesthesia. This method eliminates the rigidity of the sclera as a source of error (however, the thickness of the cornea must be used as a correction factor. See also Tonometric self-examination, page 150). At a corneal thickness of 535 μm, the measured values are the true values. At a corneal thickness of 600 μm, about 4 mm Hg must be subtracted and at 400 μm, 4 mm Hg must be added.

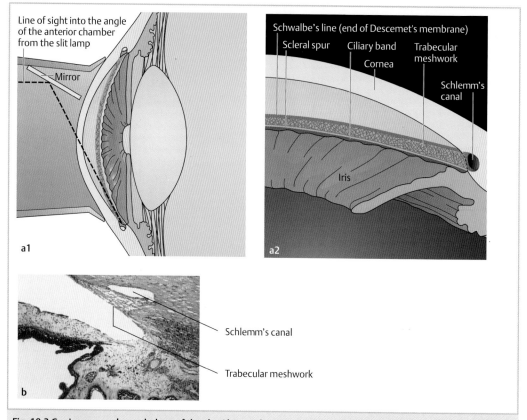

Line of sight into the angle of the anterior chamber from the slit lamp

Mirror

a1

Schwalbe's line (end of Descemet's membrane)

Scleral spur   Ciliary band   Trabecular meshwork

Cornea

Schlemm's canal

Iris

a2

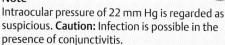

Schlemm's canal

Trabecular meshwork

b

Fig. 10.3 Gonioscopy and morphology of the chamber angle structures. (a1) Schematic diagram of gonioscopy. The angle of the anterior chamber can be visualized with a gonioscope placed on the cornea. **(a2)** Gonioscopic image of the chamber angle. **(b)** Histology of the chamber angle.

Note

Intraocular pressure of 22 mm Hg is regarded as suspicious. **Caution:** Infection is possible in the presence of conjunctivitis.

▶ **Rebound tonometry (ballistic tonometry).** In this procedure (▶ Fig. 10.4c), a thin rod with a ball-shaped tip is bounced against the cornea. An exact determination of the intraocular pressure can be made on the basis of the rebound force. Because of the very low force involved, neither surface anesthesia nor fluorescein is necessary.

▶ **Pneumatic noncontact tonometry.** The electronic tonometer directs a 3-millisecond puff of air against the cornea. The tonometer records the deflection of the cornea and calculates the intraocular pressure on the basis of this deformation.

▶ **Advantages**
• Does not require the use of a topical anesthetic.
• Noncontact measurement eliminates the risk of infection (can be used to measure intraocular pressure in the presence of conjunctivitis).

▶ **Disadvantages**
• Calibration is difficult.
• Precise measurements are possible only within low to middle range pressures.
• Cannot be used in the presence of corneal scarring.
• Examination is unpleasant for the patient.
• The air flow is noisy.
• The instrument is more expensive to purchase than an applanation tonometer.

▶ **Contour tonometry.** In this dynamic measurement, a concave pressure sensor is brought into contact with the cornea and the values are picked up by a piezoelectric crystal. At the same time, the

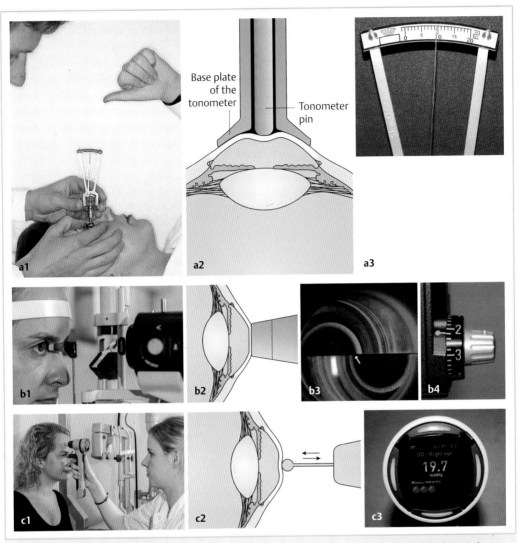

Fig. 10.4 Various possibilities for measurement of the internal pressure of the eye (tonometry). (a) Schiøtz indentation tonometry. The physician holds the patient's eyelids apart and sets the plunger on the anesthetized cornea. The patient focuses on his thumb with the other eye **(a1)**. The plunger indents the cornea **(a2)**. The higher the internal pressure of the eye, that is, the harder the eye, the less the plunger depresses the cornea and the smaller the excursion of the tonometer pointer **(a3)**. **(b)** Goldmann applanation tonometry with a slit lamp: After administration of eye drops containing fluorescein and anesthetic, a flat tonometer tip is placed on the cornea **(b1)**. The cornea is flattened on a surface of exactly 7.35 mm² (applanated, **b2**). The pressure required to achieve this is equal to the intraocular pressure. The physician looks through the slit lamp and turns the screw until both internal menisci of the fluorescein semicircles are touching **(b3,** arrow). The physician then reads the pressure **(b4,** in mm Hg). **(c)** Rebound tonometry. **(c1)** Positioning the rebound tonometer (about 1 cm from the patient's eye) and triggering five measurements. **(c2)** The plastic plunger is fired at the patient's eye. The IOP can be calculated from the rebound force. **(c3)** Reading the pressure from the display. Rebound tonometry has two considerable advantages: it can be performed without anesthetizing the corneal surface and the instruments are very light and so can be taken anywhere, such as directly to a patient's bedside.

pulse-synchronous fluctuations of the intraocular pressure can be recorded. The measurement is largely independent of the corneal thickness. Surface anesthesia is required.

▶ **Measuring the 24-hour pressure curve.** This examination is performed to analyze *fluctuations of the pressure level over a 24-hour period* in patients with suspected glaucoma (▶ Fig. 10.5).

Note

A single measurement may not be representative. Only a 24-hour curve provides reliable information about the pressure level.

Intraocular pressure fluctuates in a rhythmic pattern. The highest values frequently occur at night or in the early morning hours. In normal patients, these fluctuations in intraocular pressure rarely exceed 4 to 6 mm Hg.

Pressure is measured on the ward at 6:00 a.m., noon, 6:00 p.m., 9:00 p.m., and midnight. Outpatient 24-hour pressure curves without nighttime and early morning measurements are less reliable.

Note

In glaucoma patients receiving eye drop treatment, special attention should be given to the time of application. Pressure is measured immediately prior to applying the eye drops. In this manner, measurements are obtained when the effect of the eye drops is weakest.

▶ **Tonometric self-examination.** Recent developments have made it possible for patients to measure intraocular pressure themselves at home in a manner similar to self-monitoring of blood pressure and blood glucose (▶ Fig. 10.6a). The patient tonometer makes it possible to obtain a 24-hour pressure curve from any number of measurements obtained in normal everyday conditions. A patient tonometer can be prescribed for suitable patients (such as those with an increased risk of acute glaucoma). However, using the device requires a certain degree of skill. Patients who have problems applying eye drops are best advised not to attempt to use a patient tonometer. Younger and well-motivated patients are the best candidates for tonometric self-examination (▶ Fig. 10.6c).

▶ **Partner tonometry.** A portable pneumatic noncontact tonometer recently became available that is suitable for tonometry at home (▶ Fig. 10.6b). As the alignment of the tonometer is the only thing that needs to be done by the partner and the measurement itself is examiner-independent, the results are considered to be reliable. The disadvantage at present is the extremely high cost of the device. For details, see Pneumatic noncontact tonometry (see p. 148).

▶ **Sources of error in tonometry.** Corneal thickness needs to be taken into account in applanation tonometry. Tonometric measurements are too low in patients with thin corneas and too high in those with thick corneas. The correction factor is about 2 to 3 mm Hg per 50 µm corneal thickness (given a regular corneal thickness of 539 µm). This means that in an eye with a corneal thickness of 590 µm,

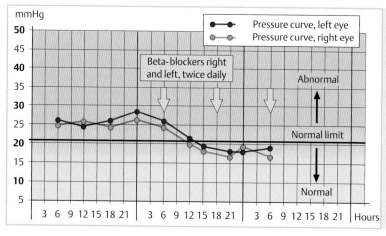

Fig. 10.5 Twenty-four-hour pressure curve. The colored dots represent the times of the measurements. The time of the initial application of antiglaucoma eye drops is marked (arrow). The time, frequency, and side of the eye drop application are also identified.

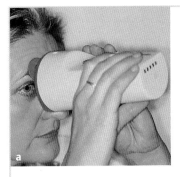

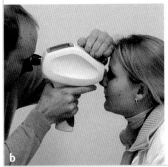

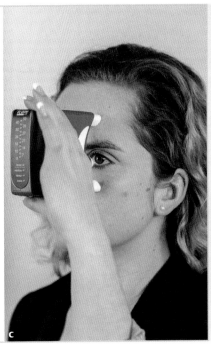

Fig. 10.6 Tonometry without an ophthalmologist. (a) Tonometric self-examination, based on the principle of applanation tonometry. The patient places the tonometer on his or her forehead and uses the fixation light to align it to the proper position. The head of the tonometer then automatically presses against the cornea, measures the intraocular pressure, and retracts. The pressure is indicated in a digital display. **(b)** Partner tonometry, based on the principle of pneumatic noncontact tonometry. The hand-held pneumotonometer can be used at home by the patient's partner, who is seen here carrying out the alignment. **(c)** Tonometric self-examination based on the principle of rebound tonometry. No anesthesia is required for this procedure.

the real intraocular pressure is about 2 to 3 mmHg lower than the measured value.

10.3.5 Optic Disc Ophthalmoscopy

The optic disc has a physiologic excavation known as the optic cup. In the presence of persistently elevated intraocular pressure, the optic cup becomes enlarged and can be evaluated by ophthalmoscopy.

Stereoscopic examination of the optic disc through a slit lamp biomicroscope fitted with a contact lens provides a three-dimensional image. The optic cup can be examined stereoscopically with the pupil dilated.

> **Note**
> The optic nerve is the eye's "glaucoma memory." Evaluating this structure will tell the examiner whether damage due to glaucoma is present and how far advanced it is.

▶ **Normal optic cup (▶ Fig. 10.7).** The normal anatomy can vary widely. Large normal optic cups are nearly always *round* and differ from the *vertical elongation* of the optic cup seen in eyes with glaucoma.

▶ **Documenting the optic disc. Recording findings in sketches** is suitable for routine documentation and follow-up examination of the optic disc. **Photographing the optic disc with a fundus camera** permits longer-term follow-up. *Stereoscopic photography* also provides a *three-dimensional image.* Optic disc measurement and tomography can provide *precise measurements of the optic nerve.*

▶ **Optic disc measurement.** The area of the optic disc, optic cup, and neuroretinal rim (vital optic disc tissue) can be measured by planimetry on *two-dimensional photographs* of the optic nerve.

▶ **Optic disc tomography.** Modern laser scanning ophthalmoscopes and optical coherence tomography (OCT) permit *three-dimensional documentation* of the optic nerve (▶ Fig. 10.8).

▶ **Glaucomatous changes in the optic nerve.** Glaucoma produces typical *changes in the shape of the optic cup.* Progressive destruction of nerve fibers, fibrous and vascular tissue, and glial tissue will be observable. This tissue atrophy leads to an *increase in the size of the optic cup* and to *pale discoloration of the optic* disc (▶ Fig. 10.9).

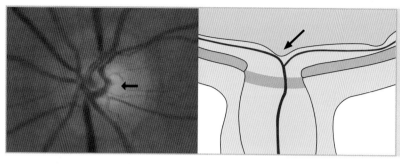

Fig. 10.7 Normal optic disc. The optic disc is sharply demarcated. It is level with the retina, and its color indicates vital tissue. The small central optic cup (arrow) is discernible as a brighter area.

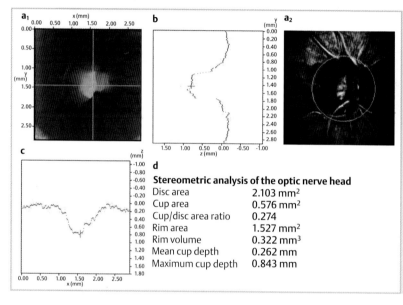

Fig. 10.8 Optic disc tomography. A laser beam scans the optic disc (a1 and a2) to produce a vertical map (b) and horizontal map (c) of the height and depth of the optic disc. The computer then calculates crucial data for the optic disc and presents a stereometric analysis (d).

Stereometric analysis of the optic nerve head

Disc area	2.103 mm²
Cup area	0.576 mm²
Cup/disc area ratio	0.274
Rim area	1.527 mm²
Rim volume	0.322 mm³
Mean cup depth	0.262 mm
Maximum cup depth	0.843 mm

Note

Progressive glaucomatous changes in the optic disc are closely associated with increasing visual field defects (see ▶ Fig. 10.10).

10.3.6 Visual Field Testing

Detecting glaucoma as early as possible requires documenting glaucomatous visual field defects at the earliest possible stage (see p. 249). It is known that glaucomatous visual field defects initially become manifest in the superior paracentral nasal visual field or, less frequently, in the inferior field, as relative scotomas that later progress to absolute scotomas (▶ Fig. 10.10).

In the detection of these early visual field defects, *static computer perimetry* (measurement of sensitivity to light differences) is superior to all kinetic methods. With computer-controlled, semiautomatic grid perimetry instruments (Octopus, Humphrey Field Analyzer) the central 30° visual field is examined (modern campimetry) (▶ Fig. 10.11).

Reproducible visual field findings are important in follow-up to exclude any enlargement of the defects.

Note

A visual field defect is not the beginning of glaucoma but the beginning of the end.

10.3.7 Examination of the Retinal Nerve Fiber Layer

The retinal nerve fibers have a characteristic arrangement that explains the typical visual field defects that occur in primary open angle glaucoma.

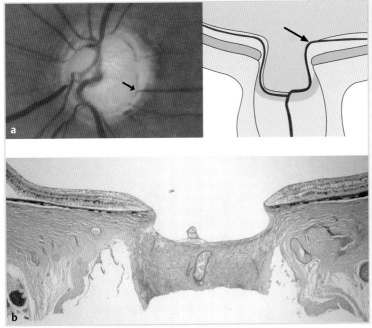

Fig. 10.9 Glaucomatous lesions in the optic nerve. (a) The optic disc is sharply demarcated and pale (a sign of tissue atrophy). The optic cup is enlarged and almost completely covers the disc. The blood vessels abruptly plunge into the deep cup, indicated by their typical bayonet-shaped kinks in the image (arrow). **(b)** Histologic appearance of an optic nerve damaged by glaucoma.

In addition to the early progressive optic nerve and visual field defects, *arc-shaped defects* also occur in the nerve fiber layer. These defects can be observed in light without red components (▶ Fig. 10.12).

10.4 Primary Glaucoma

10.4.1 Primary Chronic Open Angle Glaucoma

Definition
Primary open angle glaucoma begins in middle-aged and elderly patients with minimal symptoms that worsen progressively. The angle of the anterior chamber characteristically remains open throughout the clinical course of the disorder.

▶ **Epidemiology.** Primary open angle glaucoma is *by far the most common form of glaucoma* and accounts for over 90% of adult glaucomas. The incidence of the disorder significantly increases beyond the age of 40 years, reaching a peak between the ages of 60 and 70. Its prevalence among 40-year-olds is 0.9% as compared to 4.7% among patients over the age of 50.

There appears to be a *genetic predisposition* for primary open angle glaucoma. Over one-third of glaucoma patients have relatives with the same disorder.

Note
Patients with a positive family history are at greater risk of developing the disorder.

▶ **Etiology.** (See also Physiology and pathophysiology of aqueous humor circulation in Chapter 10.2.)

The cause of primary open angle glaucoma is not known, although it is known that **drainage of the aqueous humor is impeded**. The primary lesion occurs in the neuroretinal tissue of the optic nerve as compression neuropathy of the optic nerve.

▶ **Symptoms.** The majority of patients with primary open angle glaucoma do not experience any subjective symptoms for years. However, a small number of patients experience occasional **unspecific symptoms** such as headache, a burning sensation in the eyes, or blurred or decreased vision that the patient may attribute to lack of eyeglasses or insufficient correction. The patient may also perceive rings of color around light sources at night, which has traditionally been regarded as a symptom of angle closure glaucoma.

Peripheral optic cup in a temporal and inferior location (with damage to the optic nerve fibers in this area)

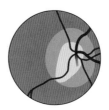

Increase in the size of the optic cup with thinning of the vital rim. The lamina cribrosa is visible

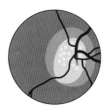

Advanced generalized thinning of the neuroretinal rim with an increasingly visible lamina cribrosa and nasal displacement of the blood vessels

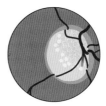

Total glaucomatous atrophy of the optic nerve. Complete atrophy of the neuroretinal rim, kettle-shaped optic cup, bayonet kinks in the blood vessels on the margin of the optic disc, some of which disappear. The lamina cribrosa is diffusely visible. Only remnants of the atrophic tissue of the optic disc remain. The optic disc is surrounded by a ring of chorioretinal atrophy (glaucomatous halo) due to pressure atrophy of the choroid and lysis of the retinal pigmented epithelium

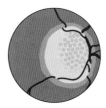

Fig. 10.10 Overview of glaucomatous visual field defects.

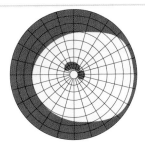

An enlarged blind spot and a superior paracentral nasal scotoma. The paracentral scotomas precede the enlargement of the blind spot

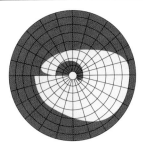

Narrowing of the peripheral superior paracentral visual field. The insular paracentral scotomas converge and extend to the blind spot

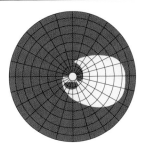

Further loss of superior nasal visual field. Circumscribed horizontal penetration of Bjerrum's scotoma into the nasal half of the field of vision. A new inferior nasal scotoma is a sign of a superior temporal nerve fiber lesion

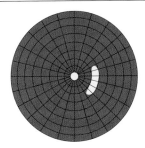

A small central and peripheral residual field of vision remains. The arc-shaped scotoma has expanded into a ring-shaped scotoma surrounding the focal point. As the focal point degenerates, the center of vision disappears and only a peripheral residual field of vision is left

Fig. 10.10 (continued)

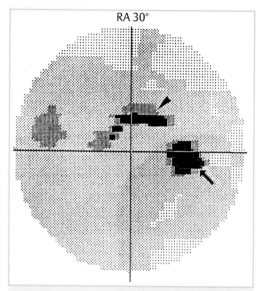

RA 30°

Fig. 10.11 Thirty-degree visual field test for glaucoma screening. The central field of vision is examined for scotomas using an automatic perimeter, as studies of early glaucoma have shown that the initial defects occur in this area (see ▶ Fig. 10.10). The figure shows the visual field defect in the early stages of glaucoma. The blind spot is slightly enlarged (arrow), and an arc-shaped paracentral Bjerrum's scotoma is present (arrowhead). The standardized examination conditions in automatic perimetry do not only allow early detection of glaucoma; the reproducible results are also helpful for prompt diagnosis of deteriorating findings.

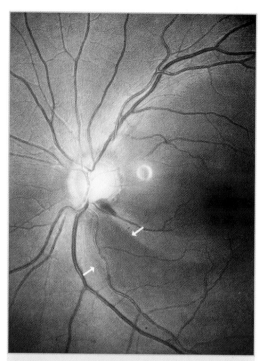

Fig. 10.12 Examination of the retinal nerve fiber layer. The arc-shaped nerve fiber defect (between the arrows) is a sign of an early glaucomatous optic nerve lesion. In addition, the hemorrhage at the disc is a suspicious sign.

Note

Primary open angle glaucoma often does not exhibit typical symptoms for years. Regular examination by an ophthalmologist is crucial for early diagnosis.

Primary open angle glaucoma can be far advanced before the patient notices an extensive visual field defect in one or both eyes.

It is crucial to diagnose the disorder as early as possible because the prognosis for glaucoma detected in its early stages is far better than for advanced glaucoma. Where increased intraocular pressure remains undiagnosed or untreated for years, glaucomatous optic nerve damage and the associated visual field defect will increase to the point of blindness.

▶ **Diagnostic considerations**

▶ **Measurement of intraocular pressure.** Elevated intraocular pressure in a routine ophthalmic examination is an alarming sign (above 22 mm Hg).

▶ **Twenty-four-hour pressure curve.** Fluctuations in intraocular pressure of over 5 to 6 mm Hg may occur over a 24-hour period.

▶ **Gonioscopy.** The angle of the anterior chamber is open and appears as normal as the angle in patients without glaucoma.

▶ **Ophthalmoscopy.** Examination of the optic nerve reveals whether glaucomatous cupping has already occurred and how far advanced the glaucoma is. Where the optic disc and visual field are normal, ophthalmoscopic examination of the posterior pole under green light may reveal fascicular nerve fiber defects as early abnormal findings.

▶ **Perimetry.** Noise field perimetry is suitable as a *screening test* because it makes the patient aware of scotomas and makes it possible to detect and describe them. The patient is shown a flickering monitor displaying what resembles image noise on a television set. The patient will not see the flickering points in the region of the scotoma. After this test, the defect should be quantified by more specific methods. Automatic grid perimetry is suitable for the *early stages* of glaucoma. Special programs (such as the G1 program on the Octopus perimeter and the 30-2 program on the Humphrey perimeter devices) reveal the earliest glaucomatous changes. In *advanced glaucoma,* kinetic hand perimetry with the Goldmann perimeter device is a useful preliminary examination to evaluate the remaining field of vision. See Chapter 14.2 on visual pathway examination methods.

▶ **Differential diagnosis.** Two disorders are important in this context.

▶ **Ocular hypertension.** Patients with ocular hypertension have significantly increased intraocular pressure over a period of years without signs of glaucomatous optic nerve damage or visual field defects. Some patients in this group will continue to have elevated intraocular pressure but will not develop glaucomatous lesions; the others will develop primary open angle glaucoma. (The risk factors are IOP >25 mm Hg, central corneal thickness <565 μm, papillary excavation >0.3.) The probability that a patient will develop definitive glaucoma increases the higher the intraocular pressure, the younger the patient, and the more compelling the evidence of a history of glaucoma in the family.

▶ **Low-tension glaucoma.** Patients with low-tension glaucoma exhibit typical progressive glaucomatous changes in the optic disc and visual field without elevated intraocular pressure. These patients are very difficult to treat because management cannot focus on the control of intraocular pressure. Often these patients will have a history of hemodynamic crises such as gastrointestinal or uterine bleeding with significant loss of blood, low blood pressure, and peripheral vascular spasms (cold hands and feet). A continuous 24-hour blood pressure profile often shows phases of low blood pressure during the night that would otherwise be undetected. These time intervals of low perfusion lead to optic neuropathy (▶ Fig. 10.13). Patients with glaucoma may also experience further worsening of the visual field due to a drop in blood pressure. Antihypertensive drugs must be discontinued or the dosage must be adjusted.

Note
Caution should be exercised when using cardiovascular and antihypertensive drugs in patients with glaucoma.

▶ **Treatment**
▶ **Indications for initiating treatment**
- *Glaucomatous changes in the optic cup.* Medical treatment should be initiated where there are signs of glaucomatous changes in the optic cup or when there is a difference of more than 20% between the optic cups of the two eyes.
- Any *intraocular pressure exceeding 25 mm Hg* should be treated.
- *Increasing glaucomatous changes in the optic cup or increasing visual field defects in spite of anti-*

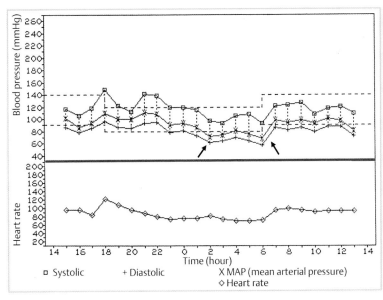

Fig. 10.13 Nocturnal hypotony phases in a 24-hour blood pressure profile. The 24-hour blood pressure profile shows a hypotony phase from midnight to 6 a.m. with a pressure drop under standard value, with low perfusion of the optic nerve head in this time period (arrows).

glaucomatous medication. Regardless of the pressure measured, these changes show that the current pressure level is too high for the optic nerve and that additional medication is indicated. A target IOP should be defined about 30% under the initial level. In addition to reducing the pressure, minimization of the daily pressure fluctuations is attempted. This also applies to patients with advanced glaucomatous damage and threshold pressure levels (around 22 mm Hg). The strongest possible medications are indicated in these cases, to lower pressure as much as possible (10–12 mm Hg).

- *Early stages.* It is often difficult to determine whether therapy is indicated in the early stages, especially where intraocular pressure is elevated slightly above threshold values. Patients with low-tension glaucoma exhibit increasing cupping of the optic disc even at normal pressures (less than 22 mm Hg), whereas patients with elevated intraocular pressure (25–33 mm Hg) may exhibit an unchanged optic nerve for years.

Patients with suspected glaucoma and risk factors such as a family history of the disorder, middle myopia, glaucoma in the other eye, or differences between the optic cup in the two eyes should be monitored closely. Follow-up examinations should be performed three to four times a year, especially for patients not undergoing treatment.

▶ **Therapeutic goals.** The aim is to reduce the intraocular pressure to the level of the target pressure. The target pressure needs to be determined individually for each patient as a specific IOP level low enough to prevent the progression of visual field loss and glaucomatous optic nerve damage. The definition of the target pressure may be a continuing process that takes several office visits.

▶ **Medication.** *Available options in medication for glaucoma* (see also ▶ Fig. 10.14):

- Inhibit aqueous humor production.
- Increase trabecular outflow.
- Increase uveoscleral outflow.

Table 10.3 Selection of useful combinations of glaucoma medications

Current medication		Carboanhydrase inhibitors (Dorzolamide, Brinzolamide)	β-Blockers (Timolol, Betaxolol, Carteolol, Levobunolol, Metipranolol)	α₂-Agonists (Clonidine, Apraclonidine, Bromonidine)	Prostaglandin derivatives (Latanoprost, Bimatoprost, Travoprost, Tafluprost)	Miotic agents (parasympathomimetics) (Pilocarpine, Carbachol)
+ Practical − Not practical						
Miotic agents (parasympathomimetics)	Pilocarpine Carbachol	+	+	+	–	
Prostaglandin derivative	Latanoprost Bimatoprost Travoprost Tafluprost	+	+	+		–
α₂-Agonists (sympathomimetics)	Clonidine Apraclonidine Bromonidine	+	+		+	+
β-Blockers (sympatholytics)	Timolol Betaxolol Carteolol Levobunolol Metipranolol	+		+	+	+
Carboanhydrase inhibitors	Dorzolamide Brinzolamide		+	+	+	+

The various active ingredients and substance groups available for medical treatment of glaucoma are listed in ▶ Fig. 10.14 and ▶ Table 10.3. For details of the individual active substances see ▶ Table 10.4.

Note
Medical therapy is the treatment of choice for primary open angle glaucoma. Surgery is indicated only where medical therapy fails.

- *Principles of medical treatment of primary open angle glaucoma:*
  - The choice of medication depends on the efficacy, side effects and contraindications of different drugs. At first, a single drug treatment should be targeted with an IOP-reducing effect of at least 20% of the untreated level.
  - The following options are available for initial local drug treatment (in alphabetical order):
    - Alpha-2-agonists.
    - Beta blockers.
    - Carboanhydrase inhibitors.
    - Prostaglandin analogs.

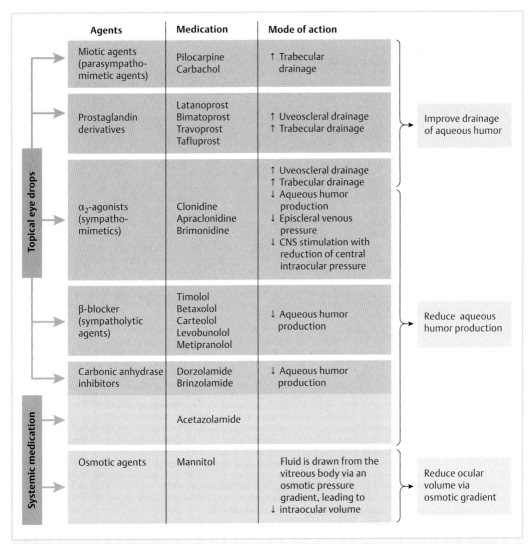

	Agents	Medication	Mode of action	
Topical eye drops	Miotic agents (parasympatho-mimetic agents)	Pilocarpine Carbachol	↑ Trabecular drainage	
	Prostaglandin derivatives	Latanoprost Bimatoprost Travoprost Tafluprost	↑ Uveoscleral drainage ↑ Trabecular drainage	Improve drainage of aqueous humor
	α₂-agonists (sympatho-mimetics)	Clonidine Apraclonidine Brimonidine	↑ Uveoscleral drainage ↑ Trabecular drainage ↓ Aqueous humor production ↓ Episcleral venous pressure ↓ CNS stimulation with reduction of central intraocular pressure	
	β-blocker (sympatholytic agents)	Timolol Betaxolol Carteolol Levobunolol Metipranolol	↓ Aqueous humor production	Reduce aqueous humor production
	Carbonic anhydrase inhibitors	Dorzolamide Brinzolamide	↓ Aqueous humor production	
Systemic medication		Acetazolamide		
	Osmotic agents	Mannitol	Fluid is drawn from the vitreous body via an osmotic pressure gradient, leading to ↓ intraocular volume	Reduce ocular volume via osmotic gradient

Fig. 10.14 Options in the medical treatment of glaucoma. For details of the individual active substances see ▶ Table 10.4.

- In selected cases, parasympathomimetic agents and nonselective adrenergic agents.
- Osmotic agents or carbonic anhydrase inhibitors (administered orally or intravenously) inhibit the production of aqueous humor. They can be administered temporarily in addition to topical medications. Their side effects usually make them unsuitable for prolonged treatment. The general rule is to try to use the weakest possible medications required to achieve normal pressure over a 24-hour period: as much as necessary, and as little as possible.

- With monotherapy, after more than 2 years of treatment, no adequate IOP reduction is achieved in 40 to 75% of glaucoma patients.
- With insufficient IOP reduction, the monotherapy is changed first, before another medication is added.
- The use of combination preparations is recommended, since patient compliance is higher if the number of eye drops to be applied is lower.
- The effectiveness of any pressure-reducing therapy should be verified by pressure analysis on the ward or on an outpatient basis.
- The effect of the eye drops should not interfere with the patient's ability to work. The tolerance,

Table 10.4 Medication for glaucoma

Active ingredients and preparations (examples)	Mode of action	Indications	Side effects
Parasympathomimetic agents			
• Pilocarpine • Carbachol	• Improve drainage of aqueous humor in primary open angle glaucoma. The effect is probably purely mechanical via contraction of the ciliary muscle and tension on the trabecular meshwork and scleral spur • In **acute angle closure glaucoma,** the forced narrowing of the pupil and the extraction of the iris from the angle of the anterior chamber are most important	• Primary open angle glaucoma • Acute angle closure glaucoma	• Younger patients frequently do not tolerate the temporary myopia due to contraction of the ciliary muscle • Miosis with worsening of the night vision and narrowing of the peripheral field of vision
α2-Agonists (sympathomimetics)			
• Clonidine	• Reduces intraocular pressure by about 20%, primarily by vasoconstriction without influencing the size of the pupil and accommodation	• Particularly suitable for young patients with primary open angle glaucoma	• Lowers blood pressure. Should be used only in low concentrations (1/16% and 1/8%) because the effect on intraocular pressure is the same as with higher concentrations but the side effects are significantly less • Dry mouth
• Apraclonidine	• Also reduces aqueous humor production • In contrast to clonidine, this agent does not reduce systemic blood pressure	• Very good reduction of intraocular pressure in decompensated glaucoma (acute, but not long term)	• Beware of cardiovascular disease
• Brimonidine	• Improves drainage of aqueous humor by reducing episcleral venous pressure and reducing aqueous humor production by decreasing ciliary body perfusion • Reduces pressure by about 27%	• As with apraclonidine	• As with apraclonidine • Allergic reaction rate lower than apraclonidine • Lowers blood pressure • Neuroprotective potential

Table 10.4 Medication for glaucoma (continued)

Active ingredients and preparations (examples)	Mode of action	Indications	Side effects
β-Blockers (sympatholytics)			
• Timolol • Betaxolol • Carteolol • Levobunolol • Metipranolol	• Reduces intraocular pressure by decreasing production of aqueous humor without influencing the size of the pupil and accommodation	• Primary open angle glaucoma • Secondary open angle glaucoma • Secondary angle closure glaucoma	• Bradycardia • Arrythmia • Heart failure • Syncope • Bronchospasm • Hypotony **Contraindications:** Beta blockers should be used with caution in patients with obstructive lung disease, cardiac insufficiency, or cardiac arrhythmia and only after consulting an internist. Absorption from topical application can produce systemic side effects
Prostaglandin derivatives			
• Latanoprost • Travoprost • Bimatoprost	• Increase in uveoscleral aqueous humor drainage • Excellent pressure reduction 30%	• Suitable for all patients with primary open angle glaucoma. Adjunctive therapy with beta blockers, epinephrine derivatives, pilocarpine, and carbonic anhydrase inhibitors	• No known systemic side effects • Local changes in the color of the iris in 16% of patients • Lashes grow in length and thickness • Conjunctival hyperemia • Cystoid macular edema
Carbonic anhydrase inhibitors			
• Dorzolamide • Brinzolamide • Acetazolamide (systemic) max. 1.0 g/day • Dichlorphenamide (systemic)	• Reduce aqueous humor production. The enzyme carbonic anhydrase contributes to the production of aqueous humor via active secretion of bicarbonate • Increase local circulation	• Acute glaucoma • Surgical procedures that can increase intraocular pressure	• Systemic: prolonged therapy causes malaise, nausea, depression, anorexia, weight loss, and decreased libido in 40–50% of glaucoma patients • Low potassium and/or sodium levels
Osmotic agents			
• Mannitol	• Decrease intraocular pressure presumably by producing an osmotic pressure gradient by means of the hyperosmotic substances released into the bloodstream. This draws water from the fluid-filled spaces, especially from the vitreous body and aqueous humor	• Exclusively indicated in acute increases of intraocular pressure such as angle closure glaucoma due to its short duration of action (only a few hours)	• Contraindications: • Renal disease • Cardiac insufficiency • Lung edema

effects, and side effects of the eye drops should be repeatedly verified on an individual basis during the course of treatment.

• Not all combinations of antiglaucoma drugs are useful (▶ Table 10.3).

▶ **Surgical treatment of primary open angle glaucoma**
• **Indications**
  ○ Treatment with medication is inadequate.

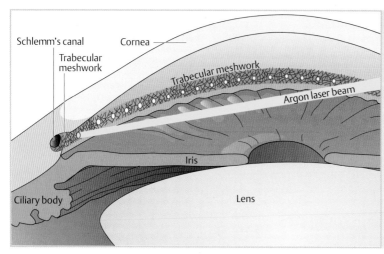

Schlemm's canal
Trabecular meshwork
Cornea
Trabecular meshwork
Argon laser beam
Iris
Ciliary body
Lens

Fig. 10.15 Laser trabeculoplasty. A laser beam is focused on the trabecular meshwork through a gonioscope and slit lamp. Approximately 100 laser burns are placed in a circle in the trabecular meshwork to improve drainage of the aqueous humor.

○ The patient does not tolerate medication. Reactions include allergy, reduced vision due to narrowing of the pupil, pain, and ciliary spasms, and ptosis.

○ The patient is not a suitable candidate for medication therapy due to a lack of compliance or a lack of dexterity in applying eye drops, (e.g. trembling in Parkinson's disease).

• **Laser trabeculoplasty**

○ *Principle:* Laser burns in the trabecular meshwork cause tissue contraction that widens the intervening spaces and improves outflow through the trabecular meshwork. An argon laser (ALT: argon laser trabeculoplasty) or a 532-nm neodymium YAG laser (SLT: selective trabeculoplasty) is suitable for trabeculoplasty.

○ *Technique:* Fifty to 100 focal laser burns are placed in the anterior trabecular meshwork (▶ Fig. 10.15).

○ *Comment:* Laser surgery in the angle of the anterior chamber is possible only if the angle is open. The surgery itself is largely painless, can be performed as an outpatient procedure, and involves few possible complications. These may include bleeding from vascular structures near the angle and synechiae between the iris and individual laser burns. Laser trabeculoplasty can bring improvement with intraocular pressures up to 30 mm Hg. It decreases intraocular pressure by about 6 to 8 mm Hg for about 2 years. Laser trabeculoplasty is only effective in about every second patient. The full effect occurs about 4 to 6 weeks postoperatively.

• **Filtration surgery**

○ *Principle:* The aqueous humor is drained through the anterior chamber through a sub-conjunctival scleral opening, circumventing the trabecular meshwork. Formation of a thin-walled filtration bleb is a sign of sufficient drainage of aqueous humor.

○ *Technique* (▶ Fig. 10.16): First, a conjunctival flap is raised, which may be either fornix-based or limbal-based. The short-time application of an antiproliferative substance (mitomycin C) inhibits wound healing postoperatively and keeps the filtration way open. Then a partial-thickness scleral flap is raised. Access to the anterior chamber is gained via a *goniotomy performed with a 1.5-mm trephine at the sclerocorneal junction or via a rectangular trabeculectomy* performed with a scalpel and dissecting scissors. A peripheral iridectomy is then performed through this opening. The scleral flap is then loosely closed and covered with conjunctiva.

○ *Comment:* A permanent reduction in intraocular pressure is achieved in 80 to 85% of these operations.

• **Cyclodialysis**

○ *Principle:* The aqueous humor is drained through an opening into the suprachoroidal space.

○ *Technique:* A full-thickness scleral incision is made down to the ciliary body 4 mm posterior to the limbus. The sclera is then separated from the ciliary body with a retractor and retracted anteriorly into the anterior chamber. The ciliary body atrophies in the area of the incision, which also helps to decrease the production of aqueous humor.

○ *Comment:* This procedure is less common today than it was in the 1980s. One reason for this is that it is difficult to gauge accurately the

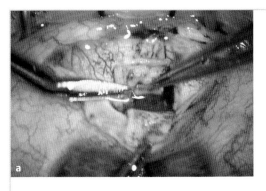
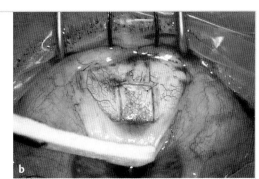
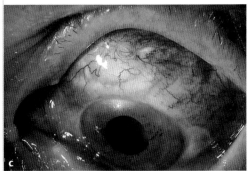

Fig. 10.16 Filtration surgery. (a) The trabecular meshwork is excised with dissecting scissors. **(b)** The partial-thickness scleral flap is closed with two sutures. **(c)** The postoperative photograph shows a prominent bleb underneath the conjunctiva.

atrophy of the ciliary body. Occasionally severe hypotonia of the globe results, which then requires surgical intervention to close the dialysis opening.

- **Cycloablation (cyclodestructive procedures)**
  - *Principle:* Atrophy is induced in portions of the ciliary body through the intact sclera to reduce intraocular pressure by decreasing the amount of tissue producing aqueous humor.
  - *Technique:*
    - *Cyclocryotherapy.* A cryoprobe is used to freeze the ciliary body at several points through the sclera. This procedure can be repeated if necessary; the interventions have a cumulative effect.
    - *Cyclodiathermy.* This method is similar to cyclocryotherapy, except that a diathermy needle is advanced through the sclera into the ciliary body to cauterize it with heat. The procedure can be performed with or without prior dissection of a partial-thickness scleral flap.
    - *Laser cycloablation* induces atrophy in the ciliary body using a YAG laser or high-energy diode laser pulses.

    - *Ultrasound disruption* induces atrophy in the ciliary body with high-frequency ultrasound waves. These last two forms of therapy have been developed to induce atrophy more effectively, more accurately, and in more controlled doses, which is less traumatic for the eye.
  - *Comment:* All these forms of cycloablation are irreversible and can cause permanent hypotonia. They therefore represent the last line of treatment options.

▶ **Prophylaxis.** No prophylactic action can be taken to prevent primary open angle glaucoma.

Note
Early diagnosis is crucial and can only be made by an ophthalmologist. By the age of 40 years at the latest, patients should have their intraocular pressure measured regularly. The ophthalmologist performs regular glaucoma screening examinations of intraocular pressure and of the pupil. Therefore, the first pair of reading eyeglasses should always be prescribed by an ophthalmologist.

▶ **Prognosis.** The prognosis depends greatly on the stage at which primary open angle glaucoma is diagnosed. As a general rule, therapy is more effective the earlier it can be initiated.

10.4.2 Primary Angle Closure Glaucoma

Definition
Acute episodic increase in intraocular pressure to several times the normal value (10–20 mm Hg) due to sudden blockage of drainage. Production of aqueous humor and trabecular resistance are normal.

▶ **Epidemiology.** The incidence among persons over the age of 60 years is 1 per 1,000. Women are three times as likely to be affected as men. Inuit are more frequently affected than other ethnic groups, whereas the disorder is rare in blacks.

▶ **Etiology.** (See also Physiology and pathophysiology of aqueous humor circulation in Chapter 10.2.) Anatomically predisposed eyes with **shallow anterior chambers** pose a relative impediment to the flow of aqueous humor through the pupil. This **pupillary block** increases the pressure in the posterior chamber (see ▶ Fig. 10.18). The pressure displaces the iris anteriorly toward the trabecular meshwork, suddenly blocking the outflow of aqueous humor (**angle closure**).Atypical glaucoma attack occurs unilaterally due to widening of the pupil either in dark surroundings and/or under emotional stress (dismay or fear). A typical situation is the evening mystery movie on television. Iatrogenic pharmacologic mydriasis and systemic psychotropic drugs can also trigger a glaucoma attack.

Note
It should be borne in mind that mydriatic agents entail a risk of triggering a glaucoma attack by widening the pupil. It is therefore important to evaluate the depth of the anterior chamber in every patient even before a routine fundus examination.

▶ Symptoms
▶ **Acute onset of intense pain.** The elevated intraocular pressure acts on the corneal nerves (the ophthalmic nerve—the first branch of the trigeminal nerve) to cause dull pain. This pain may be referred to the temples, back of the head, and jaws via the three branches of the trigeminal nerve, which can mask its ocular origin.

▶ **Nausea and vomiting.** These occur due to irritation of the vagus nerve and can simulate abdominal disorders. The generalized symptoms such as headache, vomiting, and nausea may dominate to the extent that the patient fails to notice local symptoms.

▶ **Diminished visual acuity.** Patients notice obscured vision and colored halos around lights in the affected eye. These symptoms are caused by the corneal epithelial edema precipitated by the enormous increase in pressure.

▶ **Prodromal symptoms.** Patients report transitory episodes of blurred vision or the appearance of colored halos around lights prior to the attack. These prodromal symptoms may go unnoticed or may be dismissed as unimportant by the patient in mild episodes where the eye returns to normal. Early identification of high-risk patients with shallow anterior chambers and gonioscopic findings is important, as damage to the structures of the angle may be well advanced before clinical symptoms appear.

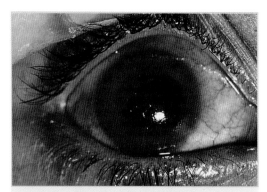

Fig. 10.17 Acute glaucoma attack: pupillary block. Typical symptoms include:
- Conjunctival and ciliary injection (red eye).
- Corneal edema.
- A dull, nonreflecting surface with a dull corneal reflex.
- Opacification of the corneal stroma that obscures the view of the fundus. The iris appears faded, and the anterior chamber is shallow.
- The pupil is oval instead of round, and is fixed and moderately dilated.
- Intraocular pressure is elevated; the eye is rock hard to palpation.
- Severe headache and gastrointestinal symptoms are present.

Note
The full clinical symptoms of acute glaucoma are not always present. The diminished visual acuity may go unnoticed if the other eye has normal vision. Patients' subjective perception of pain intensity can vary greatly.

▶ **Diagnostic considerations** (▶ Fig. 10.17)

Note
The diagnosis is made on the basis of a triad of symptoms:
- Unilateral red eye with conjunctival or ciliary injection.
- Fixed and dilated pupil.
- Hard eyeball on palpation.

▶ **Other findings**
- The cornea is dull and matt with epithelial edema.
- The anterior chamber is shallow or completely collapsed. This will be apparent when the eye is illuminated by a focused lateral light source (▶ Fig. 1.12) and on slit lamp examination. Inspection of the shallow anterior chamber will be difficult. Details of the surface of the iris will be visible, and the iris will appear faded.
- The fundus is generally obscured due to opacification of the corneal epithelium. When the fundus can be visualized as symptoms subside and the cornea clears, the spectrum of changes to the optic disc will range from a normal vital optic disc to an ill-defined hyperemic optic nerve. In the latter case, venous congestion will be present. The central artery of the retina will be seen to pulsate on the optic disc as blood can only enter the eye during the systolic phase due to the high intraocular pressure.
- Visual acuity is reduced to perception of hand motions.

▶ **Differential diagnosis.** Misdiagnosis is possible, as the wide variety of symptoms can simulate other disorders.

- **General symptoms** such as headache, vomiting, and nausea often predominate and can easily be mistaken for *appendicitis* or a *brain tumor*.
- **In iritis and iridocyclitis,** the eye is also red and the iris appears faded. However, intraocular pressure tends to be decreased rather than elevated.

▶ **Treatment**

Note
An acute glaucoma attack is an emergency, and the patient requires immediate treatment by an ophthalmologist. The underlying causes of the disorder require surgical treatment, although initial therapy is conservative.

▶ **Medication.** The goals of conservative therapy are to:

- Decrease intraocular pressure.
- Allow the cornea to clear (important for subsequent surgery).
- Relieve pain.

▶ **Timeline of IOP reduction**

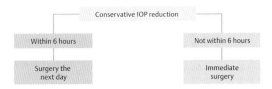

- *Principles of medication in primary angle closure glaucoma* (see ▶ Table 10.3).
- Osmotic reduction in the volume of the vitreous body is achieved via systemic *hyperosmotic solutions* (oral glycerin, 1.0–1.5 g/kg of body weight, or intravenous mannitol, 1.0–2.0 g/kg of body weight).
- Production of aqueous humor is decreased by *inhibiting carbonic anhydrase* (intravenous acetazolamide, 250–500 mg). Both steps are taken initially to reduce intraocular pressure to below 50–60 mm Hg.
- The iris is withdrawn from the angle of the anterior chamber by administering *topical miotic agents.* Pilocarpine 1% eye drops should be applied every 15 minutes. If this is not effective, pilocarpine can be applied more often—every 5 minutes—and in concentrations up to 4%. Miotic agents are not the medications of first choice because the sphincter pupillae muscle is ischemic at pressures exceeding 40 to 50 mm Hg and will not respond to miotic agents. Miotic agents also relax the zonule fibers, which causes anterior displacement of the lens that further compresses the anterior chamber. This makes it important to first initiate therapy with hyperosmotic agents to reduce the volume of the vitreous body.

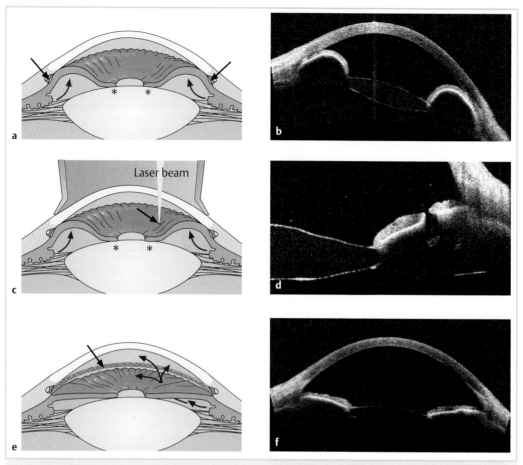

Fig. 10.18 Acute angle closure glaucoma: etiology and treatment. (a) The pupillary block (asterisks) prevents the outflow of the aqueous humor into the anterior chamber. The pressure in the posterior chamber increases (red arrows), and the peripheral iris is pressed against the trabecular meshwork. This blocks the drainage of the aqueous humor and creates an acute angle closure (black arrows). **(b)** OCT of the acute angle closure (in the pseudophakic eye). **(c)** The Nd:YAG laser focused through a contact lens (producing a circumscribed tissue tear) punctures the iris, creating a shunt between the posterior and anterior chambers (black arrow) so that the aqueous humor can flow back into the anterior chamber in spite of the pupillary block (*). **(d)** OCT of the Nd:YAG iridotomy ("small entry opening, larger exit opening"). **(e)** The aqueous humor trapped in the posterior chamber now flows through this newly created opening in the iris, equalizing the pressure in the two chambers and circumventing the pupillary block. The iris recedes into its normal position, the trabecular meshwork (black arrow) opens again, the aqueous humor can drain normally and normal intraocular pressure is restored. With Nd:YAG laser iridotomy, it is no longer possible for a pupillary block to form subsequently. **(f)** The OCT shows that the iris is flattened again and the iridocorneal angle is open.

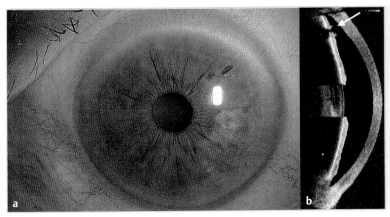

Fig. 10.19 Nd:YAG laser iridotomy. (a) The Nd:YAG laser opening in the iris (arrow) creates a shunt between the posterior and anterior chambers. **(b)** OCT imaging of Nd:YAG laser iridotomy (arrow = incision).

- Symptomatic therapy with *analgesic agents, antiemetic agents,* and *sedatives* can be initiated where necessary.

▶ **Mechanical indentation of the cornea.** Simple repetitive indentation of the central cornea with a muscle hook or glass rod for approximately 15 to 30 seconds presses the aqueous humor into the periphery of the angle of the anterior chamber, which opens the angle. If this manipulation succeeds in keeping the trabecular meshwork open for a few minutes, it will permit aqueous humor to drain and reduce intraocular pressure. This improves the response to pilocarpine and helps clear up the cornea.

▶ **Surgical management (shunt between the posterior and anterior chambers).** Once the cornea is clear, the *underlying causes of the disorder are treated surgically* by creating a shunt between the posterior and anterior chambers.

- *Nd:YAG laser iridotomy (nonincisional procedure):* The Nd:YAG laser can be used to create an opening in the peripheral iris (iridotomy) by tissue lysis without having to open the globe (▶ Fig. 10.18). The operation can be carried out with topical anesthesia (▶ Fig. 10.19).
- *Peripheral iridectomy (incisional procedure):* Where the cornea is still swollen with edema or the iris is very thick, an open procedure may be required to create a shunt. A limbal incision is made at the 12 o'clock position with the patient under topical anesthesia or general anesthesia, through which a basal iridectomy is performed. Peripheral iridectomy is the treatment of choice, when a Nd:YAG laser iridotomy is not possible.

▶ **Prophylaxis.** When the patient reports clear prodromal symptoms and the angle of the anterior chamber appears constricted, the safest prophylaxis is to perform a Nd:YAG laser iridotomy or peripheral iridectomy. If one eye has already suffered an acute attack, the fellow eye should be treated initially every 4 to 6 hours with pilocarpine 1% to minimize the risk of a glaucoma attack. The second eye should then be treated with a Nd:YAG laser to prevent glaucoma once surgical stabilization of the first eye has been achieved.

▶ **Prognosis.** One can usually readily release a pupillary block and lower intraocular pressure in an initial attack with medication and permanently prevent further attacks with surgery. However, recurrent acute angle closure glaucoma or angle closure persisting for longer than 48 hours can produce peripheral synechiae between the root of the iris and the trabecular meshwork opposite it. These persisting cases of angle closure glaucoma cannot be cured by Nd:YAG laser iridotomy or iridectomy, and the angle closure will persist despite surgery. Filtration surgery is indicated in these cases (see p. 162).

Note
When intraocular pressure is controlled and the cornea is clear, gonioscopy is indicated to demonstrate that the angle is open again and to exclude persistent angle closure.

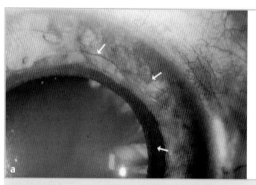
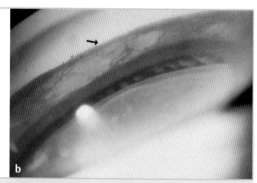

Fig. 10.20 Neovascular glaucoma: secondary angle closure glaucoma with rubeosis iridis. **(a)** Rubeosis iridis. Neovascularization (two upper arrows) is visible on the surface of the iris. Contraction everts the posterior pigmented epithelium of the iris onto the anterior surface of the iris (lower arrow) in a condition known as ectropion uveae. **(b)** Gonioscopy. The angle of the anterior chamber is closed, and the trabecular meshwork is no longer visible (arrow). Rubeosis iridis has drawn the angle of the anterior chamber together like a zipper.

10.5 Secondary Glaucomas

Definition
These glaucomas are caused by other ocular diseases or factors such as inflammation, trauma, bleeding, tumors, medication, and physical or chemical influences (see ▶ Table 10.1, ▶ Table 10.2).

10.5.1 Secondary Open Angle Glaucoma

Definition
The anatomic relationships between the root of the iris, the trabecular meshwork, and peripheral cornea are not disturbed. However, the trabecular meshwork is congested and the resistance to drainage is increased.

▶ **The most important forms**

▶ **Pseudoexfoliative glaucoma.** This form occurs particularly frequently in Scandinavian countries. Deposits of amorphous acellular material form throughout the anterior chamber and congest the trabecular meshwork.

▶ **Pigmentary glaucoma.** Young myopic men typically are affected. The disorder is characterized by release of pigment granules from the pigmentary epithelium of the iris that congest the trabecular meshwork.

▶ **Cortisone glaucoma.** Some 35 to 40% of the population react to 3-week topical or systemic steroid therapy with elevated intraocular pressure. Increased deposits of mucopolysaccharides in the trabecular meshwork presumably increase resistance to outflow; this is reversible when the steroids are discontinued.

▶ **Inflammatory glaucoma.** Two mechanisms contribute to the increase in intraocular pressure:

1. The *viscosity of the aqueous humor increases* as a result of the influx of protein from inflamed iris vessels.
2. The *trabecular meshwork becomes congested* with inflammatory cells and cellular debris.

▶ **Phacolytic glaucoma.** This is acute glaucoma in eyes with mature or hypermature cataracts. Denatured lens protein passes through the intact lens capsule into the anterior chamber and is phagocytosed. The trabecular meshwork becomes congested with protein-binding macrophages and the protein itself.

10.5.2 Secondary Angle Closure Glaucoma

Definition
In secondary angle closure glaucoma as in primary angle closure glaucoma, the increase in intraocular pressure is due to blockage of the trabecular meshwork. However, the primary configuration of the anterior chamber is not the decisive factor.

▶ **The most important causes**

▶ **Rubeosis iridis.** Neovascularization (▶ Fig. 10.20a) draws the angle of the anterior chamber together like a zipper (neovascular glaucoma) (▶ Fig. 10.20b). Ischemic retinal disorders such as *diabetic retinopathy* and *retinal vein occlusion* can lead to rubeosis iridis with progressive closure of the angle of the anterior chamber. Other forms of retinopathy or intraocular tumors can also cause rubeosis iridis. The prognosis for eyes with neovascular glaucoma is poor.

▶ **Trauma.** Posttraumatic presence of blood or exudate in the angle of the anterior chamber and prolonged contact between the iris and trabecular meshwork in a collapsed anterior chamber (following injury, surgery, or insufficient treatment of primary angle closure) can lead to anterior synechiae and angle closure without rubeosis iridis.

▶ **Treatment of secondary glaucomas**

Note
Medication therapy of secondary glaucomas is usually identical to the treatment of primary chronic open angle glaucoma.

Secondary glaucomas can be caused by many different factors, and the angle may be open or closed. Therefore, treatment will depend on the etiology of the glaucoma. The underlying disorder is best treated first. Glaucomas with uveitis (such as iritis or iridocyclitis) initially are treated conservatively with anti-inflammatory and antiglaucoma agents. Surgery is indicated where conservative treatment is not sufficient.

Note
The prognosis for secondary glaucomas is generally poorer than that for primary glaucomas.

10.6 Childhood Glaucomas

Definition
Any abnormal increase in intraocular pressure during the first years of life will cause dilatation of the wall of the globe, and especially of the cornea. The result is a characteristic, abnormally large eye (buphthalmos) with a progressive increase in corneal diameter. This is also referred to as hydrophthalmos or hydrophthalmia.

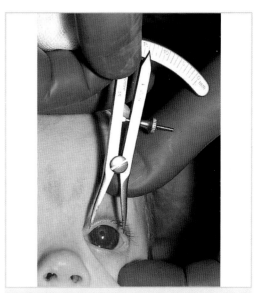

Fig. 10.21 Congenital glaucoma. Examination of a 3-month-old infant with buphthalmos under general anesthesia. The findings include a corneal diameter of 14.0 mm (the normal diameter is approximately 9.5 mm) and stromal opacification.

▶ **Epidemiology.** Glaucomas in children occur once every 12,000 to 18,000 births and account for about 1% of glaucomas. Primary congenital glaucoma is an inherited autosomal-recessive disorder. It is bilateral in approximately 70% of cases; boys are affected in approximately 70% of cases; and glaucoma manifests itself before the age of 6 months in approximately 70% of cases.

Note
There is nowadays widespread public awareness of glaucoma in adults. Unfortunately, this does not yet apply to glaucoma in children.

▶ **Etiology.** (See also Physiology and pathophysiology of aqueous humor circulation in Chapter 10.2.) The iris inserts anteriorly far in the trabecular meshwork (▶ Table 10.2). Embryonic mesodermal tissue in the form of a thin transparent membrane (Barkan's membrane) covers the trabecular meshwork and impedes the flow of aqueous humor into the canal of Schlemm. Other abnormal ocular or systemic findings are lacking.

Apart from isolated buphthalmos, other ocular changes can lead to secondary hydrophthalmos. These include:

- Hydrophthalmia with ocular developmental anomalies.
- Hydrophthalmia with systemic disease.
- Secondary buphthalmos resulting from acquired eye disorders.

Regardless of the cause of the increase in intraocular pressure, the objective signs and clinical symptoms of childhood forms of glaucoma are identical and should be apparent to any examining physician.

▶ **Symptoms.** Classic signs include photophobia, epiphora, corneal opacification, and unilateral or bilateral enlargement of the cornea. These changes may be present from birth (in congenital glaucoma) or may develop shortly after birth or during the first few years of life.

Children with this disorder are irritable, are poor eaters, and rub their eyes often. The behavior of some children may lead one to suspect mental retardation.

Note
Physicians should be alert to parents who boast about their child's "beautiful big eyes" and should measure intraocular pressure. It is essential to diagnose the disorder as early in the child's life as possible to minimize the risk of loss of or irreparable damage to the child's vision.

▶ **Diagnostic considerations.** These examinations can be performed without general anesthesia in many children. However, general anesthesia is occasionally necessary to confirm the diagnosis, especially in older children (▶ Fig. 10.21).

▶ **Measurement of intraocular pressure.** One should generally attempt to measure intraocular pressure by applanation tonometry (tonometry with a hand-held tonometer). Rebound tonometry is a real alternative in children, since there is no need to apply anesthetic drops.

▶ **Optic disc ophthalmoscopy.** The optic cup is a very sensitive indicator of intraocular pressure, particularly in the phase in which permanent visual field defects occur. Asymmetry in the optic cup can be helpful in diagnosing the disorder and in follow-up.

Note
Measurement is facilitated by giving the hungry infant a bottle during the examination. Feeding distracts the baby, and a measurement usually can be obtained easily. Such a measurement is usually far more accurate than one obtained under general anesthesia as narcotics, especially barbiturates and halothane, reduce intraocular pressure.

▶ **Special considerations.** A glaucomatous optic cup in children may well be reversible. Often it will be significantly smaller within several hours of a successful trabeculotomy.

▶ **Inspection of the cornea.** The cornea will appear whitish and opacified due to epithelial edema. Breaks in Descemet's membrane can exacerbate an epithelial or stromal edema. These lesions, known as Haab's striae, will exhibit a typical horizontal or curvilinear configuration.

The enlarged corneal diameter is a characteristic finding. The cornea measures 9.5 mm on average in normal newborn infants. Enlargement to more than 10.5 mm suggests childhood glaucoma. Chronically elevated intraocular pressure in children under the age of 3 years will lead to enlargement of the entire globe.

▶ **Gonioscopy of the angle of the anterior chamber.** Examination of the angle of the anterior chamber provides crucial etiologic information. The angle will not be fully differentiated. Embryonic tissue will be seen to occlude the trabecular meshwork.

▶ **Differential diagnosis**
▶ **Large eyes.** A large corneal diameter can occur as a harmless anomaly (megalocornea) (see p. 74).

▶ **Corneal opacification.** Diffuse corneal opacification with epithelial edema occurs in congenital hereditary endothelial dystrophy. Opacification without epithelial edema occurs in mucopolysaccharidosis (Hurler's syndrome, Scheie's syndrome, Morquio's syndrome, and Maroteaux–Lamy syndrome).

▶ **Striae in Descemet's membrane.** In contrast to the horizontal Haab's striae in congenital glaucoma, endothelial breaks can also occur as a result of injury during a forceps delivery (vertical striae), in keratoconus (see p. 72), and in deep keratitis.

Note
None of these differential diagnoses is accompanied by elevated intraocular pressure.

▶ **Treatment.** Childhood glaucomas are treated surgically. The prognosis improves the earlier surgery is performed.

▶ **Principle and procedure of goniotomy.** With a gonioscope in place on the eye, the goniotomy scalpel is advanced through the anterior chamber to the trabecular meshwork. The trabecular meshwork can now be incised as far as the canal of Schlemm over an arc of about 120° to permit drainage of the aqueous humor. Often two or three goniotomies at different locations are required to control intraocular pressure. These operations can only be performed when the cornea is clear enough to allow visualization of the structures of the anterior chamber.

▶ **Principle and procedure of trabeculotomy.** After a conjunctival flap and split-thickness scleral flap have been raised, access to the canal of Schlemm is gained through a radial incision, and the canal is probed with a trabeculotome. Then the trabeculotome is rotated into the anterior chamber (▶ Fig. 10.22). This tears through the inner wall of the canal, the trabecular meshwork, and any embryonic tissue covering it to open a drainage route for the aqueous humor.

A higher rate of success is attributed to trabeculotomy when performed as an initial procedure. This operation can also be performed when the cornea is largely opacified.

▶ **Prognosis.** Goniotomies and trabeculotomies are not always successful. Even after apparently successful initial trabecular surgery, these children require a lifetime of follow-up examinations (initially several times a year and later once every year) as elevated intraocular pressure can recur, in which case repeat goniotomy or trabeculotomy is indicated.

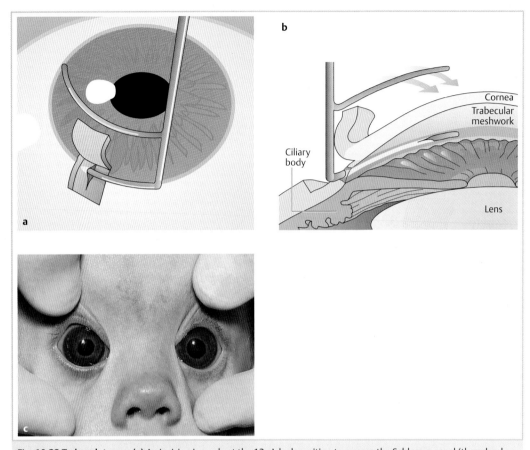

Fig. 10.22 Trabeculotomy. **(a)** An incision is made at the 12 o'clock position to expose the Schlemm canal (the scleral venous sinus), which is then probed with a trabeculotome. The trabeculotome is then rotated into the anterior chamber, tearing through the embryonic tissue occluding the angle. The aqueous humor can now readily drain into the Schlemm canal. **(b)** The surgeon can observe the rotation of the trabeculotome directly through a gonioscope placed on the eye during the operation. **(c)** The right and left eyes following successful trabeculotomy (the photograph shows the same child as in ▶ Fig. 10.21). Both eyes show a clear cornea (normal corneal light reflex) and normal intraocular pressure.

Chapter 11

Vitreous Body

11 Vitreous Body

Christoph W. Spraul and Gerhard K. Lang

11.1 Basic Knowledge

▶ **Importance of the vitreous body for the eye.** The vitreous body stabilizes the globe although the eye can remain intact without the vitreous body (see Vitrectomy, p. 183). It also prevents retinal detachment.

▶ **Embryology.** The development of the vitreous body can be divided into three phases.
• **First phase** (first month of pregnancy; fetus measures 5–13 mm from cranium to coccyx). The **primary vitreous** forms during this period. This phase is characterized by the entry of mesenchyme into the optic cup through the embryonic choroidal fissure. The main *function of the primary vitreous* is to supply the developing lens with nourishment. In keeping with this function, it consists mainly of a vascular plexus, and the *anterior and posterior tunica vasculosa lentis,* that cover the anterior and posterior surfaces of the lens. This vascular plexus is supplied by the hyaloid artery and its branches (▶ Fig. 11.1). This vascular system and the primary vitreous regress as the posterior lens capsule develops at the end of the second month of pregnancy.
• **Second phase** (second month of pregnancy; fetus measures 14–70 mm from cranium to coccyx). The **secondary vitreous** forms during this period. This avascular vitreous body consisting of fine undulating collagen fibers develops from what later becomes the retina. In normal development it expands to compress the central primary vitreous into a residual central canal (**hyaloid canal** or **Cloquet's canal**).
• **Third phase** (third month of pregnancy; fetus measures 71–110 mm from cranium to coccyx). The **tertiary vitreous** develops from existing structures in the secondary vitreous. The secondary vitreous remains. The *zonule fibers* that form the suspensory ligament of the lens develop during this period.

▶ **Composition of the vitreous body.** The gelatinous vitreous body consists of 98% water and 2% collagen and hyaluronic acid. It fills the vitreous chamber, which accounts for approximately two-thirds of the total volume of the eye.

▶ **Stabilization and confines of the vitreous body.** With their high negative electrostatic potential, the hyaluronic acid molecules fill the three-dimensional collagen fiber network and provide mechanical stability. *Condensation of peripheral collagen fibrils* creates a **boundary membrane** (**hyaloid membrane**), which is *not a basement*

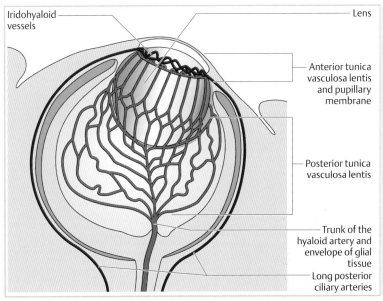

Iridohyaloid vessels

Lens

Anterior tunica vasculosa lentis and pupillary membrane

Posterior tunica vasculosa lentis

Trunk of the hyaloid artery and envelope of glial tissue

Long posterior ciliary arteries

Fig. 11.1 Transitory embryonic vascular supply. The anterior tunica vasculosa lentis (dark red) forms anastomoses with the posterior tunica vasculosa lentis (light red) through the iridohyaloid vessels.

membrane. It is attached to adjacent structures at the following locations (▶ Fig. 11.2):
- At the **ligament of Wieger** along the posterior capsule of the lens.
- At the **vitreous base** at the ora serrata.
- At the **funnel of Martegiani** (approximately 10 μm wide) surrounding the periphery of the optic disc.

The connections between the vitreous body and retina are generally loose, although there may be firm focal adhesions. These firmer focal attachments cause problems during vitreous detachment (see p. 208) because they do not permit the vitreous body to become completely detached. The focal adhesions between the vitreous body and retina produce focal traction forces that act on the retina and can cause retinal tears and detachment.

▶ **Neurovascular supply.** The vitreous body contains neither blood vessels nor nerves. As a result, pathogens can multiply undisturbed for a relatively long time before the onset of an immune response from adjacent structures.

11.2 Examination Methods

The anterior third of the vitreous body can be readily examined with a **slit lamp**. An additional **contact lens** (see p. 192) or **hand-held condensing lens** (+60, +78, and +90 diopters) is required to examine the posterior portions. **Indirect ophthal-** moscopy (see p. 192) or **retroillumination** (Brückner's test, see p. 104) is usually used to examine the vitreous body in its entirety. Opacities will appear as dark shadows. **Ultrasound examination** of the vitreous body is performed in cases such as a mature cataract where visualization by other methods is not possible.

11.3 Aging Changes

11.3.1 Synchysis

The regular arrangement of collagen fibers gradually deteriorates in middle age. The fibers condense to flattened filamentous structures. This process, known as liquefaction, creates small fluid-filled lacunae in the central vitreous body that initially are largely asymptomatic (patients may report floaters). However, once liquefaction has progressed beyond a certain point, the vitreous body can collapse and detach from the retina.

11.3.2 Vitreous Detachment

Definition
Complete or partial detachment of the vitreous body from its underlying tissue. The most common form is *posterior vitreous detachment* (see ▶ Fig. 11.3a); *anterior* or *basal vitreous detachment* is much rarer.

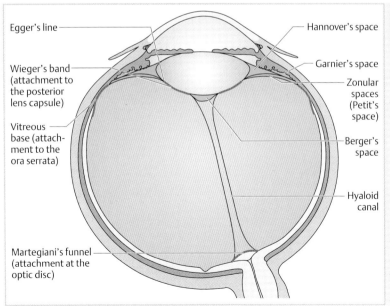

Egger's line

Wieger's band (attachment to the posterior lens capsule)

Vitreous base (attachment to the ora serrata)

Martegiani's funnel (attachment at the optic disc)

Hannover's space

Garnier's space

Zonular spaces (Petit's space)

Berger's space

Hyaloid canal

Fig. 11.2 Attachments of the vitreous body and adjacent spaces. The attachments of the vitreous body are identified by thick red lines and listed on the left. Spaces adjacent to the vitreous body are shown in green and listed on the right.

▶ **Epidemiology.** Six percent of patients between the ages of 54 and 65 years and 65% of patients between the ages of 65 and 85 years have posterior vitreous detachment. Patients with axial myopia (see p. 278) have a predisposition to early vitreous detachment. Presumably the vitreous body collapses earlier in these patients because it has to fill a "longer" eye with a larger volume.

▶ **Etiology.** Liquefaction causes collapse of the vitreous body. This usually begins posteriorly where the attachments to the underlying tissue are least well developed. Detachment in the anterior region (*anterior vitreous detachment*) or in the region of the vitreous base (*basal vitreous detachment*) usually only occurs where strong forces act on the globe as in ocular trauma.

▶ **Symptoms and findings.** *Collapse of the vitreous body* leads to vitreous densities that the patient perceives as mobile opacities. These floaters (also known as flies or cobwebs) may take the form of circular or serpentine lines or points. Detachment of the vitreous body is always pain-free. The symptoms may be so slight that patients do not even notice this detachment. The vitreous body may detach partially or completely from the retina. An increased risk of retinal detachment is present only with *partial vitreous detachment*. In this case, the vitreous body and retina remain attached, with the result that eye movements in this region will place traction on the retina. The patient perceives this phenomenon as **flashes of light**. If the traction on the retina becomes too strong, it can tear (see development of a retinal foramen in ▶ Fig. 11.3b, c). This increases the risk of retinal detachment (see

p. 208) and vitreous bleeding (see p. 179) from injured vessels.

Note
Floaters and especially flashes of light require thorough examination of the ocular fundus to exclude a retinal tear.

▶ **Diagnostic considerations.** The symptoms of vitreous detachment require examination of the entire fundus of the eye to exclude a retinal defect. Examination reveals streaks or clouding in the vitreous body or, if there is hemorrhage, residual fresh blood in the vitreous body or around the retina. In cases such as lens opacification or vitreous hemorrhage where visualization is not possible, an ultrasound examination is required to evaluate the vitreous body and retina.

Note
Vitreous detachment in the region of the attachment at the optic disc (*funnel of Martegiani*) will appear as a smoky ring (*Weiss ring*) under ophthalmoscopy (▶ Fig. 11.4).

▶ **Treatment.** The symptoms of vitreous detachment resolve spontaneously once the vitreous body is completely detached. However, the complications that can accompany partial vitreous detachment require treatment. These include vitreous body bleeding, retinal tears, and retinal detachment. For treatment see Chapter 12.4.

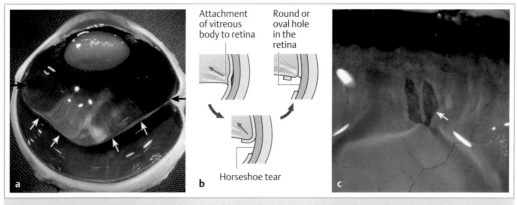

Fig. 11.3 Retinal tears in posterior vitreous detachment. **(a)** Complete posterior vitreous detachment (arrows). **(b)** This can produce traction at the posterior attachment of the base of the vitreous body (red arrows) to the retina, causing retinal tears. **(c)** Manifest retinal foramen (arrow) (cadaver eye).

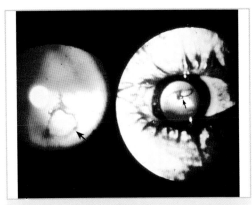

Fig. 11.4 Weiss ring. The smoky ring appears when the vitreous body detaches from its attachment at the optic disc at the funnel of Martegiani (arrow).

11.4 Abnormal Changes in the Vitreous Body

11.4.1 Persistent Fetal Vasculature (Developmental Anomalies)

The embryonic vascular system in the vitreous body and lens normally disappears completely, leaving only the *hyaloid canal*. Persistence of the vascular system is referred to as **persistent fetal vasculature.** The following section describes the varying degrees of severity of this syndrome as they relate to the vitreous body. Persistence of the anterior tunica vasculosa lentis leads to a persistent pupillary membrane.

Mittendorf's Dot

Mittendorf's dot is a small, visually asymptomatic opacity in the posterior lens capsule located approximately 0.5 mm medial to the center. This is the site where the hyaloid artery enters the embryonic lens. This harmless alteration occurs in up to 2% of the total population. Normal lens fiber development *can* be disturbed where *large* portions of the hyaloid arterial system remain, although this occurs very rarely. These patients develop posterior polar cataracts (see p. 112).

Bergmeister's Papilla

For details of Bergmeister's papilla, see page 236.

Persistent Hyaloid Artery

Isolated persistence of the hyaloid artery is rare. Usually this phenomenon is accompanied by persistence of the hyperplastic primary vitreous (see the next section). A persistent hyaloid artery will appear as a whitish cord in the hyaloid canal proceeding from the optic disc and extending to the posterior capsule of the lens. Isolated persistence of the hyaloid artery is asymptomatic and does not require treatment.

Persistent Hyperplastic Primary Vitreous (PHPV)

Definition
Persistence of the embryonic primary vitreous (hyaloid arterial system including the posterior tunica vasculosa lentis).

▶ **Epidemiology.** This developmental anomaly is very rare.

▶ **Symptoms and findings.** Usually the disorder is *unilateral.*

▶ **Anterior variant of PHPV.** With this *more frequent* variant, a *white pupil* (leukocoria or amaurotic cat's eye) typically will be discovered shortly after birth. This is caused by the whitish plate of connective tissue posterior to the lens. Depending on the severity, it will be accompanied by more or less severe changes in the lens leading to more or less severely impaired vision. In extreme cases, the lens resembles an opacified membrane (*membranous cataract*). In rare cases, fatty tissue will develop (*lipomatous pseudophakia*), and even more rarely *cartilage will develop in the lens.* Retrolenticular scarring draws the ciliary processes toward center, and they will be visible in the pupil. Growth of the eye is retarded. This results in *microphthalmos* unless drainage of the aqueous humor is also impaired, in which case *buphthalmos* (*hydrophthalmos*) will be present.

▶ **Posterior variant of PHPV.** Retinal detachment and *retinal dysplasia* can occur where primarily posterior embryonic structures persist. The whitish plate of connective tissue will only be visible where anterior changes associated with persistent hyperplastic primary vitreous are also present. The reduction in visual acuity will vary depending on the severity of the retinal changes.

► **Diagnostic considerations.** A definitive diagnosis is usually possible on the basis of the characteristic clinical picture (see Symptoms and findings above) and additional ultrasound studies (when the posterior segment is obscured by lens opacities).

► **Differential diagnosis.** Other causes of leukocoria (► Table 11.1) should be excluded. Retinoblastoma, the most important differential diagnosis, can usually be excluded on the basis of ultrasound or CT studies. In the presence of a retinoblastoma, these studies will reveal an intraocular mass with calcifications. In contrast to PHPV, *microphthalmos* will not be present.

Note
Leukocoria should be regarded as a retinoblastoma until proven otherwise.

► **Treatment.** The disorder is not usually treated, as neither conservative therapy nor surgery can improve visual acuity. Surgery is indicated only where complications such as progressive collapse of the anterior chamber, secondary increase in intraocular pressure, vitreous hemorrhage, and retinal detachment are present or imminent. The only goal is to save the eye and maintain existing visual acuity.

► **Clinical course and prognosis.** The clinical course and prognosis depend primarily on the severity of the disorder. However, adequate surgical intervention can often save the eye and stabilize visual acuity even if at a very low level.

11.4.2 Abnormal Opacities of the Vitreous Body

Asteroid Hyalosis

These usually unilateral opacities of the vitreous body (75% of cases) are not all that infrequent. They are thought to be linked to diabetes mellitus and hypercholesterolemia. The disorder is characterized by white calcific deposits that are associated with the collagen fibers of the vitreous body and therefore are not very mobile (► Fig. 11.5). Most patients are not bothered by these opacities. However, the examiner's view of the fundus can be significantly obscured by "snow flurries" of white opacities. Interestingly, these opacities do not interfere with fluorescein angiography. Vitrectomy (see p. 183) to remove the opacities is rarely necessary and is performed only when the opacities adversely affect the patient—i.e., when visual acuity is diminished.

Synchysis Scintillans

These *very rare* opacities of the vitreous body usually occur unilaterally following recurrent intraocular inflammation or bleeding. In contrast to asteroid hyalosis, these opacities are free-floating cholesterol crystals in the vitreous chamber that respond to gravity. Whetstone-shaped crystals are histologically typical. Surgery is only indicated in rare cases in which the opacities impair visual acuity.

Table 11.1 Differential diagnosis of leukocoria

Possible causes	Differential criteria
Congenital cataract (4–8:20,000)	Early infancy, unilateral or bilateral, normal globe size
Retinoblastoma (1:20,000)	Infancy, normal globe size, unilateral (two-thirds) or bilateral (one-third), calcifications in tumor
Retinopathy of prematurity, grade V (1:20,000)	Early infancy, usually bilateral, no microphthalmos, preterm birth with oxygen therapy
Exudative retinitis (Coats's disease)	Childhood, unilateral
Persistent hyperplastic primary vitreous	Usually unilateral, usually microphthalmos, connatal, centrally displaced ciliary processes
Tumors	Astrocytoma, medulloepithelioma
Exudative retinal detachment	In toxocariasis, angiomatosis retinae (von Hippel–Lindau tumor), diffuse choroidal hemangioma
Other causes	Norrie's disease, incontinentia pigmenti (Bloch–Sulzberger disease), juvenile retinoschisis, retinal dysplasia, vitreous abscess, myelinized nerve fibers, coloboma of the optic disc (morning glory disc), foreign bodies in the vitreous chamber

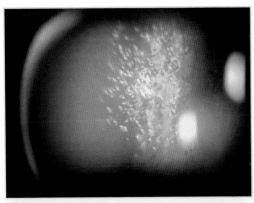

Fig. 11.5 Asteroid hyalosis. The vitreous humor is infiltrated with whitish-yellow, only slightly mobile deposits that significantly impede examination of the ocular fundus.

Vitreous Amyloidosis

This *rare* inherited autosomal-dominant disorder begins at the age of about 20 years, progresses for decades, and finally leads to diminished visual acuity. Amyloidosis causes characteristic amyloid deposits around the collagen fibers of the vitreous body except for the hyaloid canal, which remains unaffected. The amyloid exhibits histologically typical staining. The disorder can be treated by vitrectomy.

11.4.3 Vitreous Hemorrhage

Definition
Bleeding into the vitreous chamber or a space created by vitreous detachment.

▶ **Epidemiology.** The annual incidence of this disorder is 7 cases per 100,000.

▶ **Etiology.** A vitreous hemorrhage may involve one of three possible **pathogenetic mechanisms** (▶ Fig. 11.6):
1. Bleeding from *normal retinal vessels*, which can occur as a result of mechanical vascular damage in acute vitreous detachment or retinal tear.
2. Bleeding from *retinal vessels with abnormal changes*, which can occur as a result of retinal neovascularization in ischemic retinopathy or retinal macroaneurysms.

3. *Influx of blood from the retina or other sources* such as the subretinal space or the anterior segments of the eye.

More frequent causes of vitreous hemorrhage include
• Posterior vitreous detachment with or without retinal tears (38%).
• Proliferative diabetic retinopathy (32%).
• Branch retinal vein occlusion (11 %).
• Age-related macular degeneration (2%).
• Retinal macroaneurysm (2%).

Less frequent causes of vitreous hemorrhage include
• Arteriosclerosis.
• Retinal periphlebitis.
• Terson syndrome (subarachnoid hemorrhage, increase in intraocular pressure, acutely impaired drainage of blood from the eye, dilatation and rupture of retinal vessels, retinal and vitreous hemorrhage).
• Penetrating trauma.
• Retinal vascular tumors.

▶ **Symptoms.** Patients often report the sudden occurrence of black opacities that they may describe as "*swarms of black bugs*" or "*black rain.*" These are distinct from the brighter and less dense floaters seen in synchysis and vitreous detachment. Severe vitreous hemorrhage can significantly reduce *visual acuity.* Approximately 10 μL of blood is sufficient to reduce visual acuity to the perception of hand movements in front of the eye.

▶ **Diagnostic considerations.** *Hemorrhages into the vitreous body itself* do not exhibit any characteristic limitations but spread *diffusely* (the blood cannot form a fluid meniscus in the *gelatinous* vitreous body) and coagulation occurs quickly (▶ Fig. 11.7a). Vitreous hemorrhages require examination with an ophthalmoscope or contact lens. The contact lens also permits examination of the retina at a higher resolution so that the examiner is better able to diagnose small retinal tears than with an ophthalmoscope. Ultrasound studies are indicated where severe bleeding significantly obscures the fundus examination. *Bleeding in the tissues adjacent to the vitreous body*—i.e., in the retrohyaloid space, Berger's space, or Petit's space (see ▶ Fig. 11.2)—can produce a *characteristic fluid meniscus.* This meniscus will be visible under slit lamp examination (▶ Fig. 11.7b).

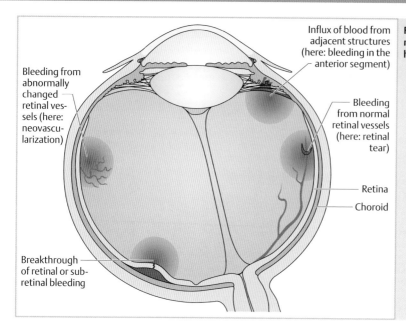

Fig. 11.6 Pathogenetic mechanisms of vitreous hemorrhage.

Influx of blood from adjacent structures (here: bleeding in the anterior segment)

Bleeding from abnormally changed retinal vessels (here: neovascularization)

Bleeding from normal retinal vessels (here: retinal tear)

Retina

Choroid

Breakthrough of retinal or sub-retinal bleeding

▶ **Treatment.** Patients with acute vitreous hemorrhage should be placed in an *upright resting position.* This has two beneficial effects:
- The bleeding usually does not continue to spread into the vitreous body.
- The blood in the retrohyaloid space will settle more quickly.

Next, the *cause of the vitreous hemorrhage* should be treated—for example, a retinal tear can be treated with a laser. Vitrectomy will be required to drain any vitreous hemorrhage that is not absorbed.

▶ **Clinical course and prognosis.** Absorption of a vitreous hemorrhage is a long process. The clinical course will depend on the location, cause, and severity of the bleeding. Bleeding in the vitreous body itself is absorbed particularly slowly.

11.4.4 Vitreitis and Endophthalmitis

Definition
This refers to acute or chronic intraocular inflammation due to microbial or immunologic causes. In the strict sense, any intraocular inflammation is endophthalmitis. However, in clinical usage and throughout this book, endophthalmitis refers only to inflammation caused by a microbial action that also involves the vitreous body (vitreitis). On the other hand, isolated vitreitis without involvement of the other intraocular structures is inconceivable due to the avascularity of the vitreous chamber.

▶ **Epidemiology.** Microbial vitreitis or endophthalmitis occurs most frequently as a result of penetrating trauma to the globe. Rarely (in 0.5% of cases), it is a complication of incisive intraocular surgery.

▶ **Etiology.** Because the vitreous body consists of only a few cellular elements (hyalocytes), inflammation of the vitreous body is only possible when the inflammatory cells can gain access to the vitreous chamber from the uveal tract or retinal blood vessels. This may occur via one of the following mechanisms:

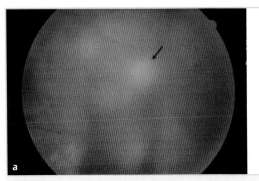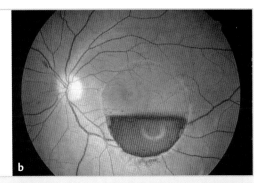

Fig. 11.7 Forms of vitreous hemorrhage. (a) Diffuse vitreous hemorrhage. The view of the fundus is obscured by the vitreous hemorrhage; details are clouded or completely obscured. The arrow indicates the optic disc. (b) Retrohyaloid bleeding with formation of a fluid meniscus. The image shows bleeding into a space created by a circular vitreous detachment. Gravity has caused the erythrocytes to sink and form a pool with a horizontal surface.

- **Microbial pathogens**—i.e., bacteria, fungi, or viruses, enter the vitreous chamber either through direct contamination (for example, via penetrating trauma or incisive intraocular surgery) or metastatically as a result of sepsis. The virulence of the pathogens and the patient's individual immune status determine whether an *acute, subacute,* or *chronic* inflammation will develop. Bacterial inflammation is far more frequent than viral or fungal inflammation. However, the metastatic form of endophthalmitis is observed in immunocompromised patients. Usually the inflammation is fungal (mycotic endophthalmitis), and most often it is caused by one of the *Candida* species.
- **Inflammatory (microbial or autoimmune) processes, in structures adjacent to the vitreous body,** such as uveitis or retinitis, can precipitate a secondary reaction in the vitreous chamber.

> **Note**
> Acute endophthalmitis is a serious clinical syndrome that can result in loss of the eye within a few hours.

▶ **Symptoms**
▶ **Acute vitreous inflammation or endophthalmitis.** Characteristic symptoms include acute loss of visual acuity accompanied by deep dull ocular pain that responds only minimally to analgesic agents. Severe reddening of the conjunctiva is present. In contrast to bacterial or viral endophthalmitis, mycotic endophthalmitis begins as a subacute disorder characterized by slowly worsening chronic visual impairment. Days or weeks later, this will also be accompanied by severe pain.

▶ **Chronic vitreous inflammation or endophthalmitis.** The clinical course is far less severe, and the loss of visual acuity is often moderate.

▶ **Diagnostic considerations.** The patient's history and the presence of typical symptoms provide important information.

▶ **Acute vitreous inflammation or endophthalmitis.** Slit lamp examination will reveal massive conjunctival and ciliary injection accompanied by hypopyon (collection of pus in the anterior chamber). Ophthalmoscopy will reveal yellowish-green discoloration of the vitreous body occasionally referred to as a *vitreous body abscess.* If the view is obscured, ultrasound studies can help to evaluate the *extent of the involvement of the vitreous body in endophthalmitis.* Roth's spots (white retinal spots surrounded by hemorrhage) and circumscribed retinochoroiditis with a vitreous infiltrate will be observed in the initial stages (during the first few days) of *mycotic endophthalmitis.* In advanced stages, the vitreous infiltrate has a creamy whitish appearance, and retinal detachment can occur.

▶ **Chronic vitreous inflammation or endophthalmitis.** Inspection will usually reveal only moderate conjunctival and ciliary injection. Slit lamp examination will reveal infiltration of the vitreous body by inflammatory cells.

A conjunctival smear, a sample of vitreous aspirate, and (where sepsis is suspected) blood cultures should be obtained for microbiological examination to identify the pathogen. Negative microbial results do not exclude possible microbial inflammation; the clinical findings are decisive. See Chapter 12.7 for diagnosis of retinitis and uveitis.

▶ **Differential diagnosis.** The diagnosis is made by clinical examination in most patients. Intraocular lymphoma should be excluded in chronic forms of the disorder that fail to respond to antibiotic therapy.

▶ **Treatment. Microbial inflammations** require pathogen-specific systemic, topical, and intravitreal therapy, where possible according to the strain's documented resistance to antibiotics. *Mycotic endophthalmitis* is usually treated with amphotericin B and steroids. Immediate vitrectomy is a therapeutic option whose indications have yet to be clearly defined.

Secondary vitreous reactions in the presence of underlying retinitis or uveitis should be addressed by treating the underlying disorder.

▶ **Prophylaxis.** Intraocular surgery requires extreme care to avoid intraocular contamination with pathogens. Immunocompromised patients (such as AIDS patients or substance abusers) and patients with indwelling catheters should undergo regular examination by an ophthalmologist.

Note
Decreased visual acuity and eye pain in substance abusers and patients with indwelling catheters suggest *Candida* endophthalmitis.

▶ **Clinical course and prognosis.** The prognosis for **acute microbial endophthalmitis** depends on the virulence of the pathogen and how quickly effective antimicrobial therapy can be initiated. Extremely virulent pathogens such as *Pseudomonas* and delayed initiation of treatment (not within a few hours) worsen the prognosis for visual acuity. With postoperative inflammation and poor initial visual acuity, an immediate vitrectomy can improve the clinical course of the disorder. The prognosis is usually far better for **chronic forms** and secondary vitreitis in uveitis/vitreitis.

11.4.5 Vitreoretinal Dystrophies

Juvenile Retinoschisis

Juvenile retinoschisis is an inherited X-linked recessive disorder that *affects only males*. A retinal schisis at the macula, sometimes referred to clinically as a "spoke phenomenon," usually develops between the ages of 20 and 30 years. This is associated with a significant loss of visual acuity. A peripheral retinal schisis is also present in about one-half of these cases. This splitting of the retina is presumably due to traction of the vitreous body. This *splitting occurs in the nerve fiber layer* in contrast to typical senile retinoschisis (see p. 211), in which *splitting occurs in the outer plexiform layer.*

Wagner's Disease

This disorder is also inherited (autosomal-dominant) and involves central liquefaction of the vitreous body. This "visual void" in the vitreous chamber and fibrillary condensation of the vitreous stroma associated with a cataract characterize *vitreoretinal degeneration in Wagner's disease.*

11.5 The Role of the Vitreous Body in Various Ocular Changes and after Cataract Surgery

11.5.1 Retinal Detachment

The close connection between the vitreous body and retina can result in retinal tears in vitreous detachment, which in turn can lead to **rhegmatogenous retinal detachment** (from the Greek word *rhegma* meaning "breakage") (see p. 208).

These retinal defects provide an opening for cells from the retinal pigment epithelium to enter the vitreous chamber. These pigment cells migrate along the surface of the retina. As they do so, they act similarly to myofibroblasts and lead to the formation of subretinal and epiretinal membranes and cause *contraction of the surface of the retina.* This clinical picture is referred to as **proliferative vitreoretinopathy** (PVR). The rigid retinal folds and vitreous membranes in proliferative vitreoretinopathy significantly complicate reattachment of the retina. Usually this requires modern techniques of vitreous surgery.

11.5.2 Retinal Vascular Proliferation

Retinal vascular proliferation can occur in retinal ischemia in disorders such as diabetic retinopathy, retinopathy in preterm infants, central or branch retinal vein occlusion, and sickle-cell retinopathy. *Growth of this retinal neovascularization into the vitreous chamber* usually occurs only where vitreous detachment is absent or partial because these proliferations require a substrate to grow on. Preretinal proliferations often lead to *vitreous hemorrhage.* Fibrotic changes produce traction of the retina resulting in a *tractional* retinal detachment (see p. 208).

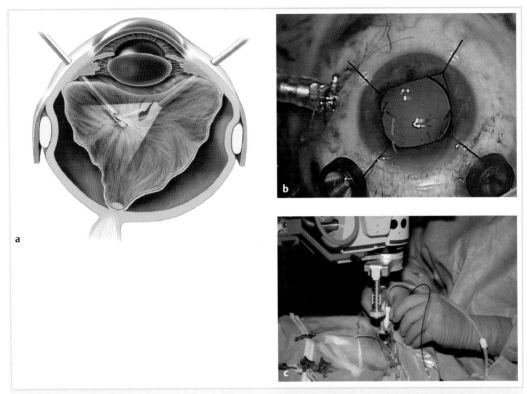

Fig. 11.8 Pars plana vitrectomy. (a) A vitrectome (suction cutting instrument, left) and a light source (right) are pictured; both of these are introduced into the vitreous humor through the pars plana. **(b)** Operative site of the pars plana vitrectomy: the pupil is widened with iris hooks; the infusion cannula is sutured in at the upper left. The two blue plastic parts are self-sealing working trocars through which the vitrectome and the light source are introduced. **(c)** Operative site with operating microscope, BIOM (wide-angle objective) and surgeon's hand position.

11.5.3 Cataract Surgery

Increased postoperative inflammation in the anterior segment can progress through the *hyaloid canal* to the posterior pole of the eye and a cystoid macular edema can develop. (Hruby–Irvine–Gass syndrome is the development of cystoid macular edema following intracapsular cataract extraction with incarceration of the vitreous body in the wound.) This complication occurs particularly frequently following cataract surgery in which the posterior lens capsule was opened with partial loss of vitreous body.

11.6 Surgical Treatment: Vitrectomy

Definition
Surgical removal and replacement of the vitreous body with Ringer's solution, gas, or silicone oil.

▶ **Indication.** The primary indications include:
- Unabsorbed vitreous hemorrhage.
- Removal of epiretinal membranes from the macula ("macular pucker" or epiretinal gliosis).
- Tractional retinal detachment.
- Proliferative vitreoretinopathy.
- Removal of intravitreal displaced lenses or foreign bodies.
- Severe postoperative or posttraumatic inflammatory vitreous changes.

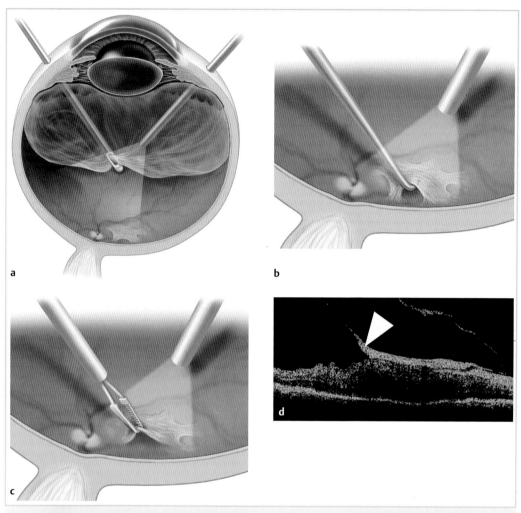

Fig. 11.9. Pars plana vitrectomy and removal of an epiretinal gliosis (membrane on the macula, "macular pucker"), graphical depiction of the operation. **(a)** Removing the vitreous humor. **(b)** Identifying and preparing the membrane. **(c)** Stripping the membrane from the retina with forceps. **(d)** OCT representation of the epiretinal gliosis membrane (arrowhead) that is surgically stripped from the retina.

▶ **Procedure.** The vitreous body cannot simply be aspirated from the eye as the vitreoretinal attachments would also cause retinal detachment. The procedure requires *successive, piecemeal cutting and aspiration with a vitrectome* (a specialized cutting and aspirating instrument). Cutting and aspiration of the vitreous body is performed with the aid of simultaneous infusion to prevent the globe from collapsing. The surgical site is illuminated by a fiberoptic light source. The three instruments (infusion cannula, light source, and vitrectome), all 1 mm in diameter, are introduced into the globe through the pars plana, which is why the procedure is referred to as a *pars plana vitrectomy* (PPV) (▶ Fig. 11.8). This site entails the least risk of iatrogenic retinal detachment. The surgeon holds the vitrectome in one hand and the light source in the other. The procedure is performed under an operating microscope with special contact lenses placed on the corneal surface. Once the vitreous body and any vitreous membranes have been removed, the retina can be treated intraoperatively with a laser (for example, to treat proliferative diabetic retinopathy or to repair a retinal tear). In many cases, such as with an unabsorbed vitreous hemorrhage, it is sufficient to fill the eye with Ringer's solution following vitrectomy, and there is no need for gas or silicone oil.

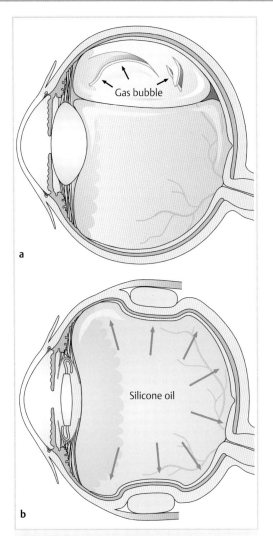

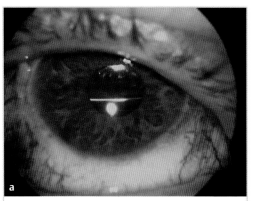

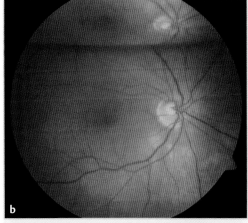

Fig. 11.11 Use of gas after pars plana vitrectomy. (a) Eye filled with gas after pars plana vitrectomy, gas level in the lower third of the pupil is visible. **(b)** In ophthalmoscopic examination of the fundus, the papilla is reflected at the surface of the gas bubble.

Fig. 11.10 Use of gas and silicone oil in vitreoretinal surgery. (a) An intraocular gas bubble exerts pressure primarily in the superior area (arrows) due to its buoyancy. This must be considered when positioning the patient postoperatively; the patient should be positioned in such a way that the foramen lies in this region. **(b)** Completely filling the globe with silicone oil fixes the retina to its underlying tissue at practically every location (arrows). This requires initial complete removal of the vitreous humor as part of the vitrectomy.

One of the most frequent indications for the pars plana vitrectomy is removal of epiretinal membranes. Gliotic tissue resting on the macula leads to metamorphopsia (distortions) and loss of vision. Removal of the membrane from the macula can restore vision and eliminate distortions (▶ Fig. 11.9).

Filling the eye with Ringer's solution is not sufficient to treat a **complicated retinal detachment** with epiretinal or subretinal membranes and contraction of the surface of the retina (so-called proliferative vitreoretinopathy, see p. 182). In these cases, the detached retina must be flattened from anterior to posterior and held with a tamponade of fluid with a very high specific gravity such as a perfluorocarbon liquid. These "heavy" liquids can also be used to float artificial lenses that have become displaced in the vitreous body. The artificial lenses have a lower specific gravity than these liquids and will float on them. At the end of the operation, these heavy liquids must be replaced with gases, such as a mixture of air and sulfur hexafluoride, that are spontaneously absorbed within a few days or with silicone oil (which must be removed in a second operation). Postoperative patient positioning should reflect the fact that maximum gas pressure will be in the superior region (▶ Fig. 11.10a) due to its buoyancy. Complicated retinal detachments will require a prolonged internal tamponade. Silicone oil has proved effective for this purpose as it completely fills the vitreous chamber and exerts permanent pressure on the entire retina (▶ Fig. 11.11). However, silicone oil inevitably causes cataract formation and occasionally corneal changes and glaucoma. It must therefore be removed in a second operation about three months later.

▶ **Complications.** Vitrectomy nearly always leads to subsequent lens opacification, and rarely to retinal tears, bleeding, or endophthalmitis.

Chapter 12

Retina

12 Retina

Gabriele E. Lang and Gerhard K. Lang

12.1 Basic Knowledge

The retina is the *innermost* of three successive layers of the globe. It consists of two parts:

- A **photoreceptive part (pars optica retinae)**, consisting of the first 9 of the 11 layers listed below.
- A **nonreceptive part (pars ceca retinae)** forming the epithelium of the ciliary body and iris. The pars optica retinae merges (along a ragged border) with the pars ceca retinae at the *ora serrata.*

▶ **Embryology.** The retina develops from a *diverticulum of the forebrain* (proencephalon). Optic vesicles develop that then invaginate to form a double-walled bowl, the optic cup. The outer wall becomes the pigment epithelium, and the inner wall later differentiates into the nine layers of the retina. The retina remains linked to the forebrain throughout life through a structure known as the retinohypothalamic tract (see p. 249).

▶ **Thickness of the retina.** See ▶ Fig. 12.1.

▶ **Layers of the retina.** Moving inward along the path of incident light, the individual layers of the retina are as follows (▶ Fig. 12.2):

1. Internal limiting membrane (glial cell fibers separating the retina from the vitreous body).
2. Nerve fiber layer (axons of the third neuron).
3. Ganglion cell layer (cell nuclei of the multipolar ganglion cells of the third neuron; "data acquisition system").
4. Inner plexiform layer (synapses between the axons of the second neuron and dendrites of the third neuron).
5. Inner nuclear layer (cell nuclei of the bipolar nerve cells of the second neuron, horizontal cells, and amacrine cells).
6. Outer plexiform layer (synapses between the axons of the first neuron and dendrites of the second neuron).
7. Outer nuclear layer (cell nuclei of the rods and cones = first neuron).
8. Outer limiting membrane (sievelike plate of processes of glial cells through which rods and cones project).
9. Layer of rods and cones (the actual photoreceptors).
10. Retinal pigment epithelium (a single cubic layer of heavily pigmented epithelial cells).

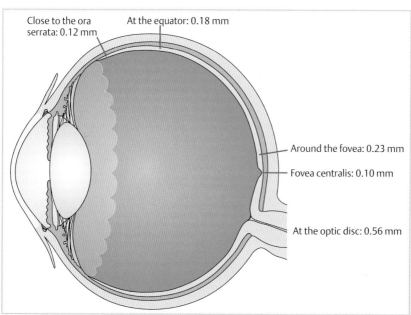

Close to the ora serrata: 0.12 mm

At the equator: 0.18 mm

Around the fovea: 0.23 mm

Fovea centralis: 0.10 mm

At the optic disc: 0.56 mm

Fig. 12.1 Thickness of the retina. Retinal tears most often occur close to the ora serrata.

11. Bruch's membrane (basal membrane of the choroid separating the retina from the choroid).

▶ **Macula lutea.** The macula lutea is a flattened oval area in the center of the retina approximately 3 to 4 mm (15°) temporal to and *slightly below* the optic disc (see ▶ Fig. 12.8). Located in its center is the avascular fovea centralis, the point at which visual perception is sharpest. Its diameter is roughly equal to that of the optic disc (1.5–1.9 mm). The macula appears *yellow* when examined under green light, hence the name macula lutea (yellow spot). The fovea centralis contains only

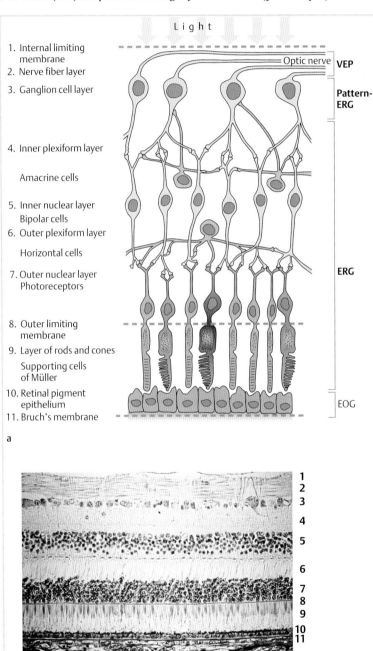

Light

1. Internal limiting membrane
2. Nerve fiber layer
3. Ganglion cell layer
4. Inner plexiform layer
   Amacrine cells
5. Inner nuclear layer
   Bipolar cells
6. Outer plexiform layer
   Horizontal cells
7. Outer nuclear layer
   Photoreceptors
8. Outer limiting membrane
9. Layer of rods and cones
   Supporting cells of Müller
10. Retinal pigment epithelium
11. Bruch's membrane

Optic nerve — VEP
Pattern-ERG
ERG
EOG

a

b

1 2 3 4 5 6 7 8 9 10 11

Fig. 12.2 Histology and function of the layers of the retina. **(a)** Layers of the retina and examination methods used to diagnose abnormal processes in the respective layers (EOG, electro-oculogram, see p. 197); ERG, electroretinogram, see p. 197); VEP, visual evoked potential, see p. 235). **(b)** The corresponding histologic image of the 11 layers of the retina.

189

cones (no rods) each with its own neural supply, which explains why this region has such distinct vision. Light stimuli in this region can directly act on the sensory cells (first neuron) because the bipolar cells (second neuron) and ganglion cells (third neuron) are displaced peripherally.

▶ **Vascular supply to the retina.** The **inner layers** of the retina (the internal limiting membrane through the inner nuclear layer) are supplied by the central artery of the retina. This originates at the ophthalmic artery, enters the eye with the optic nerve, and branches on the inner surface of the retina. The central artery is a genuine artery with a diameter of 0.1 mm. It is a terminal artery without anastomoses and divides into four main branches (see ▶ Fig.12.8).

Note
Because the central artery is a terminal artery, occlusion will lead to retinal infarction (see p. 203).

The **outer layers** (outer plexiform layer through the pigment epithelium) contain no capillaries. They are nourished by diffusion primarily from the richly supplied capillary layer of the choroid. The **retinal arteries** are normally *bright red*, have bright reflex strips (see ▶ Fig. 12.8) that become paler with advancing age, and do not show a pulse. The **retinal veins** are *dark red* with a narrow reflex strip, and may show spontaneous pulsation on the optic disc (normal).

Note
Pulsation in the retinal veins is normal; pulsation in the retinal arteries is abnormal.

The walls of the vessels are transparent so that only the blood will be visible on ophthalmoscopy. In terms of their structure and size, the retinal vessels are arterioles and venules, although they are often referred to as arteries and veins. **Venous diameter** is normally 1.5 times greater than **arterial diameter**. Capillaries are not visible.

▶ **Nerve supply to the retina.** The neurosensory retina has no sensory supply.

Note
Disorders of the retina are painless because of the absence of sensory supply.

▶ **Light path through the retinal layers.** When electromagnetic radiation in the visible light spectrum (wavelengths of 380–760 nm) strikes the retina, it is absorbed by the photopigments of the outer layer. Electric signals are created in a multiple-step photochemical reaction. They reach the photoreceptor synapses as action potentials where they are relayed to the second neuron. The signals are relayed to the third and fourth neurons and finally reach the visual cortex.

Note
Light must pass through three layers of cell nuclei before it reaches the photosensitive rods and cones. This inverted position of the photoreceptors is due to the manner in which the retina develops from a diverticulum of the forebrain.

▶ **Sensitivity of the retina to light intensity.** The retina has two types of photoreceptors, the rods and the cones. The 110 to 125 million **rods** allow *mesopic* and *scotopic* vision (twilight and night vision). They are about 500 times more photosensitive than the cones and contain the photopigment rhodopsin.

Note
Twilight vision decreases after the age of 50, particularly in patients with additional age-related miosis, cataract, and decreased visual acuity. Glaucoma patients undergoing treatment with miotic agents should therefore be advised of the danger of operating motor vehicles in twilight or at night.

The 6 to 7 million **cones** in the macula are responsible for *photopic* vision (daytime vision), resolution, and color perception. There are **three types of cones**:

- Blue cones.
- Green cones.
- Red cones.

Their retinal photopigments are the same, but their opsins are different. Beyond a certain **visual field luminance**, a transition from dark adaptation to light adaptation occurs. Luminance refers to the luminous flux per unit solid angle per unit projected area, measured in candelas per square meter (cd/m^2). The cones are responsible for vision up to a luminance of 10 cd/m^2, the rods up to 0.01 cd/m^2

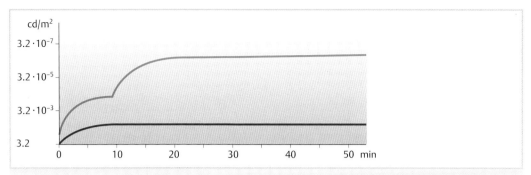

Fig. 12.3 Normal and abnormal dark adaptation curves. Horizontal axis: adaptation time in minutes. Vertical axis: luminance of the respective test marker in candelas per square meter. The blue curve shows normal progression, with Kohlrausch's typical discontinuity indicating the transition from cone to rod vision. The red curve in retinitis pigmentosa (see p. 220) is considerably less steep.

(twilight vision is 0.01–10 cd/m²; night vision is less than 0.01 cd/m²).

Adaptation is the adjustment of the sensitivity of the retina to varying degrees of light intensity. This is done by dilation or contraction of the pupil and shifting between cone and rod vision. In this manner, the human eye is able to see in daylight and at night. In *light adaptation,* the rhodopsin is bleached out so that rod vision is impaired in favor of cone vision. Light adaptation occurs far more quickly than dark adaptation. In *dark adaptation,* the rhodopsin quickly regenerates within 5 minutes (immediate adaptation), and within 30 minutes to 1 hour there is a further improvement in night vision (long-term adaptation). An *adaptometer* can be used to determine the light intensity threshold. First the patient is adapted to bright light for 10 minutes. Then the examining room is darkened and the light intensity threshold is measured with light test markers. These measurements can be used to obtain an adaptation curve (▶ Fig. 12.3).

▶ **Sensitivity to glare.** Glare refers to *disturbing brightness within the visual field sufficiently greater than the luminance to which the eyes are adapted* such as the headlights of oncoming traffic or intense reflected sunlight. Because the retina is adapted to a lesser luminance, vision is impaired in these cases. Often the glare will cause blinking or elicit an eye-closing reflex. Sensitivity to glare can be measured with a special device. Patients are shown a series of visual symbols in rapid succession that they must recognize despite intense glare. The sensitivity to glare or the speed of adaptation and readaptation of the eye is important in determining whether the patient is fit to operate a motor vehicle.

12.2 Examination Methods

12.2.1 Visual Acuity

See Chapter 1.4 for details of testing visual acuity.

12.2.2 Examination of the Fundus

▶ **Direct ophthalmoscopy.** Direct ophthalmoscopy produces an upright image (▶ Fig. 12.4a). A direct ophthalmoscope is positioned close to the patient's eye. The examiner sees a 16-power magnified image of the fundus.

▶ **Advantages.** The high magnification permits *evaluation of small retinal findings* such as diagnosing retinal microaneurysms. The dial of the ophthalmoscope contains various different plus and minus lenses and can be adjusted as necessary. These lenses compensate for refractive errors in both the patient and the examiner. They may also be used to measure the *prominence of retinal changes,* such as the prominence of the optic disc in papilledema or the prominence of a tumor. The base of the lesion is brought into focus first and then the peak of the lesion. A difference of 3 diopters from base to peak corresponds to a prominence of 1 mm. Direct ophthalmoscopy produces an erect image of the fundus, which is significantly easier to work with than an inverted image, and is therefore a suitable technique even for less experienced examiners and nonophthalmologists.

▶ **Disadvantages**. The image of the fundus is highly magnified but shows *only a small portion of the fundus.* Rotating the ophthalmoscope can only partially compensate for this disadvantage. Direct

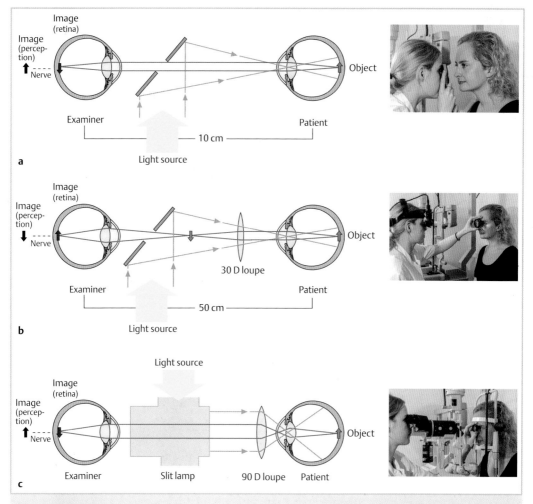

Fig. 12.4 Ophthalmoscopy. (a) Direct ophthalmoscopy: the examiner is carrying out retinoscopy of the left eye with the direct ophthalmoscope (compare with ▶ Fig. 1.10). She sees an upright image of the retina (compare the ray path). **(b)** Indirect binocular ophthalmoscopy with loupe and light source integrated in the head-mounted ophthalmoscope. The result is an upside-down fundus image, which is also mirror-inverted, created through the interposed loupe that the examiner is holding some centimeters away from the eye. **(c)** Indirect binocular ophthalmoscopy using the slit lamp with an integrated light source. The principle is the same as that described in **(b)**, only the setup for the examination is static here while in **(b)** it is mobile, so that it can be used, for example, for examinations on the ward.

ophthalmoscopy also produces only a two-dimensional image.

▶ **Indirect ophthalmoscopy.** Indirect ophthalmoscopy produces an upside-down image (▶ Fig. 12.4b). A condensing lens (+14 to +30 diopters) is held approximately 13 cm from the patient's eye. The fundus appears in 2- to 6-power magnification; the examiner sees a virtual inverted image of the fundus at the focal point of the loupe. Light sources are available for monocular or binocular examination (▶ Fig. 12.4c).

▶ **Advantages.** This technique provides a good stereoscopic, optimally illuminated overview of the entire fundus in binocular systems.

▶ **Disadvantages.** Magnification is significantly less than in direct ophthalmoscopy. Indirect ophthalmoscopy requires practice and experience.

▶ **Diagnostic contact lens examination.** The fundus may also be examined with a slit lamp when an additional magnifying lens such as a three-mirror lens (▶ Fig. 12.5) or a 78- to 90-diopter lens is used.

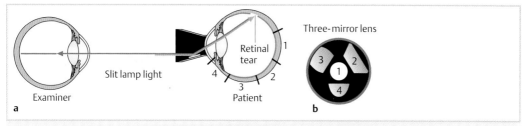

Fig. 12.5 (a,b) Examination of the fundus with a three-mirror lens. Principle of the examination. The lens is placed directly on the eye after application of a topical anesthetic. The Goldmann three-mirror lens visualizes different areas of the retina: 1, the posterior pole; 2, the central part of the peripheral retina; 3, the outer peripheral retina (important for diagnosing retinal tears); and 4, the gonioscopy mirror (see p. 147) for examining the chamber angle.

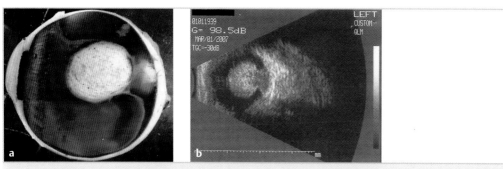

Fig. 12.6 Malignant melanoma of the retina with penetration through the Bruch membrane. **(a)** Eye incised through the tumor, after enucleation and fixation. **(b)** Echograph of the same eye with tumor base at the retina and tumor penetration through the Bruch membrane (the so-called collar-button phenomenon).

▶ **Advantages.** This technique produces a highly magnified three-dimensional image yet still provides the examiner with a good overview of the entire fundus. The three-mirror lens also visualizes "blind areas" of the eye such as the angle of the anterior chamber. Contact lens examination combines the advantages of direct ophthalmoscopy and indirect ophthalmoscopy and is therefore the *gold standard* for diagnosing retinal disorders.

Note

Where significant opacification of the optic media (as in a mature cataract) prevents direct visualization of the retina with the techniques mentioned above, the examiner can evaluate the pattern of the retinal vasculature. The sclera is directly illuminated in all four quadrants by moving a light source back and forth directly over the sclera. Patients with intact retinas will be able to perceive the shadow of their own vasculature on the retina (entoptic phenomenon). They will see what looks like the veins on a leaf in fall. Patients who are able to perceive this phenomenon have potential retinal vision of at least 20/200.

▶ **Ultrasonography.** Ultrasound studies are indicated where opacification of the optic media such as cataract or vitreous hemorrhage prevent direct inspection of the fundus or where retinal and choroidal findings are inconclusive. Intraocular tissues vary in how they reflect ultrasonic waves. The retina is highly reflective, whereas the vitreous body is normally nearly anechoic. Ultrasound studies can therefore demonstrate retinal detachment and distinguish it from a change in the vitreous body. Optic disc drusen are also highly reflective. Ultrasound is also helpful in diagnosing intraocular tumors with a prominence of at least 1.5 mm. The specific echogenicity of the tissue also helps to evaluate whether a tumor is malignant, for example in distinguishing a choroidal nevus from a malignant melanoma (▶ Fig. 12.6).

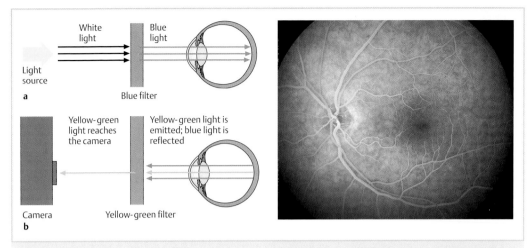

Fig. 12.7 Blue exciter and yellow-green barrier filters are placed along the optical axis of a single-lens reflex camera. (a) First, the blue filter ensures that only blue light from the light source reaches the retina. This excites the previously injected fluorescein dye in the vessels of the fundus. **(b)** The excited fluorescein emits yellow-green light, and the blue light is reflected. The yellow-green barrier filter blocks the blue components of the reflected light, so that the camera records only the image of the fluorescent dye. **(c)** A fluorescein angiographic image of a normal fundus.

> **! Note**
> Ultrasound studies can demonstrate retinal detachment where the optic media of the eye are opacified (due to causes such as cataract or vitreous hemorrhage). This is because the retina is highly reflective in contrast to the vitreous body. Ultrasound can also be used to confirm the presence of malignant choroidal processes.

▶ **Fundus photography.** Abnormal changes can be recorded with a single-lens reflex camera. This permits precise documentation of follow-up findings. Photographs obtained with a fundus camera in green light provide high-contrast images of abnormal changes to the *innermost* layers of the retina such as changes in the layer of optic nerve fibers, bleeding, or microaneurysms.

▶ **Fluorescence angiography (with fluorescein or indocyanine green).** In fluorescein angiography, 10 mL of 5% fluorescein sodium is injected into one of the patient's cubital veins. An exciter filter and a barrier filter are then placed along the optical axis of the single-lens reflex camera. The blue exciter filter ensures that only blue light from the light source reaches the retina. The yellow-green barrier filter blocks the blue components of the reflected light so that the camera records only the image of the fluorescent dye (▶ Fig. 12.7). Indocyanine green, which is excited to fluorescence by infrared

light, is also suitable for examination of retinal processes. Infrared has a longer wavelength and thus reaches deeper retinal layers than fluorescein. Since indocyanine green bonds more strongly, the retinal vessels are more clearly seen than with fluorescein.

> **! Note**
> Fluorescein angiography is used to diagnose vascular retinal disorders such as proliferative diabetic retinopathy, venous occlusion, age-related macular degeneration, and inflammatory retinal processes. Where the blood–retina barrier formed by the zonulae occludentes is disturbed, fluorescein will leak from the retinal vessels. Disorders of the choroid such as choroiditis or tumors can also be diagnosed by this method; in these cases indocyanine is better than fluorescein.

12.2.3 Normal and Abnormal Fundus Findings in General

▶ **Normal fundus.** The **retina** is *normally completely transparent without any intrinsic color.* It receives its uniform bright red coloration from the vasculature of the choroid (▶ Fig. 12.8). The **vessels of the choroid** themselves are obscured by the retinal pigment epithelium. *Loss of transparency of the*

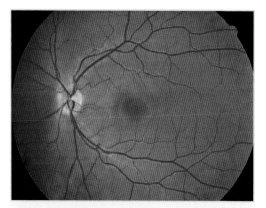

Fig. 12.8 Normal fundus. The macula lutea lies about 3 to 4 mm temporal to and slightly below the optic disc. The fundus receives its uniform bright red coloration from the vessels of the choroid. The diameter of the veins is normally 1.5 times greater than that of the arteries.

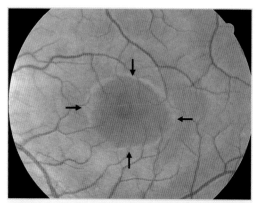

Fig. 12.9 Wall reflex surrounding the macula. A typical highly reflective fundus in a teenager (arrows: macular wall reflex). For more information see below.

Table 12.1 Forms of congenital color vision defects and frequency in males

Form	Frequency
Abnormal trichromatopsia (color weakness)	Most common form
• Deuteranomaly (green weakness)	5%
• Protanomaly (red weakness)	1%
• Tritanomaly (blue-yellow weakness)	Rare
Dichromasy (partial color blindness = one of the three cone systems necessary for color discrimination is missing)	Second most common form
• Protanopia (red blindness)	1%
• Deuteranopia (green blindness)	1%
• Tritanopia (blue–yellow blindness)	Rare

retina is a sign of an abnormal process (for example in retinal edemas, the retina appears whitish-yellow) (see ▶ Fig. 12.25). The **optic** disc is normally a *sharply defined, yellowish-orange* structure (in teenagers it is pale pink, and in young children significantly paler) that *may* exhibit a *central depression* known as the optic or physiologic cup. For details of pathologic papillary changes see Chapter 13.3. Light reflection on the inner limiting membrane will normally produce *multiple light reflexes* on the fundus. Teenagers will also exhibit a normal **foveal reflex** and **wall reflex** surrounding the macula, which is caused by the transition from the depression of the macula to the higher level of the retina (▶ Fig. 12.9).

▶ **Age-related changes.** The **optic disc** turns pale yellow with age, and often the optic cup will become shallow and will be surrounded by a region of choroidal atrophy. The **fundus** will become dull and nonreflective. Drusen can be seen in the pigment epithelium of the retina (see ▶ Fig. 12.30a) (PAS-positive deposits in the Bruch membrane) and mid-peripheral reticular pigment epithelial proliferations are found. The *arterioles will be elongated* due to loss of elasticity with *irregular filling* due to thickening of the vascular walls. *Meandering of the venules* will be present, as well as *crossing signs*— i.e., the sclerotic artery will be seen to compress the vein at the arteriovenous crossing, reducing the diameter of the column of venous blood. In extreme cases venous blood flow will be cut off almost completely.

▶ **Abnormal changes in the fundus.** As a rule, *loss of transparency of the retina* is a sign of an abnormal process. For example, in a retinal edema the retina appears whitish-yellow (see ▶ Fig. 12.21). A distinctive feature of abnormal retinal and choroidal changes is that the type and appearance of

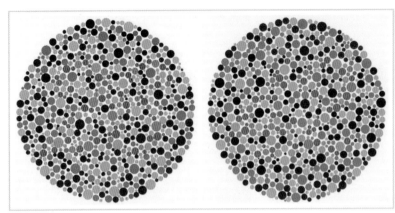

Fig. 12.10 Ishihara plates for diagnosing red–green vision defects. Patients with normal color vision can recognize the number 26 on the left and 42 on the right.

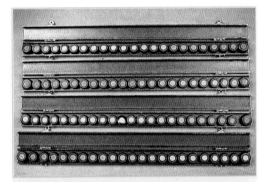

Fig. 12.11 Farnsworth–Munsell test of red–green and blue–yellow color vision defects. The patient has to sort markers of various hues in the correct order according to the colors of the rainbow.

these changes permit precise *topographic localization* of the respective abnormal process when the diagnosis is made. The ophthalmoscopic image will usually allow one to determine in which of the layers shown in ▶ Fig. 12.2 the process is occurring. For example, in ▶ Fig. 12.30a (nonexudative age-related macular degeneration) one may see that the drusen and atrophy are located in the retinal pigment epithelium; the structures above it are not affected, as is apparent from the intact vascular structures (see ▶ Fig. 12.17).

12.2.4 Color Vision Deficiencies and Testing

Color vision deficiencies may be congenital (especially in men as they are inherited and X-linked recessive) or acquired, for example in macular disorders such as Stargardt's disease (see p. 218). They can become manifest as a reduced sensitivity to certain colors (color weakness) or, much more rarely, as a complete deficiency for certain colors

(color blindness). Depending on the deficiency, certain professions are not suitable for patients with these conditions (e.g., police work, driving buses). Congenital color deficiencies most often occur in males, because the defects have X-linked recessive transmission (8% of men but only 0.4% of women have color vision defects). For a detailed list of congenital color vision defects, see ▶ Table 12.1.

Qualitative red–green vision defects are evaluated with pseudoisochromatic plates such as the Ishihara or Stilling–Velhagen plates. They contain numerals or letters composed of small color dots surrounded by confusion colors (▶ Fig. 12.10) that patients with color vision defects cannot read. Farnsworth–Munsell tests (▶ Fig. 12.11) can detect **blue–yellow color vision defects**.

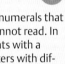

Note
Pseudoisochromatic plates contain numerals that patients with color vision defects cannot read. In the Farnsworth–Munsell test, patients with a color vision defect cannot sort markers with different hues into the right order (according to the colors of the rainbow).

The Nagel anomaloscope allows **quantitative evaluation of color vision defects**. The test plate consists of a lower yellow half whose brightness can be adjusted, and an upper half that the patient tries to match to the lower yellow color by mixing red and green. The anomaly ratio is calculated from the final adjustment. Green-blind patients will use too much green, and red-blind patients too much red when mixing the colors. Color vision defects cannot be treated.

▶ **Perimetry** For details see Chapter 14.2.

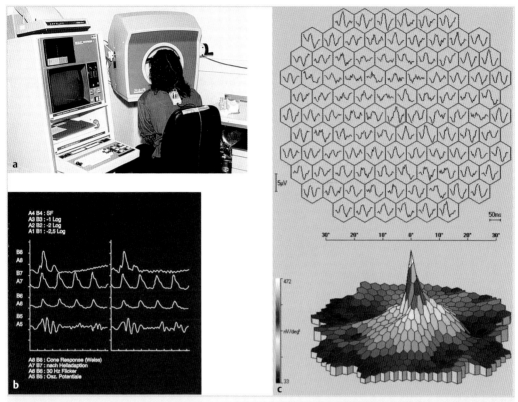

Fig. 12.12 Electroretinogram (ERG). (a) Retinal potentials are recorded with a corneal contact lens electrode and skin electrode. **(b)** Normal electroretinogram. **(c)** Multifocal electroretinography of a normal retina (different areas of the macula can be recorded separately).

12.2.5 Electrophysiologic Examination Methods

(For electroretinography, electro-oculography, and visual evoked potentials, see ▶ Fig. 12.12a)

▶ **Electroretinogram (ERG).** This examination method uses electrodes to record the electrical *response of the retina to flashes of light* (▶ Fig. 12.12a). Photopic (light-adapted) and scotopic (dark-adapted) electroretinograms are obtained. The electroretinogram (ERG) consists of a negative A wave indicating the response of the photoreceptors and a positive B wave primarily indicating the response of the bipolar cells and the supporting cells of Müller (▶ Fig. 12.12b). A **flicker ERG** (repeated flashes) isolates pure cone response; a **pattern ERG** (such as a checkerboard) and oscillating potentials can be used to evaluate the inner layers of the retina. The classic indication for an electroretinogram is retinitis pigmentosa with early loss of scotopic and photopic potentials. The ERG rep-

resents a *summation response* of the retina. A **multifocal ERG** (▶ Fig. 12.12c) can record the response of isolated areas of the retina.

This makes it possible to record retinal activity in the macular area point by point. Different areas of the macula are stimulated repeatedly. The multifocal ERG is suitable for the diagnosis of macular diseases (e.g., macular dystrophies, see p. 218, or age-related macular degeneration, see p. 214) and for differentiating between macular diseases and optic nerve head processes.

▶ **Electro-oculogram (EOG).** Electro-oculography detects *abnormal changes in the retinal pigment epithelium* such as macular vitelliform dystrophy (Best disease, see Chapter 12.2.5). This examination method utilizes the dipole of the eye in which the cornea forms the positive pole and the retinal pigment epithelium the negative pole. The standing potential across cornea and retina in comparison to the cornea is measured indirectly with two temporal electrodes (▶ Fig. 12.13). During the measuring process, the patient performs regular eye move-

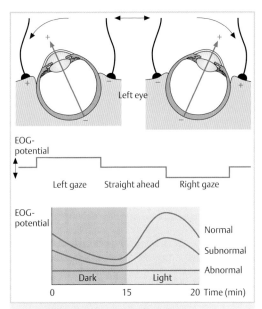

Fig. 12.13 Electro-oculogram (EOG). The eye forms a dipole in which the anterior pole is positive and the posterior pole is negative. The EOG records the change in position of the standing potential of the retina with two temporal electrodes.

ments by alternately focusing on two lights. The standing potential is normally higher in the light-adapted eye than in the dark-adapted eye. The ratio of light-adapted potential to dark-adapted potential (*Arden ratio*) is obtained to evaluate the eye; this ratio is normally greater than 1.8. The ratio is reduced in the presence of abnormal changes.

Note
The typical indication for an electro-oculogram is macular vitelliform dystrophy (Best's vitelliform dystrophy), with a significantly decreased Arden ratio.

▶ **Visual evoked potential (VEP).** This examination is used to diagnose damage along the visual pathway. The VEP is not a specific examination of the retina such as an electroretinogram or electro-oculogram. This method is briefly discussed in Chapter 13, Optic Nerve.

▶ **Optical coherence tomography (OCT).** OCT (see p. 356) is suitable for examining patients with macular diseases (macular hole, macular edema, vitreomacular traction) and for analyzing the optic nerve head (tomography of the optic nerve head in

glaucoma). In this examination method, a slit-shaped laser beam is projected onto the retina, and the reflected light is analyzed, thus producing a high-resolution cross-section of the retina. In this way, disease processes can be precisely located in a specific layer of the retina, for instance the extent of a hole in the macula: does it penetrate all the layers of the retina or only some of them? Such a precise diagnosis (see p. 356) has only been possible histologically up to now.

12.3 Vascular Disorders

12.3.1 Diabetic Retinopathy

Definition
Diabetic retinopathy is a neurovascular disease.

▶ **Epidemiology.** Diabetic retinopathy is one of the main causes of acquired blindness at the age of 30 to 60 years in industrialized countries. Approximately 90% of diabetic patients have retinopathy after 20 years. The prevalence is 7% in industrial countries.

▶ **Pathogenesis and stages of diabetic retinopathy.** Diabetic retinopathy is a microangiopathy. This results in a thickening of the basement membrane of the vessels and loss of pericytes and vascu-

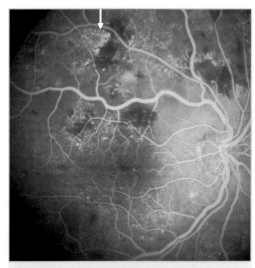

Fig. 12.14 Intraretinal microvascular anomalies. Only intraretinal changes (arrow) are present in the vessels; there is no neovascularization, although the image might suggest this. Angiography can clarify the issue because there is no dye leakage.

lar endothelial cells. Hyperglycemia plays an important role at this early stage. Later, capillary closure occurs, resulting in retinal ischemia. The further course is triggered by hypoxia. In the ischemic retina, angiogenic factors such as vascular endothelial growth factor (VEGF) and insulin-like growth factor-1 (IGF-1) are produced. They contribute to preretinal and iris new vessel formation. At any stage, a breakdown of the blood–retina barrier with increased vascular permeability can occur, leading to macular edema. Diabetes mellitus can lead to changes in almost every ocular tissue. These include symptoms of keratoconjunctivitis sicca, xanthelasma, mycotic orbital infections, transitory refractory changes, cataract, glaucoma, neuropathy of the optic nerve, and oculomotor palsy. However, *90% of visual impairments* in diabetic patients are caused by diabetic retinopathy. The most common international nomenclature used to describe the various changes in diabetic retinopathy (▶ Table 12.2) is based on the classifi-

cation of the Diabetic Retinopathy Study. A distinction is made between nonproliferative (stage 1, mild; 2, moderate; 3, severe; see ▶ Fig. 12.15) and proliferative stages with the characteristics mild, moderate, (▶ Fig. 12.16) and high risk (▶ Fig. 12.18), as well as clinically significant macular edema (▶ Fig. 12.17) and ischemic maculopathy (▶ Table 12.3).

▶ **Symptoms.** Diabetic retinopathy remains asymptomatic for a long time. Only in the late stages with macular involvement or vitreous hemorrhage will the patient notice visual impairment or suddenly go blind.

▶ **Diagnostic considerations.** Diabetic retinopathy and its various stages (see ▶ Table 12.2) are diagnosed by stereoscopic examination of the fundus with the pupil dilated. Ophthalmoscopy and evaluation of stereoscopic fundus photographs represent the gold standard. Fluorescein angiography is

Table 12.2 Retinal changes in diabetic retinopathy

Stage of retinopathy	Retinal changes
Nonproliferative diabetic retinopathy	
1. Mild	• At least one microaneurysm
2. Moderate	• Mild intraretinal microvascular abnormalities (IRMA, ▶ Fig. 12.14) in four quadrants of the retina • Moderate hemorrhages in two or three quadrants • Venous beading in one quadrant
3. Severe	• Moderate hemorrhages in four quadrants • Venous beading in two quadrants • Moderate IRMA in one quadrant
Proliferative diabetic retinopathy	
1. Mild	• New vessels elsewhere (NVE) < 0.5 of the disc area in one or more quadrants
2. Moderate	• New vessels elsewhere (NVE) ≥ 0.5 of the disc area in one or more quadrants • New vessels on disc (NVD) < 0.3–0.25 of the disc area
3. High risk	• New vessels on disc (NVD) ≥ 0.3–0.25 of the disc area • Vitreous hemorrhage with any new vessels
Rubeosis iridis (see Chapter 8.6)	• New vessels in the iris, risk of secondary angle closure glaucoma

Table 12.3 Retinal findings in diabetic maculopathy

Stage of maculopathy	Retinal findings
Clinically significant macular edema (CSME) (▶ Fig. 12.17)	• Thickening of the retina at or within 500 µm of the center of the macula • Hard exudates at or within 500 µm of the center of the macula associated with thickening of the adjacent retina • A zone or zones of thickening one disc area or larger, any part of which is within one disc diameter of the center of the macula
Ischemic maculopathy	• Enlargement of foveal avascular zone caused by capillary closure (leads to visual impairment)

used to determine whether treatment is indicated. The presence of rubeosis iridis is confirmed or excluded using a slit lamp examination with a mobile pupil—i.e., without the use of a mydriatic—and by gonioscopy of the angle of the anterior chamber. With optical coherence tomography, macular edema, hard exudates, and cystoid maculopathy can be diagnosed (see ▶ Fig. 20.5).

▶ **Differential diagnosis.** The differential diagnosis has to exclude other vascular retinal diseases, primarily hypertonic changes of the fundus (this is done by excluding the underlying disorder).

▶ **Treatment.** Drug treatment is administered intraoperatively (intravitreally) with VEGF inhibitors and steroids alone or in combination with laser

(in diabetic macular edema). Extrafoveal clinically significant macular edema—i.e., macular edema that threatens vision—is managed with focal laser treatment at the posterior pole (see ▶ Fig. 12.19). Proliferative diabetic retinopathy is treated with scatter photocoagulation performed in three to five sessions (1,200–1,600 burns, spot size on the retina

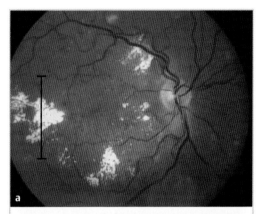
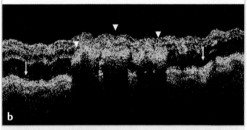

Fig. 12.17 Diabetic maculopathy. (a) Severe diabetic macular edema with hard exudates (yellow). (b) The corresponding optical coherence tomography image with macular edema (arrows) and hard exudates (arrowheads). The scan line in image (b) is shown as a black line in (a). For OCT see Chapter 20.5.

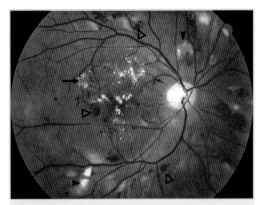

Fig. 12.15 Nonproliferative diabetic retinopathy. Microaneurysms, intraretinal hemorrhage (open arrowheads); hard exudates representing lipid deposits in the retina (arrow); and cotton-wool spots representing nerve fiber infarction (also called soft exudates) (black arrow heads).

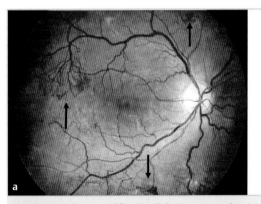
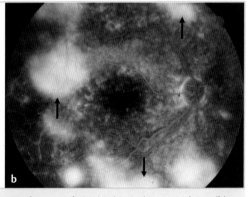

Fig. 12.16 Moderate proliferative diabetic retinopathy. (a) Preretinal neovascularization (arrows) is a typical sign. (b) The corresponding angiographic image. Fluorescein dye leakage is seen in the neovascularized area (arrows).

500 μm). Vitreous hemorrhage or tractional retinal detachment is treated with vitrectomy if applicable, with instillation of silicone oil if indicated. In rubeosis iridis, off-label treatment with VEGF inhibitors can be administered.

▶ **Prophylaxis.** Failure to perform regular ophthalmologic screening examinations in patients with diabetes mellitus is a negligent omission that exposes patients to the risk of blindness. For this reason, patients with type 2 diabetes should receive a yearly ophthalmologic examination upon diagnosis of the disorder and those with type 1 diabetes should also be examined once a year, at the latest within 5 years of the diagnosis. In the presence of

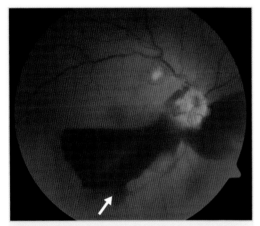

Fig. 12.18 High-risk proliferative diabetic retinopathy. The clearly visible vitreous hemorrhage seen here (arrow) is a typical sign of this stage of diabetic retinopathy. The patient will only notice deterioration of vision at this late stage.

diabetic retinopathy, examinations should be performed more frequently. Pregnant patients should be examined once every trimester.

▶ **Clinical course and prognosis.** Optimum control of blood glucose (HbA$_{1c}$ <7%) can prevent or delay retinopathy. Additional arterial hypertension also (with blood pressure being adjusted to <135/85 mm Hg) and hyperlipoproteinemia must be treated. However, diabetic retinopathy can occur despite optimum therapy. If rubeosis iridis (neovascularization in the iris) occurs in diabetic retinopathy, the risk of blindness is high, since rubeosis is a relentless and irreversible process. Without treatment, in addition to blindness resulting from rubeosis iridis, there is a danger of blindness caused by tractional retinal detachment (see p. 209). Without treatment, macular edema can also lead to severe visual impairment or blindness.

Note
The risk of blindness due to diabetic retinopathy can be reduced by optimum control of blood glucose, regular ophthalmologic examination, and timely therapy, but it cannot be completely eliminated.

12.3.2 Retinal Vein Occlusion

Definition
Vein occlusion occurs as a result of circulatory dysfunction in the central vein or one of its branches.

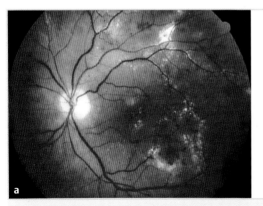
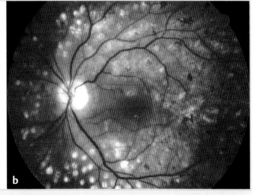

Fig. 12.19 Proliferative diabetic retinopathy before and after laser treatment. (a) Proliferative diabetic retinopathy with clinically significant macular edema before laser therapy. (b) The findings after successful laser treatment (laser burns appear whitish-brown).

▶ **Epidemiology.** Retinal vein occlusion is the second most frequent *vascular* retinal disorder after diabetic retinopathy.

> **Note**
> Frequent underlying systemic disorders of retinal vein occlusion include arterial hypertension and diabetes mellitus. Frequent underlying ocular disorders include glaucoma and retinal vasculitis, which must be specifically ruled out.

▶ **Etiology.** Occlusion of the central vein of the retina or its branches is frequently due to local thrombosis at sites where sclerotic arteries compress the veins. In **central retinal vein occlusion**, the thrombus lies at the level of the lamina cribrosa; in **branch retinal vein occlusion**, it is frequently at an arteriovenous crossing.

▶ **Symptoms.** Patients only notice a loss of visual acuity if the macula or optic disc are involved.

▶ **Diagnostic considerations and findings.** Central retinal vein occlusion can be diagnosed where linear or punctiform hemorrhages are seen to occur in all four quadrants of the retina (▶ Fig. 12.20a). Often one will find distended and increasingly meandering veins. In **branch retinal vein occlusion**, intraretinal hemorrhages will occur in the area of vascular supply; the hemorrhages may occur in only one quadrant or in two quadrants (hemispheric vein occlusion) (▶ Fig. 12.20b, c).

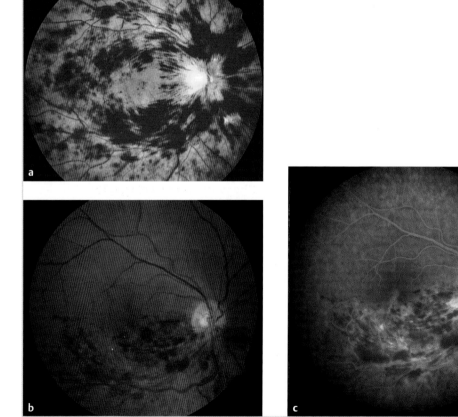

Fig. 12.20 Retinal vein occlusion. **(a)** Central retinal vein occlusion: intraretinal hemorrhages are visible in every retinal quadrant. **(b)** Occlusion of the two main inferior branches. Hemorrhages occur only in the affected areas of the retina in branch retinal vein occlusion. **(c)** Fluorescein angiography (corresponding to **(b)**) with dye leakage and blockage of fluorescence by hemorrhages.

Cotton-wool spots and retinal or optic-disc edema may also be present (simultaneous retinal and optic-disc edema is also possible). Chronic occlusions may also be accompanied by lipid deposits. Ischemic occlusion is diagnosed with the aid of fluorescein angiography (▶ Fig. 12.20c). In ischemic occlusion of central veins, regular follow-up examinations are required (every 4 weeks). This applies particularly to the first 3 months after the diagnosis is established because during this period, the risk of developing rubeosis iridis is particularly high. Overall, the 4-week checkups should be continued for a period of 6 months after establishment of the diagnosis, and quarterly after this.

▶ **Differential diagnosis.** Other forms of vascular retinal disease have to be excluded, especially diabetic retinopathy. An internist or general practitioner should be consulted to verify or exclude the possible presence of an underlying disorder.

▶ **Treatment in branch retinal vein occlusion with macular edema.** Treatment with intravitral VEGF blockers and steroids. The underlying disorders have to be treated. The patients should have follow-up examinations every 4 weeks for 6 months, and thereafter every 3 months. In central retinal vein occlusion, iris neovascularization most often develops within 3 months. Laser treatment is performed in ischemic occlusion that progresses to neovascularization or rubeosis iridis. Focal laser treatment is performed in **branch retinal vein occlusion with macular edema** when visual acuity is reduced to 20/40 or less within 3 months of occlusion.

▶ **Prophylaxis.** Early diagnosis and prompt treatment of underlying systemic and ocular disorders is important.

▶ **Clinical course and prognosis.** Visual acuity improves spontaneously in approximately one-third of all patients, remains unchanged in one-third, and deteriorates in one-third. Complications include preretinal neovascularization, retinal detachment, and rubeosis iridis with angle closure glaucoma. Pharmacotherapy has improved the prognosis.

12.3.3 Retinal Artery Occlusion

Definition
Retinal infarction due to occlusion of an artery in the lamina cribrosa or a branch retinal artery occlusion.

▶ **Epidemiology.** Retinal artery occlusions occur significantly less often than vein occlusions. (Incidence 1:10,000).

▶ **Etiology.** Emboli (▶ Table 12.4) are *frequently* the cause of central retinal artery and branch retinal artery occlusions. *Less frequent* causes include inflammatory processes such as temporal arteritis (Horton's arteritis).

Note
Horton's arteritis should be excluded where retinal artery occlusion is accompanied by headache.

▶ **Symptoms.** In **central retinal artery occlusion**, the patient generally reports *sudden, painless unilateral blindness*. In **branch retinal artery occlusion**, the patient will notice a loss of visual acuity or visual field defects.

▶ **Diagnostic considerations.** The diagnosis is made by ophthalmoscopy, fluorescein angiography and perimetry (examination of the visual field).

▶ **Central retinal arterial occlusion** (▶ Fig. 12.21). An acute and a chronic stage can be distinguished:

• In the **acute stage of central retinal artery occlusion**, the *retina* appears *grayish-white* due to edema of the layer of optic nerve fibers and is

Table 12.4 Causes of embolus in retinal artery occlusion

Type of embolus	Source of embolus
Calcium emboli (white)	Atheromatous plaques from the carotid artery or heart valves
Cholesterol emboli (yellow)	Atheromatous plaques from the carotid artery
Thrombocyte–fibrin emboli (gray)	In atrial fibrillation, myocardial infarction, or due to heart surgery
Myxoma emboli	In atrial myxoma (young patients)
Bacterial or mycotic emboli (Roth spots)	In endocarditis and septicemia

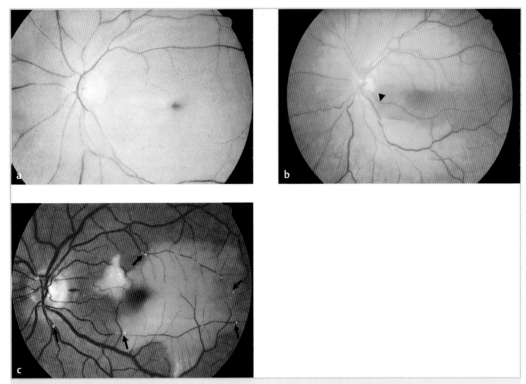

Fig. 12.21 Retinal artery occlusions. (a) Central retinal artery occlusion. The thin vessels and extensive retinal edema in which the retina loses its transparency are typical signs. Only the fovea is spared, which appears as a cherry-red spot. **(b)** Central retinal artery occlusion with perfused cilioretinal artery (arrowhead). **(c)** Branch retinal artery occlusion. Multiple emboli are visible in the affected arterial branches (arrows).

no longer transparent. Only the *fovea centralis,* which does not contain any nerve fibers, remains visible as a "*cherry-red spot*" because the red of the choroid shows through at this site (▶ Fig. 12.21a). The column of blood will be seen to be interrupted. Rarely, one will observe an embolus. Patients with a cilioretinal artery (artery originating from the ciliary arteries instead of the central retinal artery) will exhibit normal perfusion in the area of vascular supply, and their loss of visual acuity will be less (▶ Fig. 12.21b). An afferent pupillary defect is found. Perimetry reveals a severe defect in the visual field.

- *Atrophy of the optic nerve* will develop in the **chronic stage of central retinal artery occlusion**.

In both acute and chronic stages, perimetry shows a total loss of the visual field and an afferent pupillary defect.

▶ **Branch retinal artery occlusion.** A retinal edema will be found in the affected area of vascular supply (▶ Fig. 12.21c) in the acute stage. In the chronic stage the vessel is either narrowed or occluded. Perimetry (visual field testing) will reveal a total visual field defect in central retinal artery occlusion and a partial defect in branch occlusion corresponding to the area of occlusion.

▶ **Differential diagnosis.** Lipid storage diseases that can also create a cherry-red spot, such as Tay–Sachs disease, Niemann–Pick disease, or Gaucher's disease, should be excluded. These diseases can be clearly identified on the basis of their numerous additional symptoms and the fact that they afflict younger patients.

▶ **Treatment.** Emergency treatment is often unsuccessful even when initiated immediately. Ocular massage, medications that reduce intraocular pressure, or paracentesis are applied in an attempt to drain the embolus in a peripheral retinal vessel. Calcium antagonists are applied in an attempt to improve vascular supply. Work-up to identify the source of the embolus is important in order to treat

Table 12.5 Staging of hypertensive vascular changes (the Keith–Wagener–Barker classification). Source: Keith et al 1939

Stage	Characteristics
I	Constriction and tortuosity (= marked twisting) of the arterioles
II	Severe vascular constriction and Gunn's crossing sign. The column of venous blood is constricted by the sclerotic artery at an arteriovenous crossing (see ▸ Fig. 12.22a), dilated venules, silver wire arteries (see ▸ Fig. 12.22b)
III	Retinal hemorrhages, hard exudates, cotton-wool spots (see ▸ Fig. 12.22c), retinal edema
IV	Papilledema, optic atrophy

The WHO distinguishes between hypertensive retinopathy (stages I and II) and malignant hypertensive retinopathy (stages III and IV).

Table 12.6 Staging of arteriosclerotic vascular changes (the Scheie classification). Source: Scheie 1953

Stage	Characteristics
I	Widening of arteriole reflexes
II	Arteriovenous crossing sign
III	Copper-wire arteries (copper-colored arterial reflex)
IV	Silver-wire arteries (silver-colored arterial reflex)

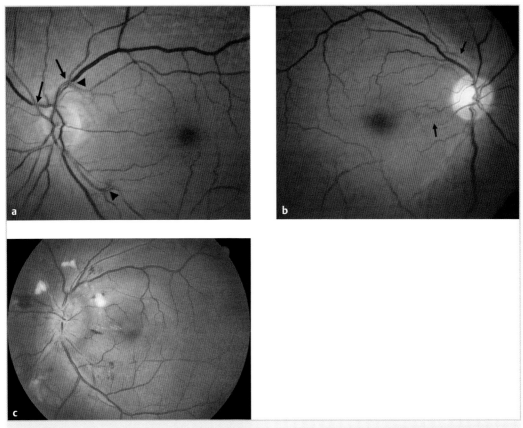

Fig. 12.22 Hypertensive fundus changes. (a) Stage II hypertensive retinopathy: Gunn's crossing sign (arrows) and typical omega division of the artery (arrowheads); the artery does not divide as usual at an acute angle. **(b)** Stage II hypertensive retinopathy: silver-colored artery reflexes (arrows). **(c)** Stage IV hypertensive retinopathy: typical findings at this stage include areas of hemorrhage, cotton-wool spots, and papilledema.

the underlying disease and prevent another embolization (such as stroke).

▶ **Prophylaxis.** Excluding or initiating prompt therapy of predisposing underlying systemic disorders is crucial.

▶ **Clinical course and prognosis.** The prognosis is poor because *irreparable damage* to the inner layers of the retina occurs *within 1 hour*. Blindness usually cannot be prevented in central retinal artery occlusion. The prognosis is better when only a branch of the artery is occluded, unless a macular branch is affected.

12.3.4 Hypertensive Retinopathy and Sclerotic Changes

Definition
Arterial changes in hypertension are primarily caused by vasospasm; in arteriosclerosis they are the result of thickening of the wall of the arteriole.

▶ **Epidemiology.** Arterial hypertension, in particular, figures prominently in clinical settings.

Note
Vascular changes due to arterial hypertension are the most frequent cause of retinal vein occlusion.

▶ **Pathogenesis.** High blood pressure can cause breakdown of the blood–retina barrier or obliteration of capillaries. This results in intraretinal hemorrhages, cotton-wool spots, retinal edema, or swelling of the optic disc.

▶ **Symptoms.** Patients with high blood pressure frequently suffer from headache or eye pain. Impaired vision or loss of visual acuity only occurs in stage III or IV hypertensive vascular changes. Arteriosclerosis does not exhibit any ocular symptoms.

▶ **Diagnostic considerations.** Hypertensive and arteriosclerotic changes in the fundus are diagnosed by ophthalmoscopy, preferably with the pupil dilated (▶ Table 12.5, ▶ Table 12.6). Changes in the retinal vasculature are frequent findings; choroidal infarctions are rare in acute hypertension (Elschnig's spots: circumscribed atrophy and pro-

liferation of pigment epithelium in the infarcted area).

▶ **Differential diagnosis.** Ophthalmoscopy should be performed to exclude other vascular retinal disorders such as diabetic retinopathy. Diabetic retinopathy is primarily characterized by parenchymal and vascular changes; a differential diagnosis is made by confirming or excluding the systemic underlying disorder.

▶ **Treatment.** Treating the underlying disorder is crucial where fundus changes due to arterial retinopathy are present. Blood pressure should be reduced to below 135/85 mm Hg. Fundus changes due to arteriosclerosis are untreatable.

▶ **Prophylaxis.** Regular blood pressure monitoring and ophthalmoscopic examination of the fundus are required to minimize the risk of complications (see below).

▶ **Clinical course and complications.** Sequelae of arteriosclerotic and hypertensive vascular changes include retinal artery and vein occlusion and the formation of macroaneurysms that can lead to vitreous hemorrhage. In the presence of papilledema, the subsequent atrophy of the optic nerve can produce lasting and occasionally severe loss of visual acuity.

▶ **Prognosis.** In some cases, the complications described above are unavoidable despite well-controlled blood pressure.

12.3.5 Coats's Disease

Definition
Congenital retinal telangiectasia with vascular anomalies that nearly always presents *unilaterally* and can lead to exudation and eventually to exudative retinal detachment.

▶ **Epidemiology.** This rare disorder manifests itself in young children and teenagers. Boys are usually affected (in about 90% of cases).

Note
Coats' disease usually occurs in young and teenage boys. It is nearly always unilateral.

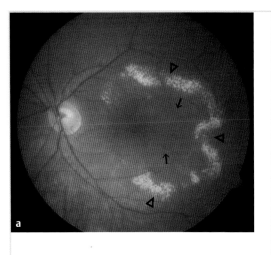
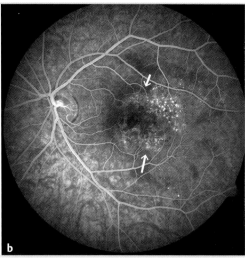

Fig. 12.23 Coats' disease. (a) Typical telangiectatic vascular changes (arrows) accompanied by exudative retinal detachment with numerous lipid deposits (arrowheads). (b) Corresponding fluorescence angiogram, telangiectatic capillaries (arrows).

▶ **Pathogenesis.** Telangiectasia and aneurysms lead to exudation and eventually to retinal detachment (see p. 208).

▶ **Symptoms.** The early stages are characterized by loss of visual acuity, the later stages by leukocoria (white pupil see ▶ Fig. 12.41a) or unilateral strabismus, although the combination of leukocoria *and* strabismus is also possible.

▶ **Diagnostic considerations and findings.** Ophthalmoscopy will reveal telangiectasia, subretinal whitish exudate with exudative retinal detachment and hemorrhages (▶ Fig. 12.23).

▶ **Differential diagnosis.** In the advanced stages of the disorder, retinoblastoma (see p. 226) should be excluded by ophthalmoscopy and retinopathy of prematurity on the basis of the patient's history. Both disorders may also cause leukocoria.

▶ **Treatment.** The treatment of choice is laser photocoagulation or cryotherapy to destroy anomalous telangiectatic capillaries.

▶ **Clinical course and prognosis.** Left untreated, the disease will eventually cause blindness due to total exudative retinal detachment. Treatment is effective in preventing blindness in about 50% of patients.

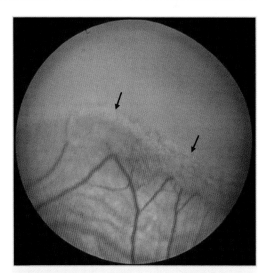

Fig. 12.24 Retinopathy of prematurity. Stage 3+, prominent ridge (arrows) with extraretinal proliferation. (Reproduced with permission from Jandek et al., Frühgeborenenretinopathie. Klin Monatsbl 2004;221:150, Thieme, Stuttgart.)

12.3.6 Retinopathy of Prematurity

Definition
A retinal disorder attributable to disruption of normal development of the retinal vasculature in preterm infants with birth weight less than 2,500 grams.

▶ **Epidemiology.** The disorder is rare. Infants with birth weight below 1,000 g are at increased risk of developing the disorder. Retinopathy of prematurity is not always preventable despite optimum care and strict monitoring of partial pressure of oxygen.

▶ **Etiology.** Preterm birth and exposure to oxygen disturbs the normal development of the retinal vasculature. Vessel obliteration occurs, followed by proliferative neovascularization (▶ Fig. 12.24). This results in vitreous hemorrhage, retinal detachment, and, in the late scarring stage, retrolental fibroplasia as vessels and connective tissue fuse with the detached retina.

▶ **Findings and symptoms.** After an initially asymptomatic clinical course, vitreous hemorrhage or retinal detachment will be accompanied by secondary strabismus. Leukocoria can occur in the retrolental fibroplasia stage. ▶ Table 12.7 shows the classification of the various stages.

   As is customary in ophthalmology, the extent of the respective abnormal change is specified by analogy with a clock face. For example, a demarcation line may be said to extend from the 1 o'clock to the 6 o'clock position. A plus stage includes dilated and tortuous vessels of the posterior pole, in addition to the other changes.

▶ **Diagnostic considerations.** The retina should be examined with the pupil dilated 4 weeks after birth at the latest. This can be done as part of the routine examination of the newborn. Follow-up examinations will depend on the degree of retinal vascularization.

▶ **Differential diagnosis.** Other causes of leukocoria such as retinoblastoma or cataract (see ▶ Table 11.1) should be considered.

▶ **Treatment.** Surgery is rarely successful in stages 4 and 5. In stage 3 (peripheral zone II), laser photocoagulation or cryotherapy is performed in the nonvascularized portion of the retina, in stage 3 (central zone II) laser or VEGF inhibitor.

▶ **Prophylaxis.** Partial pressure of oxygen should be kept as low as possible, and ophthalmologic screening examinations should be performed.

Note
Early detection of retinopathy of prematurity is particularly important.

▶ **Clinical course and prognosis.** Stage 1 and 2 retinopathy resolves spontaneously in 85% of affected children.

12.4 Degenerative Retinal Disorders

12.4.1 Retinal Detachment

Definition
Retinal detachment refers to the separation of the neurosensory retina (see ▶ Fig. 12.2) from the underlying retinal pigment epithelium, to which normally it is loosely attached.
This can be classified into four types:
- **Rhegmatogenous** retinal detachment results from a tear—i.e., a break in the retina.
- **Tractional** retinal detachment results from traction—i.e., from vitreous strands that exert tensile forces on the retina (see proliferative vitreoretinopathy and complicated retinal detachment, see p. 186).
- **Exudative** retinal detachment is caused by fluid. Blood, lipids, or serous fluid accumulation between the neurosensory retina and the retinal pigment epithelium. Coats's disease (see p. 206) is a typical example.
- **Tumor-related** retinal detachment.
Primary retinal detachment usually results from a tear. In rare cases, **secondary retinal detachment** may also result from a tear due to other disorders or injuries. Combinations of both are also possible but rare. Proliferative vitreoretinopathy frequently develops from a chronic retinal detachment (see Chapter 11, Vitreous Body, p. 182).

▶ **Epidemiology.** Although retinal detachments are relatively rarely encountered in ophthalmologic practice, they are clinically highly significant as they can lead to blindness if not treated immediately.

Table 12.7 Staging of retinopathy of prematurity

Stage	Characteristics
1	Demarcation (border between vascularized and nonvascularized retina)
2	Formation of a ridge (development of intraretinal proliferative tissue)
3	Ridge with extraretinal proliferation
4	Subtotal retinal detachment
5	Total retinal detachment

▶ **Rhegmatogenous retinal detachment (most frequent form).** Approximately 7% of adults have retinal breaks. The incidence of this finding increases with *advanced age.* The peak incidence is between the fifth and seventh decades of life. This indicates the significance of posterior vitreous detachment (separation of the vitreous body from inner surface of the retina; also age-related, see p. 175) as a cause of retinal detachment. The annual incidence of retinal detachment is 1 in 10,000 persons; the prevalence is about 0.4% in the elderly. There is a known familial disposition, and retinal detachment also occurs more frequently in conjunction with *myopia.* The prevalence of retinal detachment with emmetropia (normal vision) is 0.2% compared with 7% in the presence of severe myopia exceeding –10 diopters.

Exudative, tractional, and tumor-related retinal detachments are encountered far less frequently.

▶ **Etiology**
▶ **Rhegmatogenous retinal detachment.** This disorder develops from an *existing break in the retina.* Usually this break is in the peripheral retina, rarely in the macula (see ▶ Fig. 20.4). Two types of break are distinguished:

- *Round breaks.* A portion of the retina has been completely torn out due to a posterior vitreous detachment.
- *Horseshoe tears.* The retina is only torn (▶ Fig. 12.25).

Not every retinal break leads to retinal detachment. This will occur only where the liquefied vitreous body separates (see p. 175) and vitreous humor penetrates beneath the retina through the tear. The retinal detachment occurs when the forces of adhesion can no longer withstand this process. Tractional forces (tensile forces) of the vitreous body (usually vitreous strands) can also cause retinal detachment with or without synchysis. In this and every other type of retinal detachment, there is a *dynamic interplay of tractional and adhesive forces.*

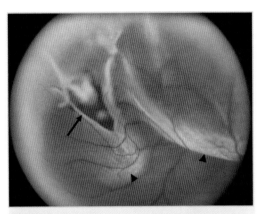

Fig. 12.25 **Horseshoe tear (arrow) and retinal detachment (whitish retina).** The image shows a typical reddish horseshoe tear in the retina (arrow) with bullous retinal detachment (arrowheads).

Whether the retina will detach depends on which of these forces is stronger.

▶ **Tractional retinal detachment.** This develops from the tensile forces exerted on the retina by preretinal fibrovascular strands, especially in proliferative retinal diseases such as diabetic retinopathy. See also proliferative vitreoretinopathy (PVR), Chapter 11.5, see p. 182).

▶ **Exudative retinal detachment.** Either the transudate from the tumor vasculature or the mass of the tumor separates the retina from its underlying tissue. Trauma may be followed by a secondary retinal detachment.

▶ **Symptoms.** Retinal detachment can remain asymptomatic for a long time. In the stage of acute posterior vitreous detachment, the patient will notice **flashes of light** (photopsia) and **floaters**, black points that move with the patient's gaze. A posterior vitreous detachment that causes a retinal tear may also cause avulsion of a retinal vessel. Blood from this vessel will then enter the vitreous body. The patient will perceive this as "**black rain**"—numerous slowly falling small black dots.

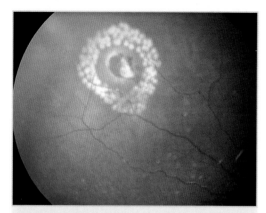

Fig. 12.26 Retinal break immediately after argon laser photocoagulation. Circular white laser burns are visible around the break.

Another symptom is a **dark shadow in the visual field** (see ▶ Fig. 20.10). This occurs when the retina detaches. The patient will perceive a falling curtain or a rising wall, depending on whether the detachment is superior or inferior. A break in the center of the retina will result in a sudden and significant **loss of visual acuity**, which will include metamorphopsia (image distortion) if the macula is involved.

Note
If the patient sees light flashes or shadows, an immediate ophthalmologic examination is necessary to rule out a retinal detachment.

▶ **Diagnostic considerations.** The lesion is diagnosed by stereoscopic examination of the fundus with the pupil dilated. The detached retina will be white and edematous and will lose its transparency. Ophthalmoscopy will reveal a bullous retinal detachment; in **rhegmatogenous retinal detachment**, a bright-red retinal break will also be visible (see ▶ Fig. 12.25). The tears in rhegmatogenous retinal detachment often occur in the superior half of the retina in a region of equatorial degeneration. In **tractional retinal detachment**, the bullous detachment will be accompanied by preretinal gray strands. In **exudative retinal detachment**, one will observe the typical picture of serous detachment; the exudative retinal detachment will generally be accompanied by massive fatty deposits and often by intraretinal bleeding.

The **tumor-related retinal detachment** (as can occur with a malignant melanoma) leads to secondary retinal detachment either above the tumor or at some distance from the tumor in the inferior peripheral retina. Ultrasound studies can help confirm the diagnosis where retinal findings are equivocal or a tumor is suspected.

Note
An inferior retinal detachment at some distance from the tumor is a sign that the tumor is malignant.

▶ **Differential diagnosis.** Degenerative **retinoschisis** (see p. 211) is the primary disorder that should be excluded as it can also involve rhegmatogenous retinal detachments in rare cases. A retinal detachment may also be confused with a choroidal detachment. Fluid accumulation in the choroid, due to inflammatory choroidal disorders such as Vogt–Koyanagi–Harada syndrome, causes the retinal pigment epithelium and neurosensory retina to bulge outward. These forms of retinal detachment have a dark brown of greenish color in contrast to the other forms of retinal detachment discussed here.

▶ **Treatment.** Retinal breaks with minimal circular retinal detachment can be treated with **laser coagulation** (▶ Fig. 12.26). The retina surrounding the break is fused to the underlying tissue whereas the break itself stays open. The scars resulting from laser coagulation therapy are sufficient to prevent any further retinal detachment. More extensive retinal detachments are usually treated with a **retinal tamponade with an elastic silicone sponge** that is sutured to the outer surface of the sclera, a so-called buckling procedure (▶ Fig. 12.27). It can be sutured either in a radial position (perpendicular to the limbus) or parallel to the limbus. This indents the wall of the globe at the retinal break and brings the portion of the retina in which the break is located back into contact with the retinal pigment epithelium. The indentation also reduces the traction of the vitreous body on the retina. An **artificial scar** is created to stabilize the restored contact between the neurosensory retina and retinal pigment epithelium. This is achieved with a cryoprobe. After a successful operation, this scar prevents recurring retinal detachment. Where there are several retinal breaks or the break cannot be located, a **silicone cerclage** is applied to the globe as a circumferential buckling procedure. The procedures described up until now apply to *uncomplicated retinal detachments*— i.e., without proliferative vitreoretinopathy. In complex retinal detachment (with and without PVR), the vitreous humor

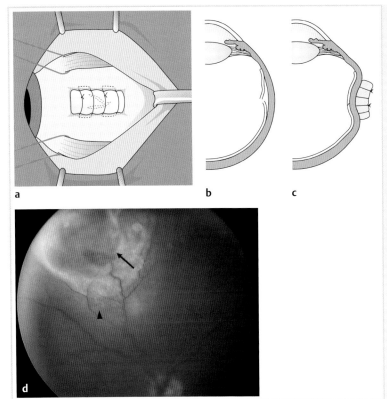

Fig. 12.27 Reattaching a detached retina with a silicone sponge tamponade. (a) The ocular muscles are retracted and the eye is brought into the proper position for the operation. The tamponade is sutured to the outer surface of the sclera. (b) Cross-section of the eye. The retinal hole is visible. (c) The tamponade is in place; the globe is indented at the site of the tamponade. The retina is reattached. (d) Wedged beneath the horseshoe tear (arrow) is a radial tamponade (arrowhead). The retina is again in contact with the underlying tissue.

is replaced and the vitreoretinal proliferations are excised. The vitreous body is replaced with Ringer's solution, gas, or silicone oil. These fluids tamponade the eye from within.

▶ **Prophylaxis.** High-risk patients above the age of 40 years with a positive family history and severe myopia should be regularly examined by an ophthalmologist, preferably once a year.

▶ **Clinical course and prognosis.** About 95% of **rhegmatogenous retinal detachments** can be treated successfully with surgery. Where there has been macular involvement (i.e., the initial detachment included the macula), a loss of visual acuity may remain. The prognosis for the **other forms of retinal detachment** is usually poor, and they are often associated with significant loss of visual acuity.

Note

In up to 20% of the patients a retinal detachment also develops in the fellow eye. A retinal tear therefore always has to be ruled out in the fellow eye as well.

12.4.2 Degenerative Retinoschisis

Definition

A frequently bilateral split in an inner and outer layer of the retina. The split is usually at the level of the outer plexiform layer (▶ Fig. 12.28).

▶ **Epidemiology.** About 25% of the general population have retinoschisis. The tendency increases with age.

▶ **Pathogenesis.** Idiopathic retinal splitting occurs, usually in the outer plexiform layer.

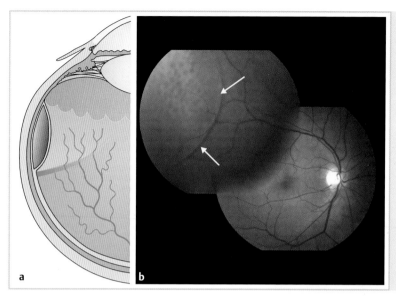

Fig. 12.28 (a, b) Retinoschisis. A split in the retina, with bullous separation of the inner layers of the retina (arrows in **b**).

▶ **Symptoms.** Retinoschisis is *primarily asymptomatic*. The patient will usually notice a reduction of visual acuity and see shadows only when the retinal split is severe and extends to the posterior pole.

▶ **Diagnostic considerations.** Ophthalmoscopic examination will reveal bullous separation of the split inner layer of the retina. The inner surface has the appearance of hammered metal. Rarely breaks will occur in the inner and outer retinal layers.

▶ **Differential diagnosis.** *Rhegmatogenous retinal detachment* should be excluded. Ophthalmoscopy will reveal a continuous break in the retina in a retinal detachment, and the retina will not appear as transparent as in retinoschisis. However, retinal breaks can also occur in retinoschisis. In the inner layer of the retina, these breaks will be very small and hardly discernible. In the outer layer, they will be very large. Complete rhegmatogenous retinal detachment can occur in retinoschisis only where there is a break in both layers.

▶ **Treatment.** Usually no treatment is required. The rare cases in which retinal detachment occurs are treated surgically using the standard procedures for retinal detachment (see p. 210).

> **Note**
> Degenerative retinoschisis differs from retinal detachment in that it usually requires no treatment.

▶ **Clinical course and prognosis.** The prognosis for degenerative retinoschisis is very good. Progressive retinal splitting or retinal detachment with a subsequent reduction in visual acuity is rare.

12.4.3 Peripheral Retinal Degenerations

Definition
Peripheral retinal degenerations refer to degenerative changes that lie parallel to the ora serrata in the peripheral portions of the retina.

There are two basic types:

- **Harmless retinal changes** such as pars plana cysts of the posterior ciliary body or peripheral chorioretinal atrophy (cobblestone degeneration).
- **Precursors of retinal detachment** such as local thinning of the retina referred to as snail track or lattice degeneration.

▶ **Epidemiology.** The prevalence of the lesions is 6 to 10%.

▶ **Pathogenesis.** Unknown.

▶ **Symptoms.** Peripheral retinal degenerations are asymptomatic.

▶ **Diagnostic considerations.** The diagnosis is made by ophthalmoscopic examination of the peripheral retina with the pupil dilated. The retina can be examined by indirect binocular ophthalmoscopy or using a three-mirror lens.

Cobblestone degenerations appear as whitish, sharply defined, localized areas of extensive atrophy of the retina, pigment epithelium, and choriocapillaris that lie between the ora serrata and the equator. **Snail track degeneration** presents with yellowish-whitish radiant dots consisting of microglia and astrocytes. **Lattice degeneration** presents with thinned retinal areas with whitish sclerotic vessels. This results in reactive focal atrophy and hypertrophy of the retinal pigment epithelium in the region of equatorial degeneration and liquefaction of the overlying vitreous body.

▶ **Differential diagnosis.** The findings are highly characteristic and easily diagnosed clinically. Rarely, vascular processes or inflammatory changes and scars from other causes must be considered in a differential diagnosis.

▶ **Treatment.** Treatment is either not required or not recommended as laser therapy does not reduce the risk of retinal detachment. Ophthalmoscopic follow-up examinations should be performed at regular intervals.

▶ **Prophylaxis.** No prophylaxis is possible.

▶ **Clinical course and prognosis.** The clinical course is usually benign. Round atrophic retinal breaks can develop in the areas of snail track and lattice degeneration. However, the long-term risk of retinal detachment is only 1%.

12.4.4 Central Serous Chorioretinopathy

Definition
Serous detachment of the retina and/or retinal pigment epithelium.

▶ **Etiology.** Serous detachment occurs through a defect in the outer blood–retina barrier "tight junctions" in the retinal pigment epithelium (▶ Fig. 12.29c). Local factors that may be related to

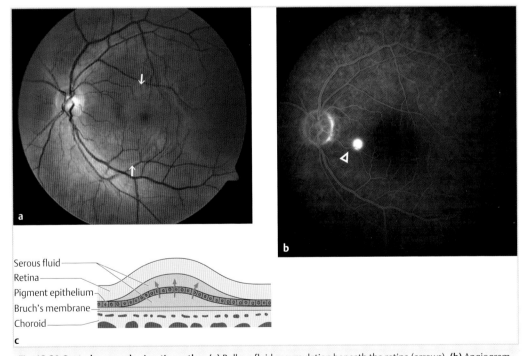

Fig. 12.29 Central serous chorioretinopathy. (a) Bullous fluid accumulation beneath the retina (arrows). **(b)** Angiogram from the same patient. The site of fluid effusion appears as a hyperfluorescent spot (arrowhead). **(c)** Schematic drawing of central serous chorioretinopathy.

physical or psychological stress are presumably involved.

▶ **Epidemiology.** The disorder primarily affects men in the third and fourth decades of life.

▶ **Symptoms.** Patients present with a loss of visual acuity, a relative central scotoma (dark spot), image distortion (metamorphopsia), or perception of objects as larger or smaller than they are (macropsia or micropsia).

▶ **Diagnostic considerations. Ophthalmoscopy** will reveal a serous retinal detachment, usually at the macula. In chronic cases, a fine brown and white pigment epithelial scar will develop at the site of the fluid effusion. Swelling in the central retina shortens the visual axis and produces hyperopia. The site of fluid effusion can be identified during the active phase with the aid of **fluorescein angiography** (▶ Fig. 12.29a ,b).

▶ **Treatment.** Usually no treatment is required for the **first occurrence** of the disorder. Retinal swelling resolves spontaneously within a few weeks. **Recurrences** can be treated with laser therapy provided the site of fluid effusion lies outside the fovea centralis or with photodynamic laser therapy (see p. 215). Carboanhydrase inhibitors, spironolactone or eplerenone can be administered off-label. Corticosteroid therapy is contraindicated as the therapy itself can lead to development of central serous chorioretinopathy in rare cases.

▶ **Clinical course and prognosis.** The prognosis is usually good. However, recurrences or chronic forms can lead to a permanent loss of visual acuity.

> **Note**
> Local stress-related factors and steroids can lead to macular edema in predisposed patients.

12.4.5 Age-Related Macular Degeneration

Definition
Progressive degeneration of the macula in elderly patients.

▶ **Epidemiology.** Age-related macular degeneration (AMD, ▶ Fig. 12.30) is the most frequent cause of blindness in patients over the age of 65 years.

The risk for people aged 85 or over is 11 to 18.5%, and the condition affects men and women similarly. AMD is much rarer in black people.

▶ **Pathogenesis.** A genetic predisposition has been confirmed, with a mutation in the *ABCR* gene (short arm of chromosome 1). Risk factors include smoking and intensive exposure to sunlight. The most important mechanisms are aging processes in the retinal pigment epithelium, which is postmitotic and has a limited regeneration ability (the retina and retinal pigment epithelium are as old as the patient). Degradation of the photoreceptor outer-segment discs leads to lipid-rich material, which accumulates in the retinal pigment epithelium together with photoreceptor outer-segment material and metabolic debris. The accumulations increase with age. The histological findings include basal laminar and linear deposits and drusen of the retinal pigment epithelium (▶ Fig. 12.30a). This results in increasing dysfunction. In addition, perfusion disturbances of the choroid develop. Presumably as a consequence of tissue hypoxia, vascular endothelial growth factor (VEGF) is expressed, which contributes substantially to the development of the late, neovascular form of AMD.

▶ **Symptoms.** Patients notice a *gradual* loss of visual acuity. In the neovascular form, in which macular edema is present, patients complain of image distortion (metamorphopsia), macropsia, or micropsia and sudden visual loss. Contrast sensitivity and color vision are also disturbed.

▶ **Findings and diagnostic considerations.** On ophthalmoscopy two main forms can be distinguished, an early and a late stage (▶ Table 12.8 and ▶ Fig. 12.30). In the late stage of AMD, choroidal neovascularization can develop. This neovascular form occurs in about 20% of the patients. Serous fluid, lipids, and blood leak through the insufficient wall of the new vessels. Finally, in the end stage, a fibrovascular scar develops, leading to irreversible severe visual loss and sometimes to blindness in 90% of patients. The diagnosis of AMD is made by stereoscopic fundus examination with a dilated pupil. The staging of AMD is carried out using fluorescein angiography (▶ Fig. 12.31). Indocyanine green angiography can provide additional information, especially regarding choroidal changes. The decision on whether to carry out laser treatment, photodynamic therapy, or intraocular VEGF inhibitor injection is based on the results of fluorescein angiography and optical coherence tomography.

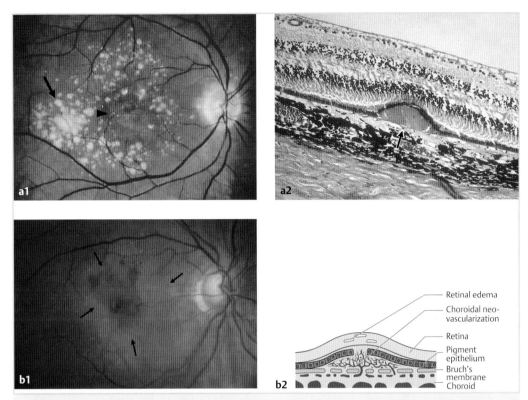

Retinal edema
Choroidal neo-
vascularization
Retina
Pigment
epithelium
Bruch's
membrane
Choroid

Fig. 12.30 Stages of age-related macular degeneration (see also ▶ Table 12.8). **(a)** Nonexudative age-related macular degeneration. Typical signs include drusen (arrow and figure on the right) and geographic central atrophy (arrowhead). **(b)** Exudative age-related macular degeneration. A typical finding is the intraretinal serous fluid (arrows and schematic drawing on the right), which is extravasating from the choroidal neovascularization.

▶ **Differential diagnosis.** Other vascular diseases of the retina, such as branch retinal vein occlusion, should be excluded with ophthalmoscopy. Malignant melanoma should be excluded using ultrasound studies (see p. 193).

▶ **Treatment.**
▶ **Pharmacological treatment.** No pharmacological treatment is yet available for non-exudative AMD, which constitutes 90% of cases. However, the Age-Related Eye Disease (ARED) study and the Lutein Antioxidant Supplementation Trial (LAST) found evidence that antioxidant supplementation has a beneficial effect on the progression of AMD and visual acuity. Pharmacotherapy of exudative AMD (= neovascular AMD = NAMD) is carried out with VEGF inhibitors (ranibizumab, aflibercept, and bevacizumab off-label).

▶ **Laser treatment.** In the late, exudative stage, choroidal neovascular membranes should be treated with thermal laser if they are located extra-

foveally and if the neovascularization can be visualized with fluorescein angiography (known as classic choroidal neovascularization). In occult choroidal neovascularization, however, the vessels cannot be seen on angiography and therefore cannot be treated with laser, but with VEGF inhibitors. The disadvantage of laser treatment is a recurrence rate of 39 to 76% within 2 years after laser therapy, as the neovascular membrane is incompletely deactivated.

▶ **Photodynamic therapy (PDT).** Photodynamic therapy is also possible in late, exudative AMD in classic and occult neovascularization, if it is located subfoveally. In contrast to laser treatment, the retina overlying the choroidal neovascularization is not damaged. PDT is a two-step procedure. Firstly, the photosensitizing dye verteporfin (Visudyne, Novartis) is infused intravenously within 10 minutes. It accumulates in the vascular endothelial cells of the choroidal neovascularization. Five minutes after the end of the infusion, the dye is acti-

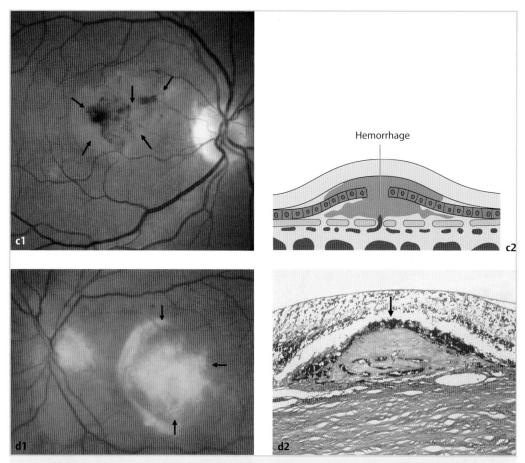

Fig. 12.30 (continued) Stages of age-related macular degeneration (see also ▶ Table 12.8). **(c)** Exudative neovascular age-related macular degeneration. A typical finding is intraretinal and subretinal hemorrhage (arrows and schematic drawing on the right). **(d)** Disciform age-related macular degeneration. A typical finding is a fibrous scar (arrows; see also the histological image on the right).

Table 12.8 Stages of age-related macular degeneration

Stage	Characteristics
1. Early	Drusen (≥63 µm), atrophy (<175 mm), and proliferation of retinal pigment epithelium
2. Late	Atrophy (≥175 µm) and proliferation of the retinal pigment epithelium (▶ Fig. 12.30a); geographic atrophy, serous detachment of the retina and/or retinal pigment epithelium, hemorrhage (▶ Fig. 12.30b, c, and see ▶ Fig. 20.5, ▶ Fig. 20.6); fibrous scar (▶ Fig. 12.30d)

vated for exactly 83 seconds using a nonthermal laser with a wavelength of 689 nm. The resulting photochemical reaction leads to photothrombosis of the neovascular membrane (the vessels close, so that they no longer leak). The treatment has to be carried out about five or six times at 3-month intervals until complete inactivation of the neovascular membrane is achieved. The goal of the treat- ment is to stabilize visual acuity (it is, however, less effective than intravitreal application of VEGF inhibitors). Surgical extraction of the neovascular membrane has not been found to be beneficial. Treatment modalities such as macular rotation or translocation may be considered in special cases. Microphotoarray implants are now also available for selected cases.

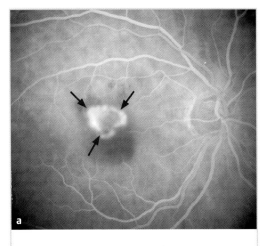

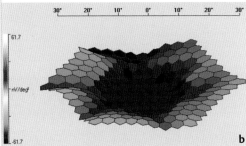

Fig. 12.31 Stages of late age-related macular degeneration. (a) Fluorescein angiogram. A classic choroidal neovascularization is visible under the fovea (arrows). This is therefore a late, exudative stage of age-related macular degeneration. **(b)** The corresponding multifocal electroretinogram (compare the ERG of a healthy retina in ▶ Fig. 12.12). The degenerated macula is hardly responding to the electrical stimulation at all.

▶ **Clinical course and prognosis.** The course of the disorder is chronic and leads to progressive loss of visual acuity. Risk factors in the progression are soft, large, and confluent drusen, foveal hyperpigmentation, and arterial hypertension. Patients can carry out self-monitoring with the Amsler grid test (▶ Fig. 12.32). Forty percent of patients with choroidal neovascularization develop neovascular AMD in the second eye. Magnifying glasses can sometimes restore up to 80% of the patients' reading ability.

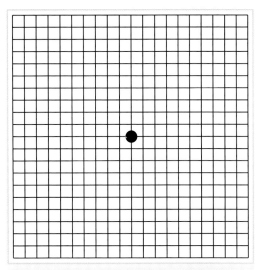

Fig. 12.32 Amsler grid. In fixation on the black fixation dot (monocular from the age of 40 years with reading glasses), all of the lines must be straight. If the lines appear wavy or warped, the macula is edematous.

12.4.6 Degenerative Myopia

Definition
The fundus in degenerative myopia is characterized by abnormal chorioretinal atrophy.

▶ **Epidemiology.** Chorioretinal atrophy due to myopia is rare.

▶ **Pathogenesis.** The atrophy usually occurs in the presence of severe myopia exceeding −6 diopters. The causes include stretching changes in the retina, choroid, and Bruch's membrane due to the elongated globe in axial myopia (see p. 278) leading to chorioretinal atrophy.

▶ **Symptoms.** Loss of visual acuity occurs where there is macular involvement.

▶ **Findings and diagnostic considerations.** Typical signs include chorioretinal atrophy around the optic disc and at the posterior pole (▶ Fig. 12.33) and defects in Bruch's membrane known as lacquer cracks. These cracks can provide openings for vascular infiltration with resulting subretinal neovascularization that can lead to retinal edema and bleeding (Fuchs's black spot). The final stage of the disorder is characterized by a disciform scar. The diagnosis is made by ophthalmoscopy. Fluorescein

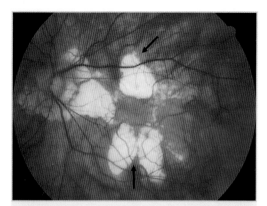

Fig. 12.33 Degenerative myopia. Extensive areas of chorioretinal atrophy (arrows).

angiography is indicated where subretinal neovascularization is suspected.

▶ **Differential diagnosis.** Choroidal scars and angioid streaks (breaks in Bruch's membrane) in pseudoxanthoma elasticum must be excluded by ophthalmoscopy. The diagnosis is unequivocal where myopia is present.

▶ **Treatment.** The causes of the disorder cannot be treated. It is important to correct myopia optimally with eyeglasses or contact lenses to avoid fostering progression of the disorder. Subretinal neovascularization outside the fovea or close to its border can be treated by intravitreal anti-VEGF therapy. An alternative in cases of juxtafoveal or extrafoveal neovascularization is laser photocoagulation. Subfoveal neovascularization is treated by VEGF inhibitors (see p. 215).

▶ **Clinical course and prognosis.** Chronic progressive myopia will result in increasing loss of visual acuity. The prognosis for subretinal neovascularization is poor. The incidence of retinal detachment is higher in myopic eyes.

12.5 Retinal Dystrophies

12.5.1 Macular Dystrophies

Definition
Macular dystrophies are disorders of the macula that usually occur bilaterally and manifest themselves between the ages of 10 and 30 years.

Stargardt's Disease

Definition
This is a macular dystrophy that proceeds from the retinal pigment epithelium.

▶ **Inheritance.** Autosomal-recessive disorder.

▶ **Epidemiology.** Stargardt's disease is rare.

▶ **Symptoms.** Progressive loss of visual acuity occurs between the ages of 10 and 20 years.

▶ **Findings and diagnostic considerations.** Initial findings are slight with whitish-yellow "fleck" lesions in the macular region (▶ Fig. 12.34a, b), which may occur in combination with lesions in the entire fundus (*fundus flavimaculatus*). The electroretinogram and electro-oculogram will be nor-

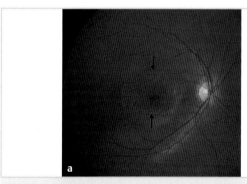
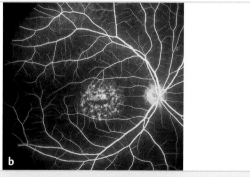

Fig. 12.34 Stargardt's disease. (a) Typical yellow maculate lesions of the macula (arrows) and atrophy of the pigment epithelium in the macula. (b) The corresponding fluorescein-angiographic finding, with spotty hyperfluorescence in the macula and blocked choroid fluorescence (dark choroid).

mal or reduced. In the later stage, the white lesions significantly increase in size and number. This will not necessarily be reflected in the ERG or EOG. Typically, retinal fluorescence is blocked in the fluorescence angiogram (the choroid appears black; ▶ Fig. 12.34b).

▶ **Differential diagnosis.** Other disorders involving white "fleck" lesions such as inherited autosomal-dominant drusen must be excluded by ophthalmoscopy. The diagnosis is confirmed by fluorescein angiography. Blockage of the choroidal fluorescein is a characteristic feature of Stargardt's disease.

▶ **Treatment.** No treatment is available. Edge-filtered eyeglasses and magnifying near vision aids can help make better use of the patient's remaining vision.

▶ **Prophylaxis.** No prophylaxis is possible. Examination of siblings and genetic counseling are indicated.

▶ **Clinical course and prognosis.** The disorder is chronically progressive. Vision in the final stages is usually 20/200 or less.

Best's Vitelliform Dystrophy

▶ **Epidemiology.** The disorder is rare, with an incidence similar to Stargardt's disease.

▶ **Inheritance.** The disorder is inherited as an autosomal-dominant trait with variable penetrance and expressivity. The gene locus is on chromosome 11 (11 q13).

▶ **Symptoms.** Clinical manifestation occurs between the ages of 5 and 15. Initially there is a subjectively slight decrease in visual acuity. In the later stages of the disorder, vision is reduced to about 20/200.

▶ **Findings and diagnostic considerations.** A typical feature of this form of macular dystrophy is that

isual acuity is negligibly diminished at the onset of the disorder. However, the *morphological findings are remarkable.* Ophthalmoscopy will reveal yellowish round vitelliform lesions in the macular region (▶ Fig. 12.35) that look like the yolk of a fried egg. (The Latin word *vitellus* means egg yolk.) Usually these lesions are bilateral and symmetrical, although eccentric lesions may also occur. ▶ Table 12.9 lists the various manifestations.

Note
The macular change resembling an egg yolk gave rise to the name vitelliform dystrophy.

▶ **Differential diagnosis.** An unequivocal diagnosis can usually be made on the basis of the clinical picture alone. Sharply reduced or absent light response in the EOG and normal ERG confirms the presence of Best's vitelliform dystrophy.

▶ **Treatment.** The causes of the disorder cannot be treated.

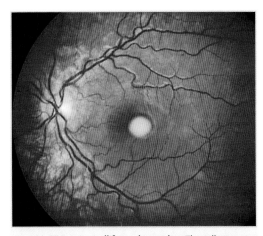

Fig. 12.35 Best's vitelliform dystrophy. The yellow, sharply demarcated lesion resembles the yolk of a fried egg.

Table 12.9 Stages of Best's vitelliform dystrophy

Stage	Characteristics
Previtelliform stage	Yellowish central pigment changes
Vitelliform stage	Sharply demarcated yellow yolk-like lesion (see ▶ Fig. 12.35)
Pseudohypopyon stage	Settling of the yellow material
Vitelliruptive stage	"Scrambling" of the yolk-like lesions with irregular yellow deposits
Scar stage	Transition to scar

▶ **Prophylaxis.** Examination of siblings and genetic counseling are indicated.

▶ **Clinical course and prognosis.** The prognosis is more favorable than for Stargardt's disease. The disorder is chronically progressive. Visual acuity in the better eye usually remains about 20/40. Secondary loss of visual acuity can result from subretinal neovascularization.

12.5.2 Retinitis Pigmentosa

Definition
This term is used to refer to a heterogeneous group of retinal disorders that lead to progressive loss of visual acuity, visual field defects, and night blindness. The name retinitis pigmentosa comes from the pigment deposits that characterize these disorders. In the classic form (see Findings and diagnostic considerations) of such disorders, these deposits progress from the periphery to the center of the retina.

▶ **Epidemiology.** The worldwide incidence of retinitis pigmentosa is estimated at between 1 in 35,000 and 1 in 7,000 persons. The estimated incidence of mutated alleles is one in 80 persons.

▶ **Forms of retinitis pigmentosa**
1. Rod–cone dystrophy (classic retinitis pigmentosa, by far the most frequent form).
2. Cone–rod dystrophy (inverse retinitis pigmentosa).
3. Sectoral retinitis pigmentosa.
4. Retinitis pigmentosa sine pigmento (form without pigment).
5. Unilateral retinitis pigmentosa.
6. Leber's congenital amaurosis (form occurring in early childhood).
7. Retinopathy punctata albescens (punctate retinitis).
8. In combination with other disorders in syndromes and metabolic disorders such as mucopolysaccharidoses, Fanconi's syndrome, mucolipidosis IV, peroxisomal disorders, Cockayne's syndrome, mitochondrial myopathies, Usher's syndrome, neuronal and ceroid lipofuscinoses, renal tubular defect syndromes, etc.

Retinitis pigmentosa occurs almost exclusively as rod–cone dystrophy. Therefore, the other extremely rare forms are not discussed here, except for the inverse form of classic retinitis pigmentosa, which is presented for purposes of comparison.

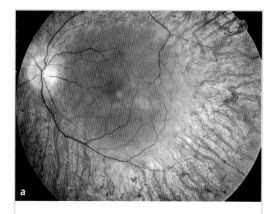

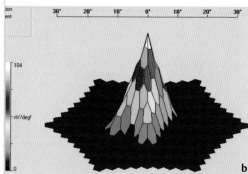

Fig. 12.36 Advanced retinitis pigmentosa. (a) Typical signs include narrowed retinal vessels, a waxy yellow appearance of the optic disc due to atrophy of the optic nerve, and "bone-spicule" proliferation of the retinal pigment epithelium. **(b)** The corresponding multifocal ERG. A typical finding is the preserved cone response.

▶ **Inheritance.** Individual genetic forms can be identified from among the heterogeneous group of disorders comprising retinitis pigmentosa. This group of disorders can involve various genotypes as well as variable phenotypic expression or different stages of a disorder with one specific genotype. There are *over 15 purely ocular forms* of retinitis pigmentosa. The most common form of inheritance is autosomal-recessive (60%), followed by autosomal-dominant (up to 25%), and X-linked (15%). Rhodopsin gene mutations (chromosome 3) and "retinal degeneration slow" (RDS) gene mutations (chromosome 6) have also been described.

▶ **Symptoms.** Initial symptoms of retinitis pigmentosa include glare, night blindness, progressive visual field defects, loss of visual acuity, and color vision defects. The age of manifestation depends on the type of inheritance.

▶ **Findings and diagnostic considerations.** The diagnosis is made by ophthalmoscopy on the basis of a classic picture.

▶ **Rod–cone dystrophy (primarily the rods are affected first).** *Proliferation of retinal pigment epithelium* is observed in the middle periphery of the retina. This will gradually spread toward the center and farther peripherally (▶ Fig. 12.36). Early deficits include color vision defects and disturbed contrast perception. *Atrophy of the optic nerve*, discernible as a waxy yellow appearance of the optic disc, will occur in the advanced stages. The *arteries will appear narrowed*, and the *fundus reflex will be extremely muted*. The patient will typically have a *"gun-barrel" visual field* with good visual acuity for a surprisingly long time, but with progressive loss of the peripheral visual field.

▶ **Cone–rod dystrophy (primarily the cones are affected first).** Here, there is early loss of visual acuity with gradual progressive loss of visual field. In both forms of retinitis pigmentosa, the diagnosis is confirmed by electroretinography. Light response in the EOG will be sharply reduced or absent early in the clinical course of the disease.

▶ **Differential diagnosis.** Differential diagnosis should consider changes collectively referred to as pseudoretinitis pigmentosa because they simulate the clinical picture of retinitis pigmentosa. The most common causes that should be excluded in this context are:

- Posttraumatic changes.
- Postinflammatory or postinfectious changes. These may include degenerative retinal pigment epithelial disease secondary to rubella with a "salt-and-pepper" fundus of punctate areas of atrophy and proliferation of retinal pigment epithelium. Other causes include syphilis, which may present with placoid lesions of pigment epithelial atrophy and proliferations.
- Tumors.
- Medications such as chloroquine, ethambutol (Myambutol, STI Pharma LLC), and thioridazine.

▶ **Treatment.** The causes of the disorder cannot be treated. Edge-filtered eyeglasses (special eyeglasses with orange or brown colored lenses that filter out certain wavelengths) and magnifying near vision aids can help make better use of the patient's remaining vision.

▶ **Prophylaxis.** No prophylaxis is possible.

▶ **Clinical course and prognosis.** Retinitis pigmentosa is chronically progressive. The clinical course depends on the specific form of the disorder; severe forms lead to blindness.

12.6 Toxic Retinopathy

Definition
Retinal changes resulting from the use of medications.

▶ **Epidemiology.** Toxic retinopathy is rare.

▶ **Pathogenesis.** The pathogenesis depends on the medication concerned.

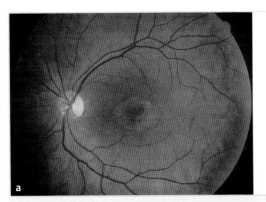 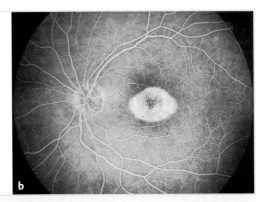

Fig. 12.37 Chloroquine toxicity (bull's eye maculopathy). (a) After prolonged medication with chloroquine, ring-shaped mild atrophy occurs, and proliferation of the retinal pigment epithelium in the macula area develops. **(b)** The corresponding fluorescein angiogram, with sharply demarcated hyperfluorescence.

221

▶ **Findings and symptoms.** Toxic retinopathy can remain asymptomatic for a long time. Loss of visual acuity occurs if the macula is affected.

Chloroquine in doses exceeding 250 g causes retinal damage. Macular edema can occur initially. Later, punctate pigment epithelial changes develop, which may progress to bull's eye maculopathy with concentric rings of hypopigmentation and hyperpigmentation in the macular region (▶ Fig. 12.37). These findings are usually bilateral and symmetrical. Other toxic retinal changes are listed in Chapter 20.1).

▶ **Diagnostic considerations.** The diagnosis is made by binocular ophthalmoscopy with the pupil dilated and confirmed by electrophysiologic studies that include an electroretinogram, electro-oculogram, and visual evoked potentials (see ▶ Fig. 12.2a).

▶ **Differential diagnosis.** Retinal pigment epithelium or retinal bleeding can result from many other retinal disorders, and may also be associated with the underlying disease for which the medication was prescribed.

▶ **Treatment.** The medication should be discontinued if possible.

▶ **Prophylaxis.** Regular ophthalmologic follow-up examinations are indicated before and during treatment that involves medications with known ocular side effects.

▶ **Clinical course and prognosis.** The clinical course depends on the specific medication and dose. Findings may improve after the medication is discontinued. However, with chloroquine in particular, findings may continue to worsen even years later.

12.7 Retinal Inflammatory Disease

12.7.1 Retinal Vasculitis

Definition
Retinal vasculitis is an inflammation of the retinal vasculature. Typical findings include cells in the vitreous body.

▶ **Epidemiology.** Retinal vasculitis is one of the more frequent ocular diseases.

▶ **Etiology.** The cause of retinal vasculitis often remains obscure. It can be caused by a pathogen or occur in association with immunologic processes (▶ Table 12.10).

▶ **Symptoms.** Patients report loss of visual acuity or black dots in their visual field. These are due to the presence of cells in the vitreous body.

▶ **Diagnostic considerations.** The ophthalmologic diagnostic work-up includes clinical examination, ophthalmoscopy, and slit lamp examination. The slit lamp examination will reveal *cells in the vitre-*

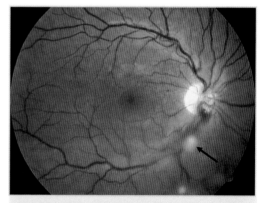

Fig. 12.38 Retinal vasculitis. Ophthalmoscopy reveals whitish preretinal vitreous infiltrates (arrow).

Table 12.10 The major causes of retinal vasculitis

Cause		
• Idiopathic	• Wegener's granulomatosis	• Borreliosis (Lyme disease)
• Eales's disease	• Polyarteritis nodosa	• Listeriosis
• Behçet's disease	• Horton's arteritis	• Brucellosis
• Multiple sclerosis	• Sarcoidosis	• Syphilis
• Lupus erythematosus	• Tuberculosis	• Viruses

ous body. Ophthalmoscopic findings will include whitish preretinal infiltrates (▶ Fig. 12.38), vascular constriction (usually involving the veins), vascular occlusion, intraretinal bleeding, and retinal edema. Fluorescein angiography can be used to evaluate the presence and activity of neovascularization. Underlying systemic disease, immunologic processes, and infections (see ▶ Table 12.10) must be excluded.

▶ **Differential diagnosis.** Other vascular diseases of the retina such as vein occlusion should be excluded. These vascular diseases can be distinguished from vascular retinitis by the *absence of cells in the vitreous body*.

▶ **Treatment.** The causes of known underlying disorders should be treated. Symptoms are treated with topical steroids and systemic steroids in the absence of contraindications. Neovascularization is treated with laser therapy.

▶ **Prophylaxis.** No prophylaxis is possible except for possible treatment of an underlying disorder.

▶ **Clinical course and prognosis.** Vascular occlusion can result in neovascularization that may lead to vitreous hemorrhage. Tractional retinal detachment is another possible complication.

12.7.2 Posterior Uveitis due to Toxoplasmosis

Definition
Focal chorioretinal inflammation caused by infection.

▶ **Epidemiology.** This clinical syndrome is encountered frequently.

▶ **Pathogenesis.** The pathogen, *Toxoplasma gondii*, is transmitted *by ingestion of tissue cysts* in raw or undercooked meat or by *oocysts* from cat feces. In congenital toxoplasmosis, the child acquires the pathogen through transplacental transmission.

▶ **Symptoms and diagnostic considerations.** As a general rule, a negative complement-fixation test does not exclude *Toxoplasma* infection where classic clinical symptoms are present. Both forms of the disorder present with characteristic *grayish-white chorioretinal focal lesions surrounded by vitreous infiltration* and *associated vasculitis* (▶ Fig. 12.39b). In **congenital toxoplasmosis** (▶ Fig. 12.39a), the

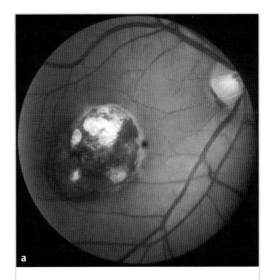

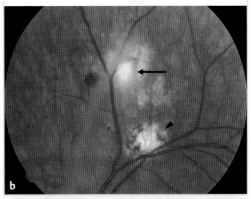

Fig. 12.39 Retinochoroidal toxoplasmosis. (a) Congenital toxoplasmosis (always located in the macula; the scar is sharply demarcated). (b) Recurrent toxoplasmosis: An acute grayish-white retinochoroidal focal lesion (arrow) and brownish-white chorioretinal scars (arrowhead). Lesions usually recur at the margin of the original scar, the so-called "mother spot."

affected children have a *macular scar* that *significantly impairs* visual acuity. This often leads to secondary strabismus. Intracerebral involvement can also result in hydrocephalus and intracranial calcifications. In the **acquired form**, visual acuity is impaired only where the macula is involved. This is rarely the case.

Note
Congenital toxoplasmosis results in a macular scar that significantly impairs visual acuity.

▶ **Differential diagnosis.** Retinochoroiditis with tuberculosis, sarcoidosis, borreliosis (Lyme disease), or syphilis should be excluded by serologic studies.

▶ **Treatment.** The treatment of choice consists of a combination of pyrimethamine, sulfonamide, folinic acid, and steroids in their respective standard doses.

▶ **Prophylaxis.** Avoid contact with raw meat and cat feces.

▶ **Clinical course and prognosis.** Posterior uveitis due to toxoplasmosis usually heals without severe loss of visual acuity where the macula is not involved. However, it can recur at any time. There is no cure for the congenital form.

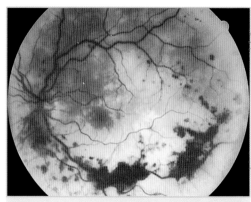

Fig. 12.40 Cytomegalovirus retinitis. Typical signs include extensive white areas of retinal necrosis and hemorrhages.

12.7.3 AIDS-Related Retinal Disorders

Definition
Retinal disorders in AIDS involve either AIDS-associated microangiopathy or infection.

▶ **Epidemiology.** In former times, up to 80% of AIDS patients were left with retinal disorders as a result of the disease. Ocular involvement is rare nowadays. Since the introduction of new antiretroviral medications, eye involvement in AIDS has decreased markedly.

▶ **Pathogenesis.** The pathogenesis of microangiopathy is still unclear. Opportunistic infections are frequently caused by viruses.

▶ **Symptoms.** Microangiopathy is usually asymptomatic. Patients with infectious retinal disorders report loss of visual acuity and visual field defects.

▶ **Diagnostic considerations.** Ophthalmoscopic findings in **AIDS-associated microangiopathy** include hemorrhages, microaneurysms, telangiectasia, and cotton-wool spots. Direct involvement of vascular endothelial cells in HIV infection or immune-complex-mediated damage to endothelial cells and vascular structures is thought to play a role.

Cytomegalovirus retinitis occurs in 20 to 40% of older patients. Peripheral retinal necrosis and intraretinal hemorrhages (▶ Fig. 12.40) are frequently observed. Vascular occlusion is rare. Secondary rhegmatogenous retinal detachment may develop. These lesions heal to produce fine granular pigment epithelial scars.

Less frequently, AIDS may involve **retinal infection** caused by **herpes simplex** and **varicella-zoster viruses**, *Toxoplasma gondii*, or *Pneumocystis carinii*. The diagnosis of a viral retinal infection in AIDS is confirmed by attempting to obtain positive serum cultures and by resistance testing.

▶ **Differential diagnosis.** Inflammatory retinal changes due to other causes should be excluded by serologic studies.

▶ **Treatment.** Microangiopathy does not require treatment. Viral retinitis is treated with ganciclovir or foscarnet. Herpes simplex and varicella-zoster viruses are treated with acyclovir.

▶ **Prophylaxis.** Ophthalmologic screening examinations are indicated in the presence of known viral infection.

▶ **Clinical course and prognosis.** The prognosis for microangiopathy is very good. Infectious retinitis will lead to blindness if left untreated. Visual acuity can often be preserved if a prompt diagnosis is made.

12.7.4 Viral Retinitis

Definition
Retinal disorder caused by viral infection.

▶ **Epidemiology.** Viral retinitis is a rare disorder.

▶ **Pathogenesis.** Infection of the retina and retinal vasculature caused by cytomegalovirus, herpes simplex, varicella-zoster, or rubella viruses. Viral retinitis frequently occurs in immunocompromised patients.

▶ **Symptoms.** Patients report loss of visual acuity and visual field defects.

▶ **Diagnostic considerations.** Slit lamp examination will reveal cells in the vitreous body. Ophthalmoscopic findings will include retinal necrosis with intraretinal hemorrhages (see ▶ Fig. 12.40). Necrosis can occur as acute lesions and spread over the entire retina like a bushfire within a few days. When the retinitis heals, it leaves behind wide-area scarring.

During pregnancy, rubella virus can cause embryopathy in the child. Ophthalmic examination will reveal typical fine granular pigment epithelial scars on the fundus that are often associated with a congenital cataract. The diagnosis is confirmed by measuring the serum virus titer. The possibility of compromised immunocompetence should be verified or excluded.

▶ **Differential diagnosis.** Posterior uveitis and vasculitis should be excluded. Those disorders can be distinguished from viral retinitis by the absence of necrosis.

▶ **Treatment.** The disorder is treated with high doses of an antiviral agent (acyclovir, ganciclovir, or foscarnet), depending on the specific pathogen.

▶ **Prophylaxis.** Ophthalmologic screening examinations are indicated in immunocompromised persons with suspected viral infection.

▶ **Clinical course and prognosis.** Viral retinitis can be arrested if diagnosed early. However, recurrences are frequent in immunocompromised patients. Blindness usually cannot be prevented in retinal necrosis syndrome.

12.7.5 Retinitis in Lyme Disease

Definition
Inflammation of the retina usually caused by *Borrelia burgdorferi*.

▶ **Epidemiology.** The incidence of this retinal disorder has increased in recent years.

▶ **Etiology.** The inflammation is caused by spirochetes, usually transmitted by bites from infected ticks.

▶ **Findings and symptoms.** Lyme disease can lead to many inflammatory ocular changes with their respective symptoms. These include conjunctivitis, keratitis, and iridocyclitis. Retinal vasculitis, retinal artery occlusion, neuroretinitis, optic neuritis, and choroiditis have also been described.

Note
Lyme disease should be excluded as a possible cause of posterior uveitis of uncertain etiology.

▶ **Diagnostic considerations.** The diagnosis is made by ophthalmoscopy and serologic studies to identify the pathogen.

▶ **Differential diagnosis.** Inflammatory ocular changes due to other causes (such as toxoplasmosis or tuberculosis) should be excluded.

▶ **Treatment.** Antibiotic treatment with tetracycline, penicillin G, or third-generation cephalosporins is indicated.

▶ **Clinical course and prognosis.** Retinal changes due to borreliosis tend to recur in spite of antibiotic treatment.

12.7.6 Parasitic Retinal Disorders

Definition
Inflammation of the retina caused by infection with parasites such as *Onchocerca volvulus* (the pathogen that causes onchocerciasis), *Toxocara canis* or *Toxocara cati* (nematode larvae that are normally intestinal parasites of dogs and cats), *Taenia solium* (pork tapeworm), and other parasites.

▶ **Epidemiology.** Onchocerciasis, like trachoma and leprosy, is one of the most frequent causes of blindness worldwide. However, like the other parasitic diseases discussed here, it is rare in Europe and North America.

▶ **Etiology.** *Onchocerca volvulus* is transmitted by the bite of black flies. This allows the larvae (microfilaria) to penetrate the skin, where they form fibrous subcutaneous nodules. There they reach maturity and produce other microfilaria, which migrate into surrounding tissue. The danger of ocular infiltration is particularly great where there are fibrous nodules close to the eye.

Toxocara canis or *Toxocara cati* (eggs of nematodes infesting dogs and cats) are transmitted to humans by ingestion of substances contaminated with the feces of these animals. The eggs hatch in the gastrointestinal tract, where they gain access to the circulatory system and may spread throughout the entire body. The choroid can become infested in this way.

Taenia solium: The pork tapeworm infestation can occur from eating pork contaminated with larvae or other substances contaminated with tapeworm eggs. Mature tapeworms can also release eggs into the intestine. The larvae travel through the bloodstream to various organs and can also infest the eye.

▶ **Diagnostic considerations and findings.** Ophthalmoscopy will reveal intraocular inflammation. Onchocerciasis has been known to be associated with posterior uveitis as well as keratitis and iritis. Histologic examination will demonstrate microfilaria in the retina. Visceral larva migrans, *Toxocara canis*, or *Toxocara cati* can cause complications involving endophthalmitis and retinal detachment. Subretinal granulomas and larval inflammation of the retina have been known to occur. The *larvae of different species of worms* can produce diffuse unilateral subacute neuroretinitis with the typical clinical picture of grayish-white intraretinal and subretinal focal lesions. *Fly larvae* can also invade the subretinal space in ophthalmomyiasis.

▶ **Differential diagnosis.** Other causes of retinal inflammation and subretinal granulomas should be excluded.

▶ **Treatment.** Laser photocoagulation or surgical removal of the worm larvae may be indicated.

▶ **Clinical course and prognosis.** It is not uncommon for these disorders to lead to blindness.

12.8 Retinal Tumors and Hamartomas

12.8.1 Retinoblastoma

Definition
Retinoblastoma is a malignant tumor of early childhood that develops from immature retinal cells.

▶ **Epidemiology.** Retinoblastoma is the most common malignant ocular tumor in children, occurring in approximately 1 in 20,000 births. In 30% of cases, it is bilateral.

▶ **Pathogenesis.** A somatic mutation is detected in about 95% of patients. In the other patients, it is inherited as an autosomal-dominant trait. Changes on chromosome 13q have been observed in germcell mutations. Retinoblastomas may then occur at several locations in the retina or bilaterally.

Note
Where retinoblastoma is inherited as an autosomal-dominant trait, the siblings of the affected child should be regularly examined by an ophthalmologist.

▶ **Symptoms.** Retinoblastoma manifests itself before the age of 3 years in 90% of affected children (▶ Fig. 12.41). Parents observe leukocoria (a whitish-yellow pupil; ▶ Fig. 12.41a) in 60% of these children, strabismus in 20%, and a reddened eye in 10%.

Note
Every child presenting with strabismus should undergo examination of the fundus with the pupil dilated to exclude a retinoblastoma.

▶ **Findings and diagnostic considerations.** A grayish-white, vascularized retinal tumor will be observed on ophthalmoscopy (▶ Fig. 12.41b). In its advanced stages, this tumor was formerly referred to as an *amaurotic cat's eye.* Infiltration of the vitreous body, anterior chamber (pseudohypopyon), and orbit may occur. A retinoblastoma that also involves the fellow eye and pineal body is referred to as a *trilateral retinoblastoma.*

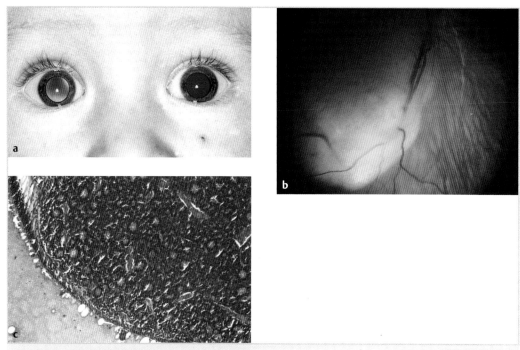

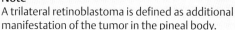

Fig. 12.41 Leukocoria in the right eye due to a retinoblastoma. **(a)** The whitish gleam of the pupil of the right eye is a typical finding in retinoblastoma. **(b)** Ophthalmoscopic finding of a retinoblastoma (gray-white tumor). **(c)** Histological finding of a retinoblastoma with Flexner–Wintersteiner rosettes.

Note

A trilateral retinoblastoma is defined as additional manifestation of the tumor in the pineal body.

Calcifications frequently occur in these tumors. Radiographs or computed tomography images that show calcifications can therefore help to confirm the diagnosis in uncertain cases.

▶ **Differential diagnosis.** Several other disorders should be excluded by ophthalmoscopy. These include

• Cataract (with leukocoria).
• Primary strabismus (with strabismus).
• Infection (with a reddened eye).

Retinal detachment, persistent hyperplastic primary vitreous (PHPV), and Coats's disease should also be excluded.

▶ **Treatment.** Tumors less than four pupil diameters in size can be managed with radiation therapy delivered by plaques of radioactive ruthenium or

iodine (brachytherapy) and cryotherapy. Larger tumors requiring enucleation of the eye can be shrunk preoperatively with chemotherapy. More recently, proton radiation is also being applied.

▶ **Prophylaxis.** Following the diagnosis, the fellow eye should be examined with the pupil dilated every 3 months for 5 years. After that, follow-up examinations can be performed at longer intervals.

▶ **Clinical course and prognosis.** Left untreated, a retinoblastoma will eventually metastasize to the brain and cause death. Patients frequently develop a second malignant tumor such as an osteosarcoma. The lethality rate of bilateral retinoblastoma is approximately 8%.

12.8.2 Astrocytoma

Definition
An astrocytoma or astrocytic hamartoma is a *benign* tumor that develops from the astrocytes of the neuroglial tissue.

▶ **Epidemiology.** Astrocytomas are rare.

▶ **Etiology.** Astrocytomas belong to the phacomatoses and are presumably congenital disorders that develop from the layer of optic nerve fibers. They may manifest themselves as purely ocular disorders or in association with tuberous sclerosis (Bourneville's disease).

▶ **Symptoms.** Patients usually have *no ocular symptoms*. Calcifying astrocytic hamartomas in the region of the basal ganglia or ventricles can cause epilepsy and mental deficiency. An astrocytoma in Bourneville disease will be associated typically with an adenoma sebaceum in the facial skin.

▶ **Findings and diagnostic considerations.** Astrocytomas are either incidental findings in ophthalmic examinations performed for other reasons, or they are diagnosed in patients presenting with reduced visual acuity. Ophthalmoscopy will reveal *single or multiple "mulberry" tumors* one to two pupil diameters in size. These will appear white and are often calcified. The tumors are inherently fluorescent when observed in blue light in fluorescein angiography (see p. 194) with a blue filter.

▶ **Differential diagnosis.** A retinoblastoma should be excluded in children. It is usually larger than an astrocytoma on ophthalmoscopy. A possible *Toxocara canis* granuloma should be confirmed or excluded by serologic studies.

▶ **Treatment.** No ophthalmologic treatment is required. The patient should be referred to a neurologist to exclude cerebral involvement.

▶ **Clinical course and prognosis.** These tumors rarely increase in size.

12.8.3 Hemangiomas

Definition
Capillary hemangiomas or hemangioblastomas occur in angiomatosis retinae (von Hippel–Lindau disease).

▶ **Epidemiology.** Hemangiomas are rare.

▶ **Etiology.** Hemangiomas belong to the class of mesodermal phacomatoses. These are *benign* congenital changes. There may be an autosomal-dominant inheritance. The gene has been localized on the short arm of chromosome 3 (3p).

▶ **Symptoms.** Loss of visual acuity will result where exudative retinal detachment develops.

▶ **Findings and diagnostic considerations.** Retinal hemangiomas are characterized by thickened tortuous arteries and veins (▶ Fig. 12.42a, b). Bilateral changes are present in 50% of patients. Approximately 70% of patients have cerebellar hemangioblastomas, about 20% have renal carcinomas, and 17% have polycythemia. These potential diseases must be specifically ruled out.

▶ **Differential diagnosis.** Coats's disease, branching retinal hemangiomas in Wyburn–Mason syndrome, and cavernous hemangiomas should be considered. Cerebral hemangiomas, renal cysts, hypernephromas, and pheochromocytomas should also be excluded.

▶ **Treatment.** Retinal hemangiomas can be treated by laser or cryocautery therapy. However, exudative retinal detachment often develops. Treatment may increase this risk.

▶ **Clinical course and prognosis.** The disorder is gradually progressive. The prognosis for visual acuity is poor in the disorder when retinal detachment develops.

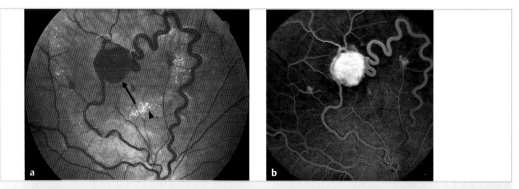

Fig. 12.42 Von Hippel–Lindau disease. (a) A hemangioblastoma (arrow) in a patient with von Hippel–Lindau disease, with enlarged retinal arteries and veins and retinal detachment with hard exudate (arrowhead). (b) The corresponding fluorescein angiogram.

Chapter 13

Optic Nerve

13 Optic Nerve

Oskar Gareis and Gerhard K. Lang

13.1 Basic Knowledge

The optic nerve extends from the posterior pole of the eye to the *optic chiasm* (▶ Fig. 13.1). After this characteristic crossing, the fibers of the optic nerve travel as the *optic tract* to the *lateral geniculate body*. Depending on the shape of the skull, the optic nerve has a total length of 35 to 55 mm.

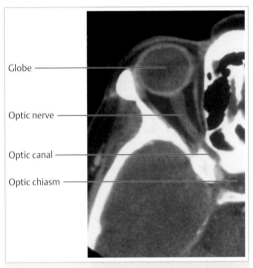

Fig. 13.1 Path of the optic nerve. CT image showing the intraorbital and intracranial portions of the optic nerve.

Globe
Optic nerve
Optic canal
Optic chiasm

The nerve consists of:
• An intraocular portion.
• An intraorbital portion.
• An intracranial portion.

13.1.1 Intraocular Portion of the Optic Nerve: Optic Disc

The intraocular portion of the optic nerve is visible on ophthalmoscopy as the **optic disc**. All the retinal nerve fibers merge into the optic nerve here, and the central retinal vessels enter and leave the eye here. The absence of photoreceptors here creates a gap in the visual field known as the *blind spot*.

▶ **Shape and size.** The optic disc (▶ Fig. 13.2) is normally *slightly vertically oval* with an average area of approximately 2.7 mm² and a horizontal diameter of approximately 1.8 mm. There is a *wide range of physiologic variability in the size of the optic disc*; its area may vary by a factor of 7, and its horizontal diameter by a factor of 2.5.

▶ **Color.** The normal physiologic color is *yellowish-orange*. The temporal half of the optic disc is usually slightly paler.

▶ **Margin.** The margin of the optic disc is *sharply defined* and readily distinguished from the surrounding retinal tissue. On the nasal side, the greater density of the nerve fibers makes the margin slightly less distinct than on the temporal side.

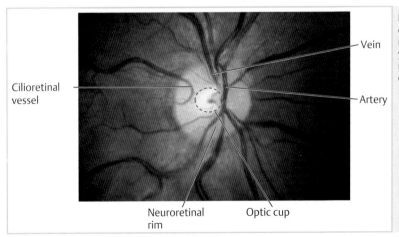

Cilioretinal vessel
Vein
Artery
Neuroretinal rim
Optic cup

Fig. 13.2 Normal optic disc. Typical signs of a normal pupil include a yellowish-orange neuroretinal rim sharply set off from the retina.

A common clinical observation is a crescent of pigment or irregular pigmentation close to the optic disc on the temporal side; sometimes the sclera will be visible through this crescent.

▶ **Prominence of the optic disc.** The normal optic disc is not prominent. The nerve fibers are practically flush with the retina.

▶ **Neuroretinal rim** (▶ Fig. 13.2). This consists of the bundles of all the optic nerve fibers as they exit through the scleral canal. The rim has a *characteristic configuration*: the narrowest portion is in the temporal horizontal region followed by the nasal horizontal area; the widest areas are the vertical inferior and superior areas.

▶ **Optic cup.** This is the *slightly eccentric cavitation* of the optic nerve that has a slightly flattened oval shape corresponding to that of the neuroretinal rim. It is the brightest part of the optic disc. No nerve fibers exit from it (▶ Fig. 13.2).

The **size of the optic cup** correlates with the size of the optic disc; the larger the optic disc, the larger the optic cup. Because enlargement of the optic cup means a loss of nerve fibers in the rim, *it is particularly important to document the size of the optic cup.* This is specified as the horizontal and vertical *ratios of cup to disc diameter* (cup–disc ratio). Due to the wide range of variability in optic disc size, it is not possible to specify absolute cup–disc ratios that indicate the presence of abnormal processes.

▶ **Central retinal artery and vein.** These structures usually enter the eye slightly nasal to the center of the optic disc. Visible pulsation in the vein is normal. However, *arterial pulsation* is *always abnormal* and occurs with disorders such as increased intraocular pressure and aortic stenosis.

▶ **Cilioretinal vessels.** These are aberrant vessels originating directly from the choroid (short posterior ciliary arteries). Resembling a cane, they usually pass along the temporal margin of the optic disc and supply the inner layers of the retina (▶ Fig. 13.2).

▶ **Blood supply to the optic disc.** The optic disc receives its blood supply from the ring of Zinn, an anastomotic ring of small branches of the short posterior ciliary arteries and the central retinal artery (▶ Fig. 13.3). Both groups of vessels originate from the ophthalmic artery, which branches from the internal carotid artery and enters the eye through the optic canal. The central retinal artery and vein branch into the optic nerve approximately 8 mm before the point at which the optic nerve exits the globe. Approximately 10 short posterior

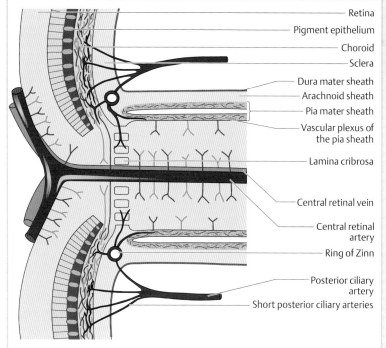

Retina
Pigment epithelium
Choroid
Sclera
Dura mater sheath
Arachnoid sheath
Pia mater sheath
Vascular plexus of the pia sheath
Lamina cribrosa
Central retinal vein
Central retinal artery
Ring of Zinn
Posterior ciliary artery
Short posterior ciliary arteries

Fig. 13.3 Vascular structures supplying the head of the optic nerve. The optic nerve is supplied with blood from both the short posterior ciliary arteries and the central retinal artery.

ciliary arteries penetrate the sclera around the optic nerve.

13.1.2 Intraorbital and Intracranial Portions of the Optic Nerve

The **intraorbital portion** begins after the nerve passes through a sievelike plate of scleral connective tissue, the lamina cribrosa. Inside the orbit, the optic nerve describes an S-shaped course that allows extreme eye movements.

After the optic nerve passes through the optic canal, the short **intracranial portion** begins and extends as far as the optic chiasm. Like the brain, the intraorbital and intracranial portions of the optic nerve are surrounded by sheaths of dura mater, pia mater, and arachnoid (see ▶ Fig. 13.3). The nerve receives its blood supply through the vascular pia mater sheath.

13.2 Examination Methods

Examination methods include:

- Ophthalmoscopy (see p. 7).
- Visual acuity testing (see p. 3).
- Perimetry test (see p. 249).
- Pupillary light reflex (see p. 137).
- Testing color vision (for example with the panel D15 test).
- Visual evoked potential (VEP).
- Optic disc tomography (see p. 198).

▶ **Panel D15 test of color vision.** This is a color marker sorting test. The patient is presented with 15 small color markers that he or she must select and sort according to a fixed blue color marker. Patients with color vision defects will typically confuse certain markers within the color series. The specific color vision defect can be diagnosed from these mistakes.

▶ **Visual evoked potential.** The VEP can be regarded as an *isolated occipital EEG*. The electrical responses in the brain to optical stimuli are transmitted by electrodes placed over the occipital lobe. Measurements include the *speed of conduction* (i.e., latency; normal values range between 90 and 110 milliseconds) and the *voltage differential* between the occipital lobe and skin electrodes (i.e., amplitude; normal values depend on the laboratory setting). The *most important indication* for VEP testing is retrobulbar optic neuritis (see p. 239) to demonstrate an extended latency period in demyelinization, such as in diffuse encephalitis.

13.3 Disorders That Obscure the Margin of the Optic Disc

13.3.1 Congenital Disorders that Obscure the Margin of the Optic Disc

There are *normal* variants of the optic disc in which the margin appears fully or partially blurred. Care should be taken to distinguish them from abnormal findings.

Oblique Entry of the Optic Nerve

Where the **optic nerve exits the eye in an oblique and nasal direction** (▶ Fig. 13.4), the nerve fibers on the nasal circumference will be elevated. The *tightly compressed nasal nerve fibers* will obscure the margin of the optic disc. Accordingly, *temporal nerve fibers are stretched,* and the neuroretinal rim cannot be clearly distinguished. Often an adjacent crescentic, whitish area, known as a temporal crescent, will be observed on the temporal side. This crescent is frequently seen in myopia (see p. 217) and is referred to as a myopic crescent. It can also be circular.

Tilted Disc

An **optic nerve that exits the eye superiorly** (▶ Fig. 13.5) is referred to as a tilted disc. The *superior circumference of the margin of the optic disc will be obscured* in a manner similar to oblique entry of the optic nerve. A number of other changes may also be observed, including an inferior crescent, situs inversus of the retinal vessels, ectasia of the fundus, myopia, and visual field defects. These findings

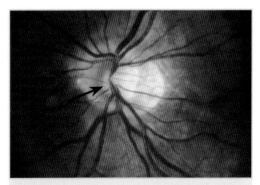

Fig. 13.4 Oblique entry of the optic nerve. Tightly compressed nasal nerve fibers cause slight elevation of the optic disc, and the margin of the disc is obscured.

may occur in various combinations and are referred to collectively as **tilted-disc syndrome**. This is *clinically highly significant* as nasal inferior ectasia of the fundus can produce temporal superior visual field defects. In contrast to bitemporal hemianopsia in chiasmal lesions, visual field defects in fundus ectasia are not confined to the midline but also affect the nasal half of the visual field. This clinical picture is regarded as a form of *rudimentary coloboma* (see p. 246).

Pseudopapilledema

Pseudopapilledema (▶ Fig. 13.6) is due to a *narrow scleral canal*. Because of the constriction, the nerve fibers are tightly compressed. The optic disc is **elevated and the full circle of the margin is obscured**. The optic cup is absent, and the retinal vessels appear tortuous. There are no abnormal morphological changes such as bleeding, nerve fiber edema,

and hyperemia; visual acuity and visual field are normal. Pseudopapilledema *can* occur with hyperopia, although it is encountered equally frequently in emmetropic or slightly myopic eyes.

Differential diagnosis: optic disc edema, optic disc drusen (▶ Table 13.1).

Myelinated Nerve Fibers

Normally, retinal nerve fibers are not myelinated. However, **myelinated areas** occasionally occur in the retina (▶ Fig. 13.7). They occur most frequently **at the margin of the optic disc**. Whitish and striated, they simulate segmental or circular blurring of the margin. Myelinated nerve fibers can *also occur on the periphery of the retina*. Because of their location in the innermost layer of the retina, they tend to obscure the retinal vessels. Myelinated nerve fibers normally cause no loss of function. Only extensive findings can lead to small scotomas.

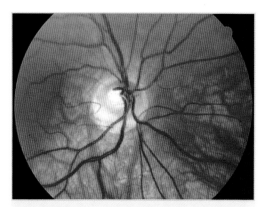

Fig. 13.5 Tilted disc. Oblique entry of the optic nerve superiorly, with an inferior crescent and inferior segmental ectasia of the fundus.

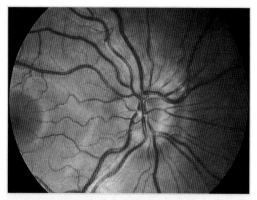

Fig. 13.6 Pseudopapilledema. Circular blurring of the margin of the optic disc, with absence of the optic cup.

Table 13.1 Differential diagnosis of pseudopapilledema, optic disc drusen, and papilledema

Differential criterion	Pseudopapilledema	Optic disc drusen	Papilledema
Size of optic disc	Small	Small	Unaffected
Optic cup	Absent	Absent	Initially present
Spontaneous venous pulse	Possibly present	Possibly present	Absent
Veins and papillary capillaries	Normal	Normal	Obstructed
Color of optic disc	Normal	Pale	Hyperemic
Peripapillary bleeding	Absent	Very rare	Present
Peripapillary nerve fibers	Normal	Normal	Edematous
Angiography	Normal	Intrinsic fluorescence	Early leakage
Ultrasound	Atypical	Highly reflective deposits	Atypical

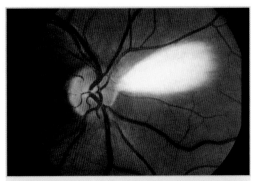

Fig. 13.7 Myelinated nerve fibers. As they are myelinated, the nerve fibers appear whitish and striated and can simulate segmental blurring of the margin.

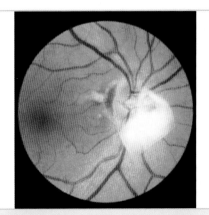

Fig. 13.8 Bergmeister's papilla. Remnants of the hyaloid artery, forming a veil-like epipapillary membrane overlying the surface of the optic disc, are seen on the nasal side (on the right in the picture).

Bergmeister's Papilla

The fetal hyaloid artery emerges from the optic disc to supply the vitreous body and lens. Glial and fibrous tissue may persist if the structure is not fully absorbed. This vestigial tissue, usually on the nasal side of the optic disc, is known as **Bergmeister's papilla.** When this tissue takes the form of a veil-like membrane overlying the surface of the optic disc, it is also referred to as an **epipapillary membrane** (▶ Fig. 13.8). Usually this condition is *asymptomatic.*

Optic Disc Drusen

Drusen are **yellowish lobular bodies in the tissue of the optic disc that are usually bilateral (in 70% of cases)**. Ophthalmoscopy can reveal superficial drusen but not drusen located deep in the scleral canal. In the presence of optic disc drusen, the disc appears *slightly elevated with blurred margins and without an optic cup* (▶ Fig. 13.9). Abnormal morphological signs such as hyperemia and nerve fiber edema will not be present. However, bleeding in lines along the disc margin or subretinal peripapillary bleeding may occur in rare cases.

A small lamina cribrosa appears to be a factor in the *etiology* of the disorder. This impedes axonal plasma flow, which predisposes the patient to axonal degeneration. This in turn produces calcifications exterior to the axons (drusen). Retinal drusen are hyaline deposits in the Bruch membrane and are a completely unrelated process.

Drusen usually **do not cause any loss of function**. Deep drusen can cause compressive atrophy of nerve fibers with resulting subsequent visual field defects.

Optic disc drusen can be diagnosed on the basis of characteristic ultrasound findings of highly reflective papillary deposits. Fluorescein angiography findings of autofluorescence prior to dye injection are also characteristic.

See ▶ Table 13.1 for *differential diagnosis.*

13.3.2 Acquired Disorders That Obscure the Margin of the Optic Disc

The normal variants and congenital changes discussed in the previous section must be distinguished from *abnormal changes to the optic disc due to nerve fiber edema*. The term optic disc edema is used in a generic sense to describe any such change. However, this term should be further specified whenever possible:

- **Optic disc edema without primary axonal damage**
  - Papilledema.
  - Hypotension papilledema (see p. 276).
- **Optic disc edema with direct axonal damage**
  - Inflammation: papillitis or retrobulbar optic neuritis.
  - Infarction with ischemic optic neuropathy (nonarteriosclerotic or arteritic).
- **Optic disc edema due to infiltration**
  - For example, due to an underlying hematologic disorder.

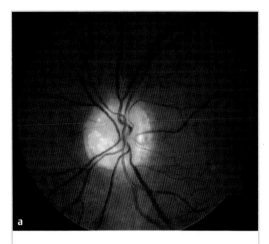

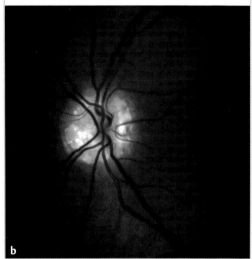

Fig. 13.9 Optic disc drusen. (a) The yellowish lobular deposits (drusen) make the optic disc appear elevated, with blurred margins and without an optic cup. (b) In this black and white photograph, the drusen light up distinctly.

Papilledema

Definition
Bilateral optic disc edema secondary to increased intracranial pressure.

▶ **Epidemiology.** Epidemiologic data from the 1950s describe papilledema in as many as 60% of patients with brain tumors. Since then, advances in neuroradiology have significantly reduced the inci-

dence of papilledema. The diagnostic importance of the disorder has decreased accordingly.

▶ **Etiology.** An adequate theory to fully explain the pathogenesis of papilledema is lacking. Current thinking centers around a mechanical model in which increased intracranial pressure and impeded axonal plasma flow through the narrowed lamina cribrosa cause nerve fiber edema. However, there is no definite correlation between intracranial pressure and prominence of the papilledema. Nor is there a definite correlation between the times at which the two processes occur. However, severe papilledema can occur within a few hours of increased intracranial pressure, such as in acute intracranial hemorrhage. Therefore, papilledema is a *conditional, unspecific sign of increased intracranial pressure* that does not provide conclusive evidence of the cause or location of a process.

In approximately 60% of cases, the increased intracranial pressure with papilledema is caused by an *intracranial tumor*; 40% of cases are due to other causes, such as hydrocephalus, meningitis, brain abscess, encephalitis, malignant hypertension, intracranial hemorrhages, or idiopathic intracranial hypertension (pseudotumor cerebri). This is a matter of elevated intracranial pressure with normal computed tomography and spinal fluid findings. The patient should be referred to a neurologist, neurosurgeon, or internist for diagnosis of the underlying causes.

Note
Every incidence of papilledema requires immediate diagnosis of the underlying causes as increased intracranial pressure is a life-threatening situation.

The incidence of papilledema in the presence of a brain tumor decreases with increasing age; in the first decade of life it is 80%, whereas in the seventh decade it is only 40%. Papilledema cannot occur where there is atrophy of the optic nerve, as papilledema requires intact nerve fibers to develop.

▶ **Special forms**
- *Foster Kennedy syndrome.* This refers to isolated atrophy of the optic nerve (see p. 243) due to direct tumor pressure on one side and papilledema due to increased intracranial pressure on the other side. Possible causes may include a meningioma of the wing of the sphenoid or frontal lobe tumor.
- *Hypotension papilledema.* This refers to a nerve fiber edema due to ocular hypotension. Possible

causes may include penetrating trauma or fistula secondary to intraocular surgery.

▶ **Symptoms and diagnostic considerations.** Visual function remains unimpaired for a long time. This significant discrepancy between morphological and functional findings is an *important characteristic in differential diagnosis.* **Early functional impairments can include reversible obscurations.** *Perimetry testing* may reveal an increase in the size of the blind spot (▶ Fig. 13.10c). Central visual field defects and concentric narrowing of the visual field are **late functional impairments** that occur with existing complex atrophy of the optic nerve (see p. 243).

Note
Papilledema is characterized by significant morphological findings and only slight visual impairment.

The following **phases** can be distinguished by *ophthalmoscopy*:

▶ **Early phase** (▶ Fig. 13.10a). First the nasal margin and then the superior and inferior margins of the optic disc (see p. 232) are obscured because of the difference in the relative densities of the nerve fibers. The optic cup *is initially preserved.* This is important in a differential diagnosis to exclude pseudopapilledema and optic disc drusen. The optic disc is hyperemic due to dilation of the capillaries, and there is no pulsation in the central reti-

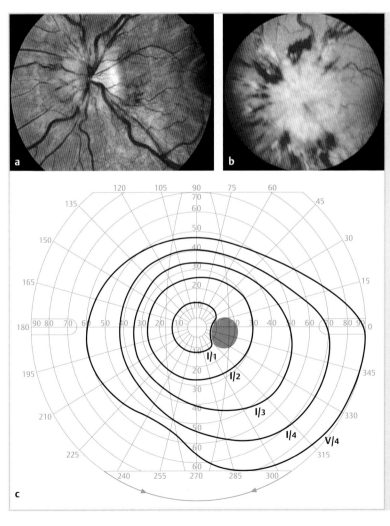

a

b

c

Fig. 13.10 Papilledema. (a) Early phase of papilledema. The nasal margin of the optic disc is partially obscured. The optic disc is hyperemic due to dilatation of the capillaries, and the optic cup is still visible. **(b)** Acute stage. The optic disc is increasingly elevated and has a gray to grayish-red color. Radial hemorrhages around the margin of the optic disc and grayish-white exudates are observed. The optic disc can no longer be clearly distinguished. **(c)** Functional findings. The enlarged blind spot (indicated by shading) is an early functional correlate to the ophthalmoscopic findings. The markers used in the test are light markers of varying size (indicated by roman numerals) and varying light intensity (indicated by arabic numerals). The larger the number, the larger the size and greater the light intensity of the respective marker.

nal vein. Edema can produce concentric peripapillary retinal folds known as Paton's folds.

▶ **Acute phase** (▶ Fig. 13.10b). This is characterized by increasing elevation of the optic disc, radial hemorrhages around the margin of the optic disc and grayish-white exudates. *The optic cup is often no longer discernible.* The color of the optic disc will be red to grayish-red.

▶ **Chronic phase.** The optic cup is obliterated. The prominence and hyperemia will be seen to subside.

▶ **Atrophic phase.** Proliferation of astrocytes results in complex or secondary atrophy of the optic nerve (see p. 243).

▶ **Differential diagnosis.** This includes pseudopapilledema, optic disc drusen (see ▶ Table 13.1), abnormalities of the optic disc without functional impairment, optic disc edema with hypertension, and optic neuritis (see below).

▶ **Treatment.** Intracranial pressure should be reduced by treating the underlying disorder (see Etiology). Once intracranial pressure has been normalized, the papilledema will resolve within a few weeks. Usually complex atrophy of the optic nerve will remain. The severity will vary according to the duration of the papilledema.

Optic Neuritis

Definition
Optic neuritis is an inflammation of the optic nerve that may occur within the globe (papillitis) or posterior to it (retrobulbar optic neuritis).

▶ **Epidemiology.** Optic neuritis occurs most frequently in adults between the ages of 20 and 45 years. Women are more frequently affected than men. Some 20 to 40% of patients with optic neuritis develop diffuse encephalitis (multiple sclerosis).

▶ **Etiology**
▶ **Papillitis:**
• *Inflammatory processes.* These include infectious diseases such as Lyme disease, malaria, and syphilis, and manifestations in the optic nerve of inflammation of the orbit, paranasal sinuses, or base of the skull.
• *Autoimmune disorders.* These include lupus erythematosus, polychondritis, regional enteritis

(Crohn's disease), ulcerative colitis, nodular panarteritis, and Wegener's granulomatosis.
• *Toxic damage* due to agents such as methanol, lead, ethambutol hydrochloride, and chloramphenicol.

In 70% of these cases, the *cause is not determined.*

▶ **Retrobulbar optic neuritis.** The primary causes of this disorder are *demyelinating diseases of the central nervous system* such as diffuse encephalitis. In 20% of cases, retrobulbar optic neuritis is an isolated early symptom of diffuse encephalitis. However, a differential diagnosis should always also consider the *other causes of papillitis mentioned above.*

▶ **Symptoms.** The **cardinal symptom** is *sudden loss of vision,* which may occasionally be accompanied by fever (*Uhthoff's symptom*). The field of vision is typically impaired by a central scotoma (▶ Fig. 13.11b), paracentral scotomas, a centrocecal scotoma involving the macula and blind spot, and wedge-shaped visual field defects up to and including complete blindness.

Other symptoms include pain that increases in extreme positions of gaze and when pressure is applied to the globe, and reduced perception of color intensity.

▶ **Diagnostic considerations.** Ophthalmoscopic findings in **papillitis** (▶ Fig. 13.11a) include edema and hyperemia of the head of the optic nerve. This flattens the optic cup and obscures the margin of the optic disc. Bleeding at the margin of the optic disc may or may not be present. The elevation of the optic disc is considerably less than in papilledema.

The optic disc will appear normal in **retrobulbar optic neuritis**.

Note
In retrobulbar optic neuritis, the patient sees nothing (due to a central scotoma), and the physician sees nothing (the fundus appears normal).

▶ **Other findings upon examination.** These include an afferent pupillary defect (see p. 138), which is mandatory; red–green color vision defect, and delayed latency in the visual evoked potential (see p. 234).

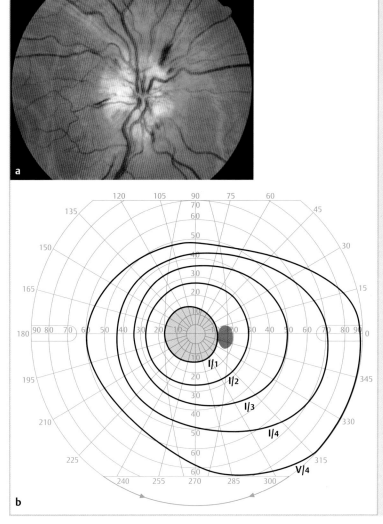

Fig. 13.11 Papillitis. (a) Papillitis in Lyme disease. The margin of the optic disc is slightly obscured by edema and hyperemia of the head of the optic nerve. The optic cup is obscured. **(b)** Central scotoma in papillitis. A central scotoma is a typical functional finding in retrobulbar optic neuritis but one that may also be observed in papillitis. In this case, a relative scotoma is present (indicated by the central grayish area)—i.e., the patient is only unable to discern markers I/1 and weaker in the central area whereas larger markers are visible (see also ▶ Fig. 13.10). The blind spot is also located next to this area.

▶ **Differential diagnosis**

▶ **Papilledema.** Initially there is no loss of function.

▶ **Ischemic optic neuropathy.** The central scotoma is lacking, and patients are usually older than 60.

▶ **Treatment.** Treatment depends on the underlying disorder. Retrobulbar optic neuritis with severe loss of vision (less than 0.1) can be treated with high-dose steroids—i.e., 1,000 mg of oral prednisolone daily for 3 days and 1 mg of oral prednisolone per kilogram of body weight on days 4 to 14. However, this treatment only leads to more rapid restoration of vision. Final visual acuity after 1 year is the same with or without high-dose steroid therapy. This treatment can, however, inhibit relapses of multiple sclerosis.

▶ **Prognosis.** The prognosis depends on the underlying disorder. Severe permanent losses of visual acuity are possible, as are significant spontaneous improvements. **Retrobulbar optic neuritis in diffuse encephalitis** usually exhibits a strong tendency toward spontaneous improvement within 4 weeks without any treatment. However, *discrete functional defects* such as reduced visual contrast and reduced perception of color intensity will *always* remain. Morphological findings *always* include a *pale optic disc* as a result of complex atrophy of the optic nerve following papillitis or partial isolated atrophy of the optic nerve following retrobulbar optic neuritis.

Anterior Ischemic Optic Neuropathy (AION)

The following forms of anterior ischemic optic neuropathy (AION) are distinguished according to the cause of the disorder:

- **Arteriosclerotic** anterior ischemic optic neuropathy.
- **Arteritic** anterior ischemic optic neuropathy.

Arteriosclerotic Anterior Ischemic Optic Neuropathy

Definition
An acute disruption of the blood supply to the optic disc—i.e., optic disc infarction, resulting from vascular changes in arteriosclerosis.

▶ **Epidemiology.** Arteriosclerotic AION is a common cause of sudden loss of visual acuity. The greatest incidence of this disorder is between the ages of 60 and 70 years. In contrast to arteritic AION, it can also occur in adults below the age of 60.

▶ **Etiology.** The causes of the disorder lie in acute disruption of the blood flow through the lateral branches of the short posterior ciliary arteries and the ring of Zinn in the setting of severe arteriosclerosis. A narrow scleral canal—i.e., a small optic disc, is a predisposing factor. The disorder known as *diabetic papillopathy* also belongs to this group of disorders, although it has a better prognosis in terms of vision.

▶ **Symptoms.** Patients report a *sudden unilateral loss of visual acuity*. This is due to segmental or complete infarction of the anterior portion of the optic nerve. Severity is variable. The patient may present with wedge-shaped visual field defects (▶ Fig. 13.12b) or horizontal visual field defects that correlate with segmental nerve fiber edemas. However, severe concentric defects progressing to total blindness can also occur. Vision may or not be impaired. An afferent pupillary defect is always present.

▶ **Diagnostic considerations.** The patient will frequently have a history of hypertension, diabetes mellitus, or hyperlipidemia.

Ophthalmoscopy will reveal edema of the optic disc, whose margin will be accordingly obscured. The margin is often obscured in a segmental pattern, which is an important criterion in differential diagnosis (▶ Fig. 13.12a). The head of the optic nerve is also hyperemic with marginal bleeding.

Note
Obscured segments of the margin of the optic disc that correlate with visual field defects are a sign of an arteriosclerotic AION.

▶ **Treatment.** Anterior ischemic optic neuropathy is nearly impossible to treat. Attempted methods include hemodilution (pentoxifylline infusions, acetylsalicylic acid, and bloodletting depending on hematocrit levels) and systemic administration of steroids to control the edema. Diagnosis of the underlying cause is important; examination by an internist and Doppler ultrasound studies of the carotid artery may be helpful. Underlying disorders such as diabetes mellitus or arterial hypertension should be treated.

▶ **Prognosis.** The prognosis is usually poor even where therapy is initiated early. Isolated atrophy of the optic nerve will appear within 3 weeks; complex atrophy of the optic nerve is less frequent but may also be observed.

Arteritic Anterior Ischemic Optic Neuropathy

Definition
An acute impairment of the blood supply to the optic disc due to inflammation of medium-sized and small arterial branches.

▶ **Epidemiology.** The annual incidence is approximately 3 cases per 100,000. The disorder occurs almost exclusively after the age of 60 years. Women are affected slightly more often than men, accounting for 55% of cases. Fifty percent of patients suffer from ocular involvement within a few days up to approximately 3 months after the onset of the disorder.

▶ **Etiology.** Giant cell arteritis is a frequently bilateral granulomatous vasculitis that primarily affects the medium-sized and small arteries. Common sites include the temporal arteries, ophthalmic artery, short posterior ciliary arteries, central retinal artery, and the proximal portion of the verte-

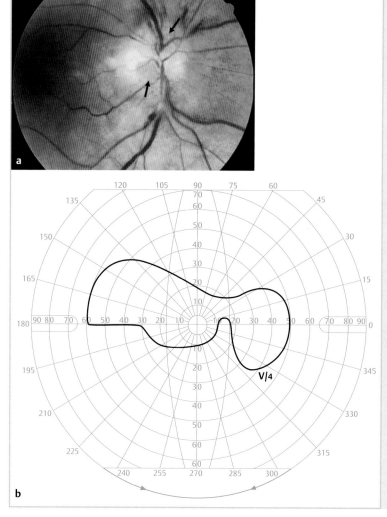

b

Fig. 13.12 Anterior ischemic optic neuropathy (AION). (a) The superior and inferior segments of the margin of the optic disc are obscured (arrows) due to edema. This is a typical morphological sign of AION. **(b)** The superior and inferior wedge-shaped visual field defects correlate with obscured segments of the margin of the optic disc. These are absolute scotomas.

bral arteries, which may be affected in varying combinations.

▶ **Symptoms.** Patients report *sudden unilateral blindness or severe visual impairment.* Other symptoms include headaches, painful scalp in the region of the temporal arteries, tenderness to palpation in the region of the temporal arteries, pain while chewing (a characteristic sign), weight loss, and reduced general health and exercise tolerance. Patients may have a history of amaurosis fugax or polymyalgia rheumatica.

▶ **Diagnostic considerations.** The **ophthalmoscopic findings** are the same as in arteriosclerotic AION (see ▶ Fig. 13.12a). **Other findings** include a

significantly increased erythrocyte sedimentation rate (precipitous sedimentation is the most important hematologic finding), an increased level of C-reactive protein (CRP), leukocytosis, and iron-deficiency anemia.

Note

Erythrocyte sedimentation rate and CRP should be measured in every patient presenting with anterior ischemic optic neuropathy.

The temporal arteries are prominent (▶ Fig. 13.13), painful to palpation, and have no pulse. The diagnosis is confirmed by a biopsy of the temporal

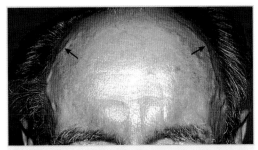

Fig. 13.13 Prominent temporal arteries in temporal arteritis. The prominent temporal arteries are painful on palpation and have no pulse.

artery. Because of the segmental pattern of vascular involvement, negative histologic findings cannot exclude giant cell arteritis.

> **Note**
> Giant cell arteritis should be considered in every patient presenting with anterior ischemic optic neuropathy.

▶ **Differential diagnosis.** Arteriosclerotic AION should be considered.

▶ **Treatment.** *Immediate* high-dosage systemic steroid therapy (initial doses up to 1,000 mg of intravenous prednisone) is indicated. Steroids are reduced as the erythrocyte sedimentation rate decreases, C-reactive protein levels drop, and clinical symptoms abate. However, a maintenance dose will be required for several months. Vascular treatment such as pentoxifylline infusions may be attempted.

> **Note**
> High-dosage systemic steroid therapy (for example, 500 mg of intravenous prednisone) is indicated to protect the fellow eye even if a giant cell arteritis is only suspected.

▶ **Prognosis.** The prognosis for the affected eye is *poor* even where therapy is initiated early. Immediate steroid therapy is absolutely indicated because in approximately 75% of cases the fellow eye is affected within a few hours and cerebral arteries may also be at risk.

Infiltrative Optic Disc Edema

Infiltration of the optic disc occurs in about 1 in 3 cases of leukosis or other blood dyscrasias. This infiltration results in optic disc edema that is usually associated with infiltration of the meninges. The optic disc edema can therefore occur from both direct leukemic infiltration and secondary to increased pressure in the meninges of the optic nerve. The prognosis for both vision and survival is poor.

13.4 Disorders in Which the Margin of the Optic Disc is Well Defined

13.4.1 Atrophy of the Optic Nerve

> **Definition**
> Irreversible loss of axons in the region of the third neuron (from the retinal layer of ganglion cells to the lateral geniculate body).

▶ **Morphology and pathologic classification.** Atrophy of the optic nerve is classified according to its morphology and pathogenesis. The following forms are distinguished **on the basis of ophthalmoscopic findings:**

- Primary atrophy of the optic nerve.
- Secondary atrophy of the optic nerve.
- Glaucomatous atrophy of the optic nerve (see p. 153).

Forms of primary atrophy of the optic nerve can be further classified according to their pathogenesis:

- *Ascending* atrophy in which the lesion is located anterior to the lamina cribrosa in the ocular portion of the optic nerve or retina.
- *Descending* atrophy in which the lesion is located posterior to the lamina cribrosa in a retrobulbar or cranial location.

▶ **Etiology**
▶ **Etiology of primary atrophy of the optic nerve.** The most important causes are as follows:

- *Ascending atrophy (after 2–4 weeks)*
  - Usually vascular, such as central retinal artery occlusion or anterior ischemic optic neuropathy.

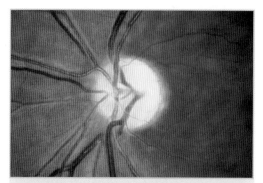

Fig. 13.14 Primary atrophy of the optic nerve. The optic disc is well defined and pale. The neuroretinal rim is atrophied, resulting in a flattened optic disc.

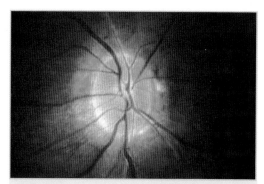

Fig. 13.16 Waxy pallor optic atrophy. Waxy pallor optic atrophy is associated with tapetoretinal degeneration

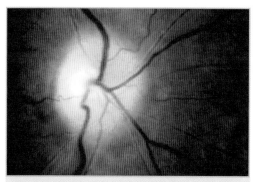

Fig. 13.15 Secondary atrophy of the optic nerve. The optic disc is elevated and pale due to proliferation of astrocytes.

- *Descending atrophy (after 4–6 weeks)*
  - Compressive, such as from an orbital or intracranial mass or hydrocephalus.
  - Traumatic, such as avulsion, compression of the optic nerve in a fracture, or hematoma in the optic nerve sheath.
  - Inflammatory, such as retrobulbar optic neuritis, arachnoiditis of the optic chiasm, or syphilis.
- *Toxic*
  - Chronic abuse of inferior quality tobacco and alcohol.
  - Lead, arsenic, or thallium.
  - Methyl alcohol.
  - Medications including ethambutol, chloramphenicol, gentamicin, isoniazid, vincristine, penicillamine.
- *Congenital or hereditary*
  - Infantile hereditary optic atrophy (an autosomal-dominant disorder with slow progressive loss of visual acuity, color vision defects, and visual field defects.

  - Juvenile hereditary optic atrophy (similar to the infantile form, only the onset is usually later, in the second decade of life).
  - Leber's optic atrophy (see p. 245).
  - Behr's infantile recessive optic atrophy.
- *Systemic disorders*
  - Hemorrhagic anemia or pernicious anemia.
  - Leukosis.

▶ **Etiology of secondary atrophy of the optic nerve.** The most important causes are

- Papilledema (see p. 237).
- Anterior ischemic optic neuropathy (see p. 241).
- Papillitis (see p. 239).

Note
The etiology of any atrophy of the optic nerve should be determined to exclude possible life-threatening intracerebral causes such as a tumor.

▶ **Symptoms.** The spectrum of functional defects in optic atrophy is broad. These range from small peripheral visual field defects in partial optic atrophy to severe concentric visual field defects or blindness in total optic atrophy.

▶ **Diagnostic considerations.** The most important examinations are a detailed history, ophthalmoscopy, and perimetry testing. Color vision testing and visual evoked potential (see p. 234) may be useful as follow-up examinations in early optic atrophy.

▶ **Primary atrophy of the optic nerve.** Ophthalmoscopy will reveal a well-defined, pale optic disc

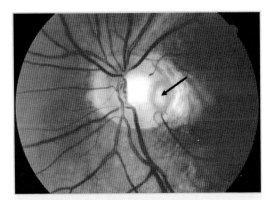

Fig. 13.17 Optic nerve pits. These are oval, grayish temporal depressions in the papillary tissue (arrow).

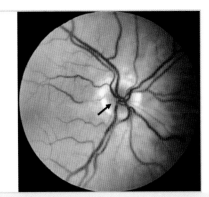

Fig. 13.19 Melanocytoma. A benign tumor of the optic disc, which represents a special form of uveal nevus (arrow).

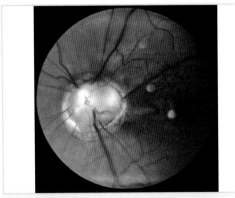

Fig. 13.18 Optic disc coloboma. The optic disc is enlarged, with a funnel-shaped depression with whitish tissue and a peripapillary pigment ring. The retinal vessels do not branch from a central venous or arterial trunk.

(▸ Fig. 13.14). The pallor can cover the entire optic disc (it will appear chalk-white in total optic atrophy), or it may be partial or segmental. The neuroretinal rim is atrophied, which causes the optic disc to flatten out. The diameter of the retinal vessels will be decreased.

▸ **Secondary atrophy of the optic nerve.** Ophthalmoscopy will reveal a pale optic disc. The disc is slightly elevated due to proliferation of astrocytes, and the margin is blurred (▸ Fig. 13.15). The optic cup will be partially or completely obscured. The retinal vessels will be constricted.

▸ **Treatment.** The disorder involves *irreversible* damage to the nerve fibers. As a result, no effective treatment is available.

▸ **Prognosis.** Early identification and timely management of a treatable cause such as a tumor or pernicious anemia can arrest the progression of the disorder. Where this is not the case, the prognosis for vision is poor.

Special Forms of Atrophy of the Optic Nerve

▸ **Leber's atrophy.** Here there is involvement of both optic nerves *without additional neurologic symptoms*. In 85% of cases, men between the ages of 20 and 30 years are affected. The disorder is due to mutations in the mitochondrial DNA.

Ophthalmoscopy will reveal optic disc edema as in papillitis followed by primary optic nerve atrophy. Initial retrobulbar optic neuritis is also possible.

Functional symptoms include a large central scotoma with a peripherally limited visual field. This will lead to significant loss of vision within a few months, although the remaining vision will not decrease any further.

There is no *treatment*.

▸ **Waxy pallor optic atrophy.** This disorder (▸ Fig. 13.16) is associated with tapetoretinal degeneration, such as retinitis pigmentosa (▸ Fig. 12.36).

Ophthalmoscopy will reveal an *optic disc with a waxlike pallor* that is shallow with a well-defined margin. There will be severe thinning of the central retinal vessels. The *cause of the waxlike yellow color is not known*.

There is no *treatment*.

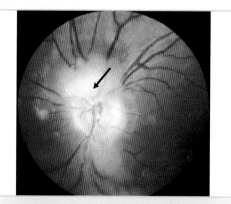

Fig. 13.20 Astrocytoma in tuberous sclerosis (Bourneville's disease). A whitish, "mulberry" tumor on the superior margin of the optic disc (arrow).

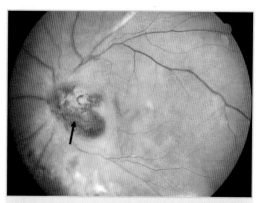

Fig. 13.21 Capillary hemangioma in von Hippel's disease. Eccentric capillary vascular deformity on the optic disc (arrow).

13.4.2 Optic Nerve Pits

An optic nerve pit (▶ Fig. 13.17) is characterized by a **round or oval grayish depression in the papillary tissue that does not compromise the margin of the optic disc**. These pits are usually found in an inferior temporal location, although they do occur elsewhere. In 85% of cases, one eye is affected. Several pits in one optic disc have been described. Serous retinal detachment occurs in 25% of cases, depending on the location of the pit. Where the detachment affects the macula, a significant loss of visual acuity will result that will prove very difficult to manage with laser surgery. Otherwise, optic nerve pits are an *incidental finding without any functional deficit*. They are considered to be rudimentary colobomas.

13.4.3 Optic Disc Coloboma (Morning Glory Disc)

An optic disc coloboma (▶ Fig. 13.18) is the result of incomplete closure of the embryonic optic cup. The optic disc is enlarged with a funnel-shaped depression with whitish tissue and a peripapillary pigment ring. The retinal vessels extend outward across the margin of the disc in a radial pattern without a central trunk vessel. Patients with optic disc coloboma often have *decreased visual acuity and visual field defects*.

13.5 Tumors

Optic nerve tumors are classified as **intraocular** or **retrobulbar tumors**. Intraocular tumors are rare.

13.5.1 Intraocular Optic Nerve Tumors

▶ **Melanocytoma.** These are benign pigmented tumors that primarily occur in blacks (▶ Fig. 13.19). The color of the tumor varies from gray to pitch black. It is often eccentric and extends beyond the margin of the optic disc. In 50% of cases, one will also observe a peripapillary choroidal nevus. Visual acuity is usually normal, although discrete changes in the visual field may be present.

▶ **Astrocytoma.** Astrocytomas appear as white reflecting "mulberry" masses that can calcify (▶ Fig. 13.20). Their size can range up to several disc diameters. The tumor is highly vascularized. Visual field defects can result where the tumor is sufficiently large to compress the optic nerve. Astrocytomas occur in tuberous sclerosis (Bourneville's disease) and neurofibromatosis (Recklinghausen's disease).

▶ **Hemangioma.** Capillary hemangiomas are eccentric, round orange-colored vascular deformities on the optic disc (von Hippel's disease) (▶ Fig. 13.21). They may occur in association with other angiomas, for example, in the cerebellum (in von Hippel–Lindau disease).

13.5.2 Retrobulbar Optic Nerve Tumors

The most common retrobulbar optic nerve tumors are **gliomas** and **meningiomas.** *Symptoms* include a usually slow loss of visual acuity with exophthalmos. *Ophthalmoscopy* will reveal descending primary atrophy of the optic nerve. *Meningioma of the sheath of the optic nerve* is typically accompanied by the formation of opticociliary shunt vessels with compression of the central retinal vessels.

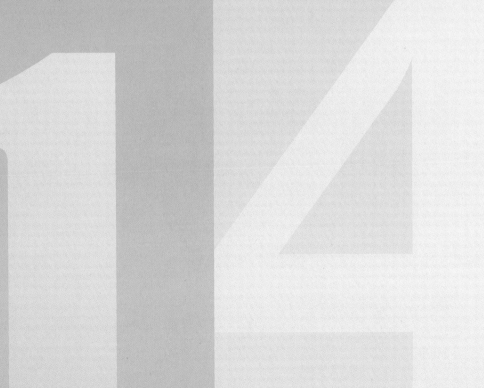

Chapter 14

Visual Pathway

14 Visual Pathway

Oskar Gareis and Gerhard K. Lang

14.1 Basic Knowledge

The anatomy of the visual pathway can be divided into six separate parts (▶ Fig. 14.1):

1. **Optic nerve.** This includes all of the optic nerve fiber bundles of the eye.
2. **Optic chiasm.** This is where the characteristic crossover of the nerve fibers of the two optic nerves occurs. The *central and peripheral fibers* from the temporal halves of the retinas *do not cross* the midline, but continue into the optic tract of the *ipsilateral side*. The *fibers of the nasal halves cross the midline* and there enter

the *contralateral* optic tract. It was formerly thought that the inferior and superior nasal fibers traveled in a small arc through the contralateral optic nerve (anterior arc of Wilbrand) or the ipsilateral optic tract (posterior arc of Wilbrand), but the arcs of Wilbrand do not exist in a normal chiasm. It is only in cases of optic atrophy that the nerve fibers are drawn to the optic nerve, due to shrinking of the tissue.

3. **Optic tract.** This includes all of the *ipsilateral optic nerve fibers and those that cross the midline.*

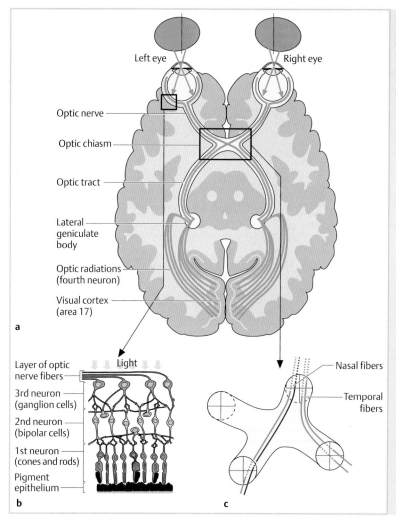

Optic nerve

Optic chiasm

Optic tract

Lateral geniculate body

Optic radiations (fourth neuron)

Visual cortex (area 17)

Left eye

Right eye

a

Layer of optic nerve fibers

3rd neuron (ganglion cells)

2nd neuron (bipolar cells)

1st neuron (cones and rods)

Pigment epithelium

Light

b

Nasal fibers

Temporal fibers

c

Fig. 14.1 Anatomy of the visual pathway. (a) Overview of the course of the visual pathway. (b) Structure of the retina. (c) The course of the nerve fibers in the optic chiasm.

4. **Lateral geniculate body.** The optic tract ends here. The third neuron connects to the fourth here, which is why atrophy of the optic nerve does not occur in lesions beyond the lateral geniculate body.
5. **Optic radiations** (geniculocalcarine tracts). The fibers of the *inferior retinal quadrants* pass through the temporal lobes; those of the *superior quadrants* pass through the parietal lobes to the occipital lobe and from there to the visual cortex.
6. **Primary visual area** (striate cortex or Brodmann's area 17 of the visual cortex): The *nerve fibers diverge* within the primary visual area; the macula lutea accounts for most of these fibers. The macula is represented on the most posterior portion of the occipital lobe. The central and intermediate peripheral regions of the visual field are represented anteriorly. The temporal crescent of the visual field, only present unilaterally, is represented farthest anteriorly.

Other connections extend from the visual cortex to associated centers and oculomotor areas (**parastriate** and **peristriate areas**). Aside from the optic tract there is also another tract known as the **retinohypothalamic tract**. This tract is older in evolutionary terms and diverges from the optic chiasm. It transmits light impulses for metabolic and hormonal stimulation to the diencephalon and pituitary gland system and influences the circadian rhythm.

14.2 Examination Methods

▶ **Visual field testing (perimetry).** This is the most important test for visual pathway lesions. Because it permits one to diagnose the location of the lesion, it is also of interest from a neurologic standpoint. The "visual field" is defined as the *field of perception of the eye at rest with the gaze directed straight ahead*. It includes all points (objects and surfaces) in space that are simultaneously visible when the eye focuses *on one point.*

The examination is performed on *one eye at a time.* The **principle** of the test is to have the patient focus on a central point in the device while the eye is in a defined state of adaptation with controlled ambient lighting (see below). Light markers appear in the hemisphere of the device. The patient signals that he or she perceives the markers by pressing a button that triggers an acoustic signal.

There are two types of perimetry.
1. **Kinetic perimetry.** Hemispheric Goldmann or Rodenstock perimeters are used for this test (▶ Fig. 14.2a). Kinetic perimetry involves *moving* points of light that travel into the hemi-

sphere from the periphery. Light markers of identical size and intensity produce concentric rings of identical perception referred to as *isopters.* The points of light decrease in size and light intensity as they move toward the center of the visual field, and the isopters become correspondingly smaller (▶ Fig. 14.2b). This corresponds with the sensitivity of the retina, which increases from the periphery to the center. The advantage of Goldmann perimetry is the personal interaction between physician and patient. This method is especially suitable for older patients who may have difficulties with a stereotyped interaction required by a computer program. *Specific indications* for kinetic perimetry include visual field defects due to neurologic causes and examinations to establish a disability (such as hemianopsia or quadrantic anopsia).
2. **Static perimetry.** This is usually performed with computerized equipment such as the *Humphrey field analyzer* (▶ Fig. 14.3a) or *Octopus 2000,* although a Goldmann or Rodenstock hemispheric perimeter can also be used for static testing of the visual field. In static perimetry, the light intensity of *immobile* light markers is increased until they are perceived. The intensity threshold continuously increases from the macula, with the highest sensitivity, to the periphery. A variety of different computer programs can be selected depending on the specific clinical setting. These include the outer margins or the 30° visual field in glaucoma (▶ Fig.14.3b).

▶ **Other examination methods**
• Pupillary findings.
• Pupillary light reflex; see Chapter 9.2.
• Visual evoked potential; see Chapter 13.2.
• CT or MRI to diagnose causes.

14.3 Disorders of the Visual Pathway

Lesions of the visual pathway can be classified according to three main locations.
1. Prechiasmal lesions (lesions of the optic nerve) involve visual field defects on the same side.
2. Chiasmal lesions (disorders of the optic chiasm) (see p. 251) typically cause bilateral temporal hemianopsia but can also cause unilateral or bilateral visual field defects.
3. Retrochiasmal lesions (disorders of visual pathway posterior to the optic chiasm—i.e., from the optic tract to the visual cortex) cause homonymous visual field defects.

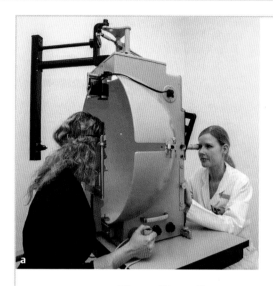

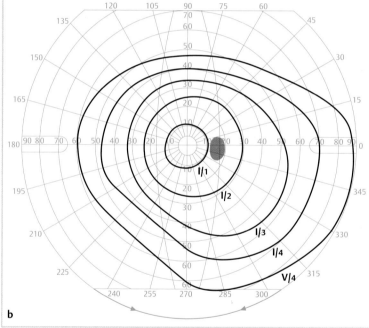

Fig. 14.2 Goldmann hemispheric perimeter and visual field findings. (a) The patient focuses with one eye on a black dot in the middle of the hemisphere. As soon as the patient notices the light marker moving in from the periphery, he or she presses a button that triggers an acoustic signal. The examiner sits behind the hemisphere. From there, the examiner controls the light marker and records which points the patient recognizes. (b) Normal visual field. Due to the anatomy of the bridge of the nose and roof of the orbit, the visual field is physiologically limited in the nasal and superior regions. The blind spot (optic disc) normally lies 10 to 20° off-center in the horizontal plane, on the right in the right eye and on the left in the left eye.

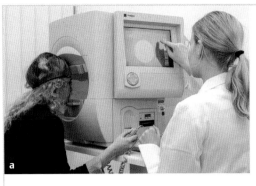

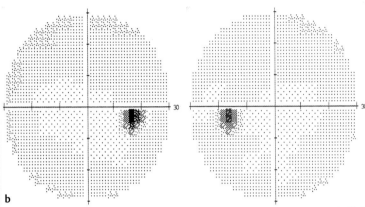

Fig. 14.3 Humphrey field analyzer and visual field findings. (a) In static perimetry, the patient also focuses on a black dot in the middle of the hemisphere. As soon as the patient perceives a light marker, he or she presses a button that triggers an acoustic signal. The result is shown on the monitor on the right. (b) Normal visual field in the left and right eyes, in the 30° range. The severity of the visual field defect is depicted with increasing gray scales. The dark area in the each graph represents the blind spot.

14.3.1 Prechiasmal Lesions

Disorders of the optic nerve (see p. 232) lead to an ipsilateral decrease in visual acuity and/or visual field defects.

14.3.2 Chiasmal Lesions

▶ **Anatomy.** The optic chiasm and the optic nerves (▶ Fig. 14.4) lie on the diaphragma sellae, a dural fold that forms the roof of the sella turcica.

The pituitary gland in the sella turcica lies **inferior to the chiasm**. The internal carotid artery defines the **lateral border of the chiasm**. The hypothalamus and anterior lobe of the cerebrum are located **superior to the chiasm**. **Within the chiasm**, the inferior nasal fibers cross inferiorly and anteriorly, and are therefore most likely to be affected by *pituitary tumors*. The superior nasal fibers cross posteriorly and superiorly within the chiasm and are therefore most likely to be affected by *craniopharyngiomas*. The macular fibers cross in various locations throughout the chiasm, including posteriorly and superiorly.

▶ **Etiology and corresponding visual field defects**
▶ **Pituitary adenomas.** These are tumors that proceed from the hormone-secreting cells of the anterior lobe of the pituitary gland. As they increase in size superiorly, they reach the anterior margin of the chiasm where they compress the inferior and nasal fibers that cross there (▶ Fig. 14.5). This leads to an *initial visual field defect* in the superior temporal quadrant that may later progress to complete bilateral temporal hemianopsia. The visual field defect usually spreads in an asymmetrical pattern. The eye with the more severe visual field defect often exhibits the lesser central visual acuity.

▶ **Craniopharyngiomas.** These slow-growing tumors develop from tissue of the pouch of Rathke (the pituitary diverticulum) along the stem of the pituitary gland. Craniopharyngiomas compress the optic chiasm posteriorly and superiorly and therefore primarily affect the superior nasal fibers that cross there (▶ Fig. 14.6). The corresponding *visual field defect* begins in the inferior temporal quadrants and then spreads into the superior temporal quadrants.

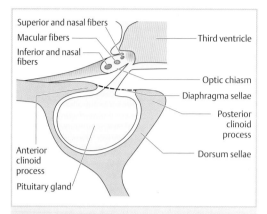

Fig. 14.4 Anatomic relationships of the optic chiasm. Sagittal section of the optic chiasm (see text for details).

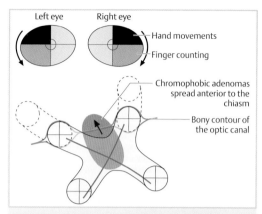

Fig. 14.5 Inferior compression of the optic chiasm by a pituitary adenoma. The visual field defect begins as a bilateral superior temporal defect and can progress to complete bilateral temporal hemianopsia. The terms "finger counting" and "hand motion" describe the patient's visual perception.

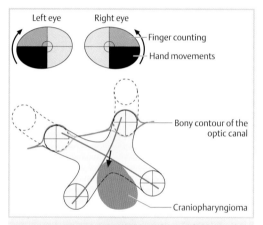

Fig. 14.6 Superior compression of the optic chiasm by a craniopharyngioma. The visual field defect starts bilaterally in the inferior temporal quadrants and can progress to complete bilateral temporal hemianopsia.

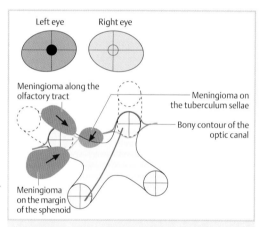

Fig. 14.7 Possible compression of the optic nerve by a meningioma. Different visual defects can arise depending on the position of the meningioma.

▶ **Meningiomas.** These are tumors that proceed from the arachnoid. They may affect various different parts of the chiasm depending on the site of their origin (▶ Fig. 14.7). When they occur on the tuberculum sellae, they can compress either the optic nerve or the chiasm. Meningiomas can also proceed from the margin of the sphenoid and compress the optic nerve. Those that originate along the olfactory tract can lead to a loss of sense of smell and to compression of the optic nerve.

▶ **Aneurysms.** Dilation of the internal carotid artery due to an aneurysm can result in lateral compression of the optic chiasm (▶ Fig. 14.8). The resulting *visual field defect* begins unilaterally but can become bilateral if the chiasm is pressed against the contralateral internal carotid artery. Initially there is ipsilateral hemianopsia extending nasally. This is followed by compression of the contralateral side with contralateral hemianopsia that also extends nasally.

▶ **Other changes in the chiasm.** Aside from the external effects on the chiasm, changes can occur within the chiasm itself. These include gliomas, demyelination, and trauma. The chiasm can also be involved in infiltrative or inflammatory changes of the basal leptomeninges (arachnoiditis of the optic chiasm). *The resulting visual field defects are highly variable.*

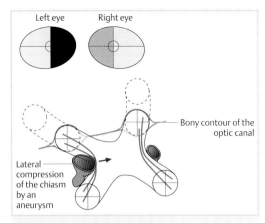

Left eye   Right eye

Bony contour of the optic canal

Lateral compression of the chiasm by an aneurysm

Fig. 14.8 Lateral compression of the optic chiasm by an aneurysm in the internal carotid artery. The visual field defect begins on the same side as hemianopsia, extending nasally, and can progress to bilateral nasal hemianopsia.

▶ **Symptoms, diagnostic considerations, and clinical picture.** The compression of the optic nerve produces **primary descending atrophy of the optic nerve**. This is associated with a more or less severe **decrease in visual acuity** and **visual field defects** (see Etiology). A visual field defect consisting of heteronymous bilateral temporal hemianopsia is referred to as **chiasm syndrome**. The visual field defects in these cases are frequently incongruent. Chiasm syndrome develops *slowly* and usually represents the late stage of a pituitary adenoma or craniopharyngioma.

Note
Heteronymous bilateral temporal hemianopsia with decreased visual acuity and unilateral or bilateral optic nerve atrophy is referred to as chiasm syndrome.

Bilateral temporal visual field defects are typical for chiasmal processes. However, the many possible locations of lesions in the region of the chiasm produce widely varying visual field defects depending on the specific etiology.

Note
Bilateral temporal visual field defects are due to chiasmal lesions. A chiasmal lesion should always be considered in the presence of any uncertain visual field defect.

Further diagnostic studies can be performed after visual acuity testing, pupillary light reaction testing, perimetry, and ophthalmoscopy of the fundus and optic disc. Such studies include radiography of the sella turcica (to detect enlargement or destruction of the sella turcica due to a pituitary adenoma), CT, MRI, carotid arteriography, and, in applicable cases, endocrinologic studies.

▶ **Treatment.** Treatment depends on the underlying cause. Neurosurgery may be indicated or medication, such as bromocriptine for a pituitary tumor.

▶ **Prognosis.** This also depends on the underlying disorder. Ocular functional deficits may subside when the disorder is promptly diagnosed and treated.

14.3.3 Retrochiasmal Lesions

▶ **Etiology.** Retrochiasmal lesions may result from a wide variety of **neurologic disorders** such as tumors, vascular insults, basal meningitis, aneurysms of the posterior communicating artery, abscesses, injuries (such as a contrecoup injury to the occipital lobe), and vasospasms (in an ocular migraine).

▶ **Symptoms, diagnostic considerations, and clinical picture.** Visual field testing in particular will provide information on the location of the lesion. **Perimetry** is therefore a crucial diagnostic study. *Bilateral simultaneous visual field defects* are common to all retrochiasmal lesions of the visual pathway. Often these defects will be incongruent.

Note
Homonymous visual field defects are the result of a retrochiasmal lesion.

▶ **Lesions of the optic tract and the lateral geniculate body.** Because the nerve fibers are concentrated in a very small space, the visual field defect that occurs typically in these lesions is homonymous hemianopsia. Lesions on the right side produce visual field defects in the left half of the visual field and vice versa. Partial primary atrophy of the optic nerve may occur as the third neuron is affected, which extends from the retina to the lateral geniculate body. An *afferent pupillary defect on the side opposite the lesion* will be present. The cause of this defect is not known.

253

▶ **Lesions of the optic radiations.** The *visual field defects* assume *many different forms* due to the wide spread of the optic radiations. Injuries to both the temporal and parietal lobes typically produce *homonymous hemianopsia*. Injuries primarily involving the temporal lobe produce homonymous *superior* quadrantic anopsia; injuries primarily involving the parietal lobe produce homonymous *inferior* quadrantic anopsia. Pupillary findings are normal because the lesion affects the fourth neuron. Approximately 30% of cases involve an *afferent pupillary defect on the side opposite the lesion*. The cause of this defect is not known.

▶ **Lesions of the visual cortex.** The visual field defects, like the lesions of the visual pathway, are *homonymous and hemianoptic*. The macula may or may not be affected depending on the extent of the lesion.

▶ **Special forms**
- **Cortical blindness.** Bilateral lesions of the visual cortex, especially injuries, can produce both temporal and nasal visual field defects with *normal pupillary light reaction* and *normal optic disc findings*.
- **Visual agnosia.** Where the association areas of the brain are damaged, as often occurs in lesions of the parietal lobe or marginal visual cortex, the patient can see but is unable to interpret or classify visual information. Examples of this include alexia (acquired inability to comprehend written words) and color agnosia (inability to distinguish colors).

▶ **Other symptoms and findings.** Depending on the underlying disorder, these may include headache, nausea, vomiting, and papilledema. A differential diagnosis requires CT and MRI studies.

▶ **Treatment.** Depending on the underlying disorder, the patient is referred to either a neurologist or neurosurgeon for treatment.

▶ **Prognosis.** The prognosis is generally poor, and the visual field defects usually do not subside.

14.3.4 Ocular Migraine

This is due to a **transient vasospasm of the posterior cerebral artery** that supplies the visual cortex.

▶ **Symptoms.** Symptoms vary. Typically there will be a unilateral homonymous and initially paracentral scintillating scotoma, a series of flashes of bright light (fortification spectra), and perceptions of dazzling colors. Headache, nausea, and vertigo also occur. Paresis of the ocular muscles (*ophthalmoplegic migraine*) may also occur.

▶ **Treatment.** Patients should be referred to a neurologist; analgesic serotonin agonist (sumatriptan).

▶ Fig. 14.9 provides a **schematic overview** of all major lesions of the visual pathway with their associated visual field defects.

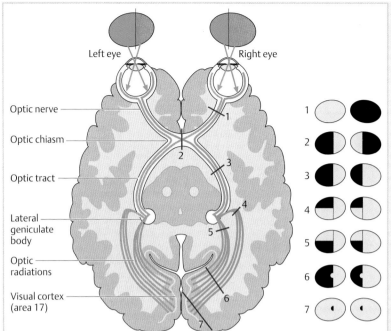

Left eye Right eye

Optic nerve

Optic chiasm

Optic tract

Lateral geniculate body

Optic radiations

Visual cortex (area 17)

1
2
3
4
5
6
7

Fig. 14.9 Visual field defects associated with the major lesions of the visual pathway.

Chapter 15

Orbital Cavity

15 Orbital Cavity

Christoph W. Spraul and Gerhard K. Lang

15.1 Basic Knowledge

▶ **Importance of the orbital cavity for the eye.** The orbital cavity is the *protective bony socket* for the globe together with the optic nerve, ocular muscles, nerves, blood vessels, and lacrimal gland. These structures are surrounded by orbital fatty tissue. The orbital cavity is shaped like a *funnel* that opens anteriorly and inferiorly. The six ocular muscles originate at the apex of the funnel around the optic nerve and insert into the globe. The globe moves within the orbital cavity as in *a joint socket.*

▶ **Bony socket.** This consists of seven bones (▶ Fig. 15.1):
- Frontal.
- Ethmoid.
- Lacrimal.
- Sphenoid.
- Maxillary.
- Palatine.
- Zygomatic.

The bony rim of the orbital cavity forms a strong ring. Its other bony surfaces include very thin plates of bone (see Adjacent structures).

▶ **Adjacent structures.** The close proximity of the orbital cavity to adjacent structures is clinically significant. The **maxillary sinus** inferior to the orbital cavity is separated from it by a plate of bone 0.5 mm thick. The **ethmoidal air cells** located medial and posterior to the orbital cavity are separated from it by a plate of bone only 0.3 mm thick *or by periosteum alone.* The following structures are also located *immediately adjacent to* the orbital cavity:
- Sphenoidal sinus.
- Middle cranial fossa.
- Region of the optic chiasm.
- Pituitary gland.
- Cavernous sinus.

Superior adjacent structures include the **anterior cranial fossa** and the **frontal sinus**. ▶ Table 15.1 lists the various bony openings into the orbital cavity and the anatomical structures that pass through them. Because of this anatomical situation, the

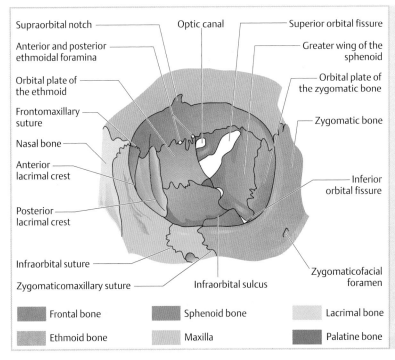

Supraorbital notch — Optic canal — Superior orbital fissure

Anterior and posterior ethmoidal foramina — Greater wing of the sphenoid

Orbital plate of the ethmoid — Orbital plate of the zygomatic bone

Frontomaxillary suture — Zygomatic bone

Nasal bone —

Anterior lacrimal crest — Inferior orbital fissure

Posterior lacrimal crest —

Infraorbital suture — Zygomaticofacial foramen

Zygomaticomaxillary suture — Infraorbital sulcus

Fig. 15.1 Anterior aspect of the left orbital cavity. Diagram of the seven orbital bones and the openings into the orbital cavity.

	Frontal bone		Sphenoid bone		Lacrimal bone
	Ethmoid bone		Maxilla		Palatine bone

Table 15.1 Openings into the orbital cavity and the structures that pass through them

Orbital openings	Structures
Optic canal	• Optic nerve • Ophthalmic artery

Superior orbital fissure	• Oculomotor nerve
	• Trochlear nerve
	• Abducens nerve
	• Ophthalmic nerve
	  ○ Lacrimal nerve
	  ○ Frontal nerve
	  ○ Nasociliary nerve
	• Superior ophthalmic veins

Inferior orbital fissure	• Infraorbital nerve • Zygomatic nerve • Inferior ophthalmic vein
Infraorbital canal	• Infraorbital nerve

orbital cavity is frequently affected by disorders of adjacent structures. For example, inflammations of the paranasal sinuses can result in orbital cellulitis (see p. 263).

The walls of the orbital cavity are lined with periosteum, which is also referred to as periorbita. Its anterior boundary is formed by the orbital septa extending from the orbital rim to the superior and inferior tarsal plates, the lateral and medial palpebral ligaments, and the eyelids.

▶ **Arterial supply.** The orbital cavity is supplied by the **ophthalmic artery**, a branch of the internal carotid artery. The ophthalmic artery communicates with the angular artery, a branch of the external carotid artery, via the supraorbital and supratrochlear arteries.

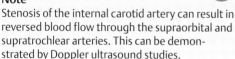

Note
Stenosis of the internal carotid artery can result in reversed blood flow through the supraorbital and supratrochlear arteries. This can be demonstrated by Doppler ultrasound studies.

▶ **Venous drainage from the orbital cavity.** The orbital cavity drains through the **inferior ophthalmic vein** into the pterygoid plexus, through the **superior ophthalmic vein** into the cavernous sinus, and through the **angular vein** into the facial veins.

15.2 Examination Methods

▶ **Cardinal symptoms.** Unilateral or bilateral **enophthalmos** (recession of the eyeball within the orbital cavity) or **exophthalmos** (protrusion of the

eyeball) are characteristic of many orbital disorders (▶ Table 15.2). These conditions should be distinguished from **pseudoexophthalmos** due to a long eyeball in severe myopia, and **pseudoenophthalmos** due to a small eyeball, such as in microphthalmos or phthisis bulbi.

The following list of examination techniques begins with the simple standard techniques and progresses to the difficult, more elaborate methods. As a general rule, orbital disorders require interdisciplinary cooperation between ENT specialists, neurologists, neurosurgeons, neuroradiologists, internists, nuclear medicine specialists, and oncologists.

▶ **Visual acuity and visual field testing.** For details see Chapter 1.4.

▶ **Ocular motility.** The pattern of disturbed ocular motility can be a **sign of the cause of the disorder**. Causes may be neurogenic, myogenic, or mechanical. For further details see Chapter 17.

▶ **Examination of the fundus.** Retrobulbar processes can press the globe inward. This often produces **choroidal folds that are visible upon ophthalmoscopy**. Compression of the optic nerve by a tumor may result in **optic nerve atrophy or edema**. Meningiomas in the sheath of the optic nerve lead to the development of **shunt vessels on the optic disc**.

▶ **Exophthalmometry.** The *Hertel mirror exophthalmometer* (▶ Fig. 15.2) measures the anterior projection of the globe beyond the orbital rim. A **change in the position of the globe with respect to the orbital rim** is a cardinal symptom of many orbital disorders (see ▶ Table 15.2).

Table 15.2 Causes for exophthalmos and enophthalmos listed according to clinical syndromes of similar etiology. Both the groups themselves and the disorders within each group are listed in descending order of incidence

Change in position	Causes
Exophthalmos (protrusion of the eyeball)	• Graves's disease (most frequent cause) **Inflammatory orbital disorders** • Orbital cellulitis (most frequent cause in children) • Orbital pseudotumor (autoimmune disorder) • Myositis of the ocular muscles (special form of pseudotumor) • Orbital abscess • Cavernous sinus thrombosis (serious clinical syndrome) • Severe tenonitis (inflammation of the Tenon capsule) • Mucocele • Mycosis (in immunocompromised patients) • Parasitic infestation of the orbital cavity (rare) **Vascular orbital disorders** • Arteriovenous fistulas (pulsating) • Orbital hematomas (usually post-traumatic) • Orbital varices (intermittent exophthalmos) **Orbital tumors** (slowly progressive) **Developmental anomalies** • Craniosynostosis (premature fusion of cranial sutures) • Meningoencephalocele (very rare) • Bone disease (rare)
Enophthalmos (recession of the eyeball)	**Orbital fractures** (most frequent cause) • Blow-out fracture not associated with an orbital hematoma **Neurogenic causes** • Horner's syndrome (sympathetic palsy) • Paresis of the oblique ocular muscles **Atrophy of orbital tissue** (symmetrical) • Senile atrophy of the orbital fat • Dehydration

Note
The difference between the two sides is more important than the absolute value. A difference greater than 3 mm between the two eyes is abnormal. Unilateral exophthalmos is recognizable without an exophthalmometer. To do so, the examiner stands behind the patient, slightly lifts the patient's upper eyelids, and looks down over the patient's forehead toward the cheek.

▶ **Visual field testing (see p. 249).** This is used to **document damage to the optic nerve** in orbital disorders.

▶ **Ultrasound studies.** Two techniques are available for this noninvasive examination.
1. The **B-mode scan** (B stands for brightness) provides a *two-dimensional image of orbital structures*. This examination is indicated in the presence of suspected orbital masses.
2. The **A-mode scan** (A stands for amplitude) permits *precise measurement of optic nerve and muscle thickness*. This examination is indicated as a follow-up study in the presence of Graves's disease (endocrine orbitopathy).

These studies may also be combined with **Doppler scans** to evaluate blood flow.

▶ **Conventional radiographic studies.** These studies usually only provide information about the **nature of bone structures**—i.e., whether a fracture is present and where it is located. Smaller fractures often cannot be diagnosed by conventional radiography and require CT scans.

▶ **Computed tomography and magnetic resonance imaging.** These examination modalities can precisely visualize orbital structures in various planes. They are **standard methods for diagnosing tumors**.

Note
In the presence of orbital trauma, initial CT studies should be performed as this method can better visualize bony structures. Where soft-tissue lesions are suspected, however, an initial MRI is recommended.

▶ **Angiography.** This is indicated in the presence of **suspected arteriovenous fistulas**.

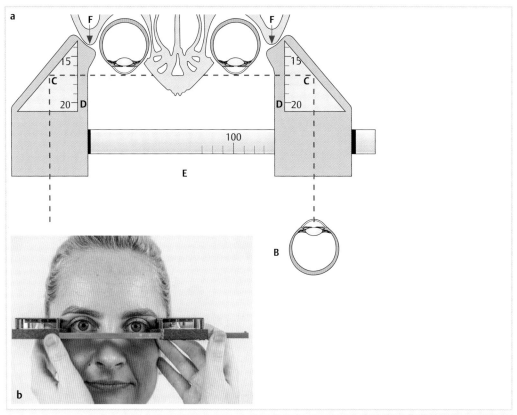

Fig. 15.2 Function and application of the Hertel mirror exophthalmometer. (a) The device measures the extraorbital prominence of the eye from the anterior surface of the cornea (dashed line) to the temporal bony rim of the orbit (F). The examiner (B) views the anterior surface of the cornea through a mirror (C). The extraorbital prominence in millimeters is then read off the integral scale (D). To obtain reproducible results, it is important to maintain a constant base setting in millimeters (here 104 mm) (E) every time the exophthalmometer is applied. **(b)** The exophthalmometer is placed on the lowest point of the temporal zygomatic bone. To avoid parallactic measurement errors, the examiner moves his or her own eye horizontally until the two integral graduations align in the projection. Once the graduations have been aligned, the examiner reads the value of the extraorbital prominence of the anterior surface of the cornea on the scale. The examiner reads the measurement with only one eye. The examiner uses his or her left eye to read the value for the patient's right eye, and vice versa.

15.3 Developmental Anomalies

Congenital developmental anomalies affecting the orbital cavity are very rare.

15.3.1 Craniofacial Dysplasia

Craniostenosis

This clinical picture involves **premature fusion of the cranial sutures**. Clinical signs often include *bilateral exophthalmos* associated with *ocular hypertelorism and exotropia* (divergent strabismus). The mechanical impairment of the optic nerve is evidenced by development of *papilledema* and requires surgical decompression to prevent atrophy of the optic nerve.

Oxycephaly

Premature fusion of the coronal suture causes the orbits to become elevated, flattened, and smaller than normal.

Craniofacial Dysostosis

Premature fusion of the coronal and sagittal sutures also results in a high skull and abnormally small orbits. This condition is also characterized by a wide root of the nose and a prominent chin.

Note
Enucleation in early childhood can result in orbital hypoplasia as the globe provides a growth stimulus for the orbital cavity. Therefore the patient should promptly receive a prosthesis.

15.3.2 Mandibulofacial Dysplasia

Oculoauriculovertebral Dysplasia

Epibulbar dermoids near the limbus are present in addition to outer ear anomalies and rudiments of a branchial passage in the cheek (see ▶ Fig. 4.18).

Mandibulofacial Dysostosis

Also known as Treacher Collins syndrome (incomplete type) or Franceschetti syndrome (complete type), this **anomaly of the first branchial arch** is characterized by orbital deformities with *antimongoloid palpebral fissures, coloboma of the lower eyelid,* low-set ears, and a hypoplastic mandible with dental deformities.

Oculomandibular Dysostosis

In addition to the typical birdlike face, this anomaly may be accompanied by bilateral microphthalmos associated with cataract, nystagmus, and strabismus.

Rubinstein–Taybi Syndrome

This craniomandibulofacial dysplasia is primarily characterized by antimongoloid palpebral fissures, ocular hypertelorism, epicanthal folds, and enophthalmos. Cataracts, iris colobomas, and infantile glaucoma have also been described.

15.3.3 Meningoencephalocele

Incomplete fusion of the cranial sutures in the orbital region can lead to evaginations of dural sac with brain tissue. Clinical findings occasionally include *pulsating exophthalmos* or, in extreme cases, a *tumorous protrusion.*

15.3.4 Osteopathies

Many of these disorders can produce orbital changes. The most common of these diseases include *Paget's disease of bone, dysostosis multiplex* (Hurler's syndrome), and *marble-bone disease of*

Albers-Schönberg (osteopetrosis) in which compressive optic neuropathy also occurs.

15.4 Orbital Involvement in Autoimmune Disorders: Graves's Disease

Definition
Autoimmune disorder with orbital involvement is frequently associated with thyroid dysfunction. Histologic examination reveals inflammatory infiltration of the orbital cavity.

▶ **Epidemiology.** Women are affected eight times as often as men. Sixty percent of patients have hyperthyroidism. Ten percent of patients with thyroid disorders develop Graves's disease during the course of their life.

Note
Graves's disease is the most frequent cause of both unilateral and bilateral exophthalmos.

▶ **Etiology.** The precise etiology of this autoimmune disorder is not clear. Histologic examination reveals lymphocytic infiltration of the orbital cavity. The ocular muscles are particularly severely affected. Fibrosis develops after the acute phase.

Note
An autonomous adenoma of the thyroid gland is not associated with Graves's disease. Some patients with Graves's disease never exhibit any thyroid dysfunction during their entire life.

▶ **Symptoms.** The onset of this generally painless disorder is usually between the ages of 20 and 45 years. Patients complain of reddened dry eyes with a sensation of pressure (symptoms of keratoconjunctivitis sicca) and of cosmetic problems. Ocular motility is also limited, and patients may experience double vision (binocular diplopia.)

▶ **Diagnostic considerations.** Cardinal symptoms include *exophthalmos,* which is unilateral in only 10% of cases, and eyelid changes that involve development of a *characteristic eyelid sign* (▶ Table 15.3 and ▶ Fig. 15.3). Thickening of the muscles (primarily the rectus inferior and medialis) and subse-

Table 15.3 Eyelid signs in Graves's disease

Eyelid sign	Explanation
Dalrymple sign	Upper eyelid is retracted with visible sclera superior to the limbus and widened palpebral fissure with developing exposure keratitis (overactive muscle of Müller)
Von Gräfe sign	Upper eyelid retracts when the eye depresses (overactive muscle of Müller)
Gifford sign	Upper eyelid is difficult to evert (due to eyelid edema)
Stellwag sign	Rare blinking
Kocher sign	Fixed gaze
Möbius sign	Convergence deficit
Enroth sign	Upper eyelid edema
Jellinek sign	Over-pigmentation of the upper eyelid
Pocher sign	Horizontal eyelid furrow
Joffroy sign	Lack of forehead wrinkling when glance is raised
Rodenbach sign	Eyelid flutters when closed

quent fibrosis lead to limited motility and double vision (binocular diplopia). Elevation is impaired; this can lead to false high values when **measuring intraocular pressure** with the gaze elevated. The ability to maintain convergence is also limited (Möbius sign).

The tentative clinical diagnosis of Graves's disease is supported by **thickening of the extraocular muscles** identified in **ultrasound or CT studies** (▶ Fig. 15.4). The further diagnostic work-up requires the cooperation of an internist, endocrinologist, and radiologist.

▶ **Differential diagnosis.** Rarer clinical syndromes such as orbital tumors and orbital pseudotumors must be excluded.

▶ **Treatment.** The main principles in treating the disease in its **acute stage** include *management of the thyroid dysfunction*, *systemic cortisone* (initially 60–100 mg of prednisone) and *radiation therapy of the orbital cavity. Surgical decompression of the orbital cavity* is indicated in **recurrent cases that do not respond to treatment** to avoid compressive optic neuropathy. **Exposure keratitis** (keratitis due to inability to close the eye) should be treated with *artificial tears* or *tarsorrhaphy* (partial or complete suture closure of the upper and lower eyelid to shorten or close the palpebral fissure). In the **chronic stage** of the disease, *eye muscle surgery* can be performed to correct strabismus.

▶ **Clinical course and prognosis.** Visual acuity will remain good if treatment is initiated promptly. In the postinflammatory phase, exophthalmos often persists despite the fact that the underlying disorder is well controlled.

15.5 Orbital Inflammation

Because of the close proximity of the orbital cavity to the paranasal sinuses, which are particularly susceptible to inflammation, orbital inflammation represents the *second most frequent* group of orbital disorders after Graves's disease. Orbital cellulitis is the *most severe* of these.

15.5.1 Orbital Cellulitis

Definition
Acute inflammation of the contents of the orbital cavity with the cardinal symptoms of limited motility and general malaise.

Note
Orbital cellulitis is the most frequent cause of exophthalmos in children.

▶ **Etiology.** Acute orbital inflammation posterior to the orbital septum is *usually* an inflammation that has spread from surrounding tissue. Over 60% of cases (as high as 84% in children) can be classified as originating in the **sinuses**, especially the ethmoidal air cells and the frontal sinus. In infants, **tooth germ inflammations** may be the cause. *Less frequently*, this clinical picture occurs in association

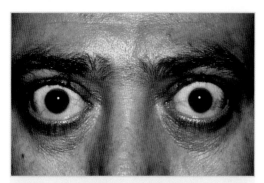

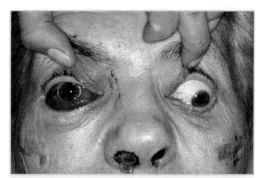

Fig. 15.3 Patient with Graves's disease, more severe in the left than in the right eye. Typical signs include exophthalmos, which here is readily apparent in the left eye, retraction of the upper eyelid with visible sclera superior to the limbus (Dalrymple sign), conjunctival injection, and fixed gaze (Kocher sign) as well as upward strabismal deviation of the left eye.

Fig. 15.5 Patient with orbital cellulitis. Typical symptoms include chemosis (conjunctival swelling), exophthalmos, and significantly limited ocular motility (the right eye does not move with the left eye).

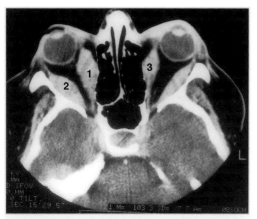

Fig. 15.4 CT image of a patient with Graves's disease. The image shows obvious thickening of the extraocular muscles in the right orbit, primarily the rectus medialis (1) and rectus lateralis (2), and of the rectus medialis (3) in the left orbit.

involvement of the paranasal sinuses, an ENT specialist should be consulted to evaluate the sinuses and initiate any necessary treatment.

The sinogenic cause was previously treated via an orbital and nasal approach.

▶ **Differential diagnosis.** *Preseptal cellulitis*, which is **more frequently encountered**, should be excluded. The inflammation in preseptal cellulitis is anterior to the orbital septum; *chemosis* and *limited motility* are absent. **Rarer clinical syndromes** that should also be considered in a differential diagnosis include an *orbital pseudotumor* (see p. 265), *orbital periostitis (see p. 266)* which may be accompanied by a subperiosteal abscess, and an *orbital abscess*.

Note

The crucial characteristic feature of orbital cellulitis for differential diagnosis is the significantly limited ocular motility ("cemented" globe). A rhabdomyosarcoma should also be considered in children.

with facial furuncles, erysipelas, hordeolum, panophthalmitis, orbital injuries, and sepsis.

▶ **Symptoms.** Patients report severe malaise, occasionally accompanied by fever and pain exacerbated by eye movement.

▶ **Diagnostic considerations.** Typical symptoms include **exophthalmos** with severe **chemosis** (conjunctival swelling), **eyelid swelling**, and significantly **limited ocular motility** ("cemented" globe; see ▶ Fig. 15.5). Patients may exhibit **leukocytosis** and an **increased erythrocyte sedimentation rate**. Where there is clinical evidence of suspected

▶ **Treatment.** This consists of **high-dose intravenous antibiotic therapy** with 1.5 g of oxacillin every 4 hours combined with one million units of penicillin G every 4 hours. Infants are treated with ceftriaxone and school-age children with oxacillin combined with cefuroxime in the appropriate doses. **Treatment of underlying sinusitis** is indicated in applicable cases.

▶ **Clinical course and complications.** Orbital inflammation can lead to **optic neuritis** with subsequent atrophy and loss of vision. Purulent thrombophlebitis of the orbital veins can result in cavernous sinus thrombosis (see below) with meningitis, cerebral abscess, or sepsis.

Note
Orbital cellulitis can progress to a life-threatening situation (cavernous sinus thrombosis).

15.5.2 Cavernous Sinus Syndrome

Definition
Rare but *severe acute* clinical syndrome with unilateral paresis of the oculomotor, trochlear, and abducens nerves associated with sensory deficits in branch 1 of the trigeminal nerve (ophthalmic nerve) in pathologic changes of the cavernous spaces of the retroorbital cavernous sinus.

▶ **Etiology.** A pathologic process (tumor/metastasis, large aneurysm of the internal carotid artery or fistula between the carotid and the cavernous sinus, sinus thrombosis, inflammatory infiltration) affecting the cavernous sinus causes pressure damage to nerves resulting in simultaneous complete or partial failure of cranial nerves III (oculomotor nerve), IV (trochlear nerve), and VI (abducens nerve), and partial failure of cranial nerve V (trigeminal nerve).

▶ **Symptoms.** Patients present with an acute clinical picture with double vision, headache, fever, and vomiting in reduced general state of health.

▶ **Clinical findings.** The most prominent symptom is the concurrent paralysis of the three eye muscles innervated by the three cranial oculomotor nerves with the related movement disorders, strabismal deviation, and double vision that culminate in total ophthalmoplegia. Damage to the parasympathetic fibers (running together with cranial nerve III) results in anisocoria with enlargement of the ipsilateral pupil. The disorders can occur unilaterally or bilaterally, depending on size and localization. If the trigeminal nerve is affected, the sensitivity of the cornea and the upper portions of the face can be decreased due to a lesion in both of its branches—the ophthalmic nerve and the maxillary nerve. In case of an acute onset and signs of a drainage disorder, such as venous congestion of the orbital content, with swelling of the eyelid and connective tissue as well as exophthalmus, a venous thrombosis and/or fistula between the carotid artery and

the cavernous sinus can be assumed. In the latter case, the exophthalmus is pulsating if the shunt volume is high. Fever and leukocytosis indicate septic thrombosis with a risk of intracranial spread with development of hemianopses and unconsciousness. In aseptic ("bland") thrombosis, the venous congestion is a threat to vision.

Note
The limited motility of the globe is primarily neurogenic and due to damage to the nerves in the cavernous sinus as opposed to the mechanical limitation of motility due to the orbital inflammation in orbital cellulitis.

▶ **Diagnostic considerations and treatment.** This lies primarily in the hands of ENT specialists, neurosurgeons, and internists. High-dose systemic antibiotic therapy and anticoagulation are indicated.

15.5.3 Orbital Pseudotumor

Definition
Lymphocytic orbital tumor *of unknown origin.*

▶ **Symptoms and findings.** Painful, moderately severe inflammatory reaction with **eyelid swelling**, **chemosis**, and unilateral or bilateral **exophthalmos**. Involvement of the ocular muscles results in **limited motility with diplopia**.

▶ **Diagnostic considerations.** The **CT and MR images** will show diffuse soft-tissue swelling. A **biopsy** is required to confirm the diagnosis.

Note
Occasionally the CT image will simulate an infiltrative tumor.

▶ **Differential diagnosis.** Various disorders should be excluded. These include **Graves's disease** (see p. 262) and **orbital cellulitis** (see p. 263), which is usually bacterial. **Special forms of orbital pseudotumor** include myositis and Tolosa–Hunt syndrome (painful total ophthalmoplegia produced by an idiopathic granuloma at the apex of the orbit).

▶ **Treatment.** High-dose **systemic cortisone** (initially 100 mg of prednisone) usually leads to remis-

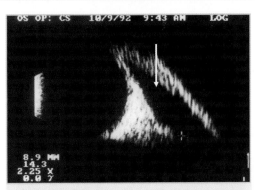

Fig. 15.6 Diagnosis of myositis. The ultrasound image (B-mode scan) shows thickening of the entire hypoechoic rectus medialis (arrow).

sion. Orbital radiation therapy or surgical intervention may be indicated in patients with no response to treatment.

15.5.4 Myositis

This a **special form of orbital pseudotumor** in which the lymphatic infiltration *primarily involves one or more ocular muscles.* Aside from significant *pain during motion,* symptoms include *limited ocular motility with double vision* (diplopia). Depending on the extent of the myositic changes, *exophthalmos with chemosis and eyelid swelling* may also be present. *Ultrasound studies* (▶ Fig. 15.6) will reveal thickening of the ocular muscles with *tenonitis* (inflammation of Tenon's capsule).

> **Note**
> In Graves's disease, only the muscle belly is thickened. In myositis, the entire muscle is thickened.

15.5.5 Orbital Periostitis

This is an **inflammation of the periosteum lining the orbital cavity,** *usually due to bacterial infection* such as actinomycosis, tuberculosis, or syphilis. *Less frequently,* the disorder is due to *osteomyelitis* or, in infants, *tooth germ inflammations.* The *clinical symptoms are similar to those of orbital cellulitis* although significantly less severe and without limitation of ocular motility.

> **Note**
> Liquefaction of the process creates an orbital abscess; large abscesses may progress to orbital cellulitis (see p. 263).

15.5.6 Mucocele

These **mucus-filled cysts** may invade the orbital cavity in *chronic sinusitis.* They displace orbital tissue and cause exophthalmos.

Treatment is required in the following cases:
- Displacement of the globe causes cosmetic or functional problems, such as lagophthalmos or limited motility.
- Compression neuropathy of the optic nerve results.
- The mucocele becomes infected (pyocele).

15.5.7 Mycoses (Mucormycosis and Aspergillomycosis)

These *rare* disorders occur primarily in immunocompromised patients, such as those with diabetes mellitus or AIDS. The disorder often spreads from *infected paranasal sinuses.* The clinical picture is similar to those of inflammatory orbital disorders.

15.6 Vascular Disorders

These changes are *rare.* The most important and most frequently encountered disorder in this group is pulsating exophthalmos.

15.6.1 Pulsating Exophthalmos

Definition
Acute exophthalmos with palpable and audible pulsations synchronous with the pulse in the presence of a *cavernous sinus fistula* or *arteriovenous aneurysm.*

▶ **Etiology.** An abnormal communication between the *cavernous sinus* and the *internal carotid artery* (a direct shunt) or *its branches* (indirect shunt) results in distention of the orbital venous network. Eighty percent of cases are attributable to trauma; less frequently the disorder is due to syphilis or arteriosclerosis.

▶ **Symptoms.** Patients report an unpleasant sound in the head that is reminiscent of a machine and synchronous with their pulse.

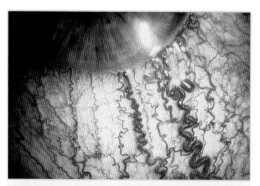

Fig. 15.7 Fistula between the carotid artery and cavernous sinus. The episcleral and conjunctival vessels are significantly dilated and describe tortuous corkscrew courses.

▶ **Diagnostic considerations.** The increased venous pressure leads to **dilatation of the episcleral and conjunctival vessels** (▶ Fig. 15.7), retinal signs of venous stasis with bleeding, exudation, and papilledema. **Intraocular pressure** is also **increased.** The increased pressure in the cavernous sinus can also result in oculomotor and abducens nerve palsy.

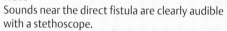

Note
Sounds near the direct fistula are clearly audible with a stethoscope.
Doppler ultrasound studies can confirm a clinical suspicion. However, only **angiography** can determine the exact location of the shunt.

▶ **Treatment.** Selective embolization can be performed in cooperation with a neuroradiologist once the shunt has been located.

Note
Small shunts may close spontaneously in response to pressure fluctuations such as can occur in air travel.

15.6.2 Intermittent Exophthalmos

This *rare* clinical picture characterized by **intermittent unilateral or bilateral exophthalmos** is caused by *varicose dilation of the orbital veins*, such as can occur following trauma or in Osler's disease (polycythemia vera). Patients report protrusion of the eyeball of varying severity. Exophthalmos is usually unilateral and is especially prone to occur when the resistance to venous drainage is increased, as can occur when the patient presses, bends over, screams, or compresses the vessels of the neck. Occasionally the exophthalmos will be associated with increased filling of the episcleral and/or conjunctival vessels. The disorder can be diagnosed in *ultrasound studies using the Valsalva maneuver.* A differential diagnosis should exclude a fistula between the carotid artery and cavernous sinus or an arteriovenous aneurysm, which is usually accompanied by a dramatic clinical picture with pulsation and increased intraocular pressure. In these clinical pictures, the ultrasound examination will reveal *generalized* dilatation of the orbital veins. Surgical removal of orbital varices entails a high risk of damaging crucial delicate neurovascular structures in the orbital cavity. However, it may be indicated in rare cases such as cosmetically unacceptable exophthalmos or where symptoms of keratoconjunctivitis sicca occur due to exposure that fails to respond to treatment.

15.6.3 Orbital Hematoma

Orbital bleeding is **usually posttraumatic** but may occur **less frequently due to coagulopathy** resulting from vitamin C deficiency, anticoagulants, or leukemia. Retrobulbar injections prior to eye surgery and acute venous stasis such as may occur in coughing fits, asphyxia, or childbirth can also cause orbital hematomas. Exophthalmos may be accompanied by *monocle or eyeglass hematoma, eyelid swelling,* and *subconjunctival hemorrhage; limited motility* is rare. Surgical decompression of the orbital cavity (trans-fornix orbital decompression or orbitotomy) is indicated where damage to the optic nerve or blockage of the central retinal artery is imminent.

15.7 Tumors

15.7.1 Orbital Tumors

All orbital tumors displace the globe and cause exophthalmos that is frequently associated with limited ocular motility. Some tumors also cause specific additional symptoms and findings. These are discussed separately for each of the tumors presented in this section.

Tumors of the lacrimal gland are discussed in Chapter 3, Lacrimal System.

Hemangioma

Hemangiomas are the *most common benign orbital tumors* in both children and adults. They usually occur in a *nasal superior* location. *Capillary* hemangiomas are more common in **children** (they swell when the child screams), and *cavernous* hemangiomas are more common in **adults**. *Treatment* is only indicated where the tumor threatens to occlude the visual axis with resulting amblyopia or where there is a risk of compressive optic neuropathy. Capillary hemangiomas in children can be treated with cortisone or low-dose radiation therapy.

Dermoid and Epidermoid Cyst

These lesions are the *most common orbital tumors in children* (▶ Fig. 15.8). Etiologically, they are choristomas—i.e., dermal or epidermal structures that have been displaced into deeper layers. However, they *usually are located anterior to the orbital septum* (and therefore are not in the actual orbit itself). Lesions located posterior to the orbital septum usually become clinically significant only in adulthood. *Treatment* consists of complete removal.

Neurinoma and Neurofibroma

These tumors are often associated with *Recklinghausen's disease (neurofibromatosis)*. If they occur in the optic canal, they must be removed before they cause compressive optic neuropathy.

Meningioma

A meningioma can proceed from the optic nerve (**meningioma of the optic nerve sheath**) or from within the cranium (**sphenoid meningioma**). Symptoms vary depending on the location of the

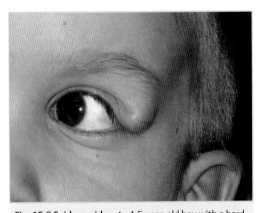

Fig. 15.8 Epidermoid cyst. A 5-year-old boy with a hard, cystic swelling not painful on pressure. The localization at the temporal edge of the orbit is typical. Usually the cyst is connected to the periosteum of the orbital margin.

tumor. Exophthalmos, limited motility, and compressive optic neuropathy can result. *Hyperostoses* are frequent findings in radiographic studies. Treatment consists of neurosurgical removal of the tumor. Like neurinomas, 16% of meningiomas are associated with *neurofibromatosis* (Recklinghausen's disease). *Meningiomas of the optic nerve sheath* are usually histologically benign but can recur if not completely removed. Interestingly, the average age of patients is 32 years; 20% are younger than 20 years.

Histiocytosis X

This is a generic term for the **proliferation of Langerhans cells** of undetermined etiology; all three of the following types can cause exophthalmos where there is orbital involvement:
- Letterer–Siwe disease (malignant).
- Hand–Schüller–Christian disease (benign).
- Eosinophilic granuloma (rare and benign).

Leukemic Infiltrations

Leukemic infiltrations occur especially in acute lymphoblastic leukemia and in a special form of myeloid leukemia (granulocytic sarcoma or chloroma). Inflammation is present in addition to exophthalmos.

Lymphoma

Lymphomas can occur in isolation or in systemic disease. Cooperation with an oncologist is required. The disorder can be treated by radiation therapy or chemotherapy. Usually these tumors are *only slightly malignant*. **The highly malignant Burkitt's lymphoma**, which has a high affinity for the orbital cavity, is a notable exception.

Rhabdomyosarcoma

This is the *commonest primary malignant tumor in children*. The tumor often grows very rapidly (a few months) then leads to exophthalmus and must be distinguished from orbital cellulitis (see p. 263) on the basis of the frequently occurring "inflammatory" components around the eyelids (which can, on very rare occasions, be associated with spontaneous bleeding). Other indicated diagnostic studies include a CT scan or magnetic resonance imaging and possibly a biopsy. With modern therapeutic regimens such as chemotherapy and radiation therapy, curative treatment is possible in many cases.

15.7.2 Metastases

In **children**, the incidence of metastasis is higher in the orbital cavity than in the choroid. In **adults**, it is exactly the opposite. The most common orbital metastases in children originate from *neuroblastomas.* Malignant tumors from adjacent tissue can also invade the orbital cavity.

15.7.3 Optic Nerve Glioma

In *children*, this is the *second most common potentially malignant orbital tumor.* In 25% of patients, the optic nerve glioma is associated with *neurofibromatosis* (Recklinghausen's disease). Fifteen percent of patients with neurofibromatosis develop optic nerve gliomas. The prognosis is good only where the tumor is completely resected.

15.7.4 Injuries

See Chapter 18, Ocular Trauma.

15.8 Orbital Surgery

Access to the orbital cavity is gained primarily through an **anterior** approach (transconjunctival or transpalpebral approaches yield good cosmetic results) or through a **lateral** approach. The lateral Krönlein approach provides better intraoperative exposure. *Transantral, transfrontal, transcranial,* and *transnasal* orbitotomies are used less frequently.

Orbital exenteration is indicated with advanced malignant tumors. This involves removal of the entire contents of the orbital cavity including the eyelids.

Chapter 16

Optics and Refractive Errors

16 Optics and Refractive Errors

Christoph W. Spraul and Gerhard K. Lang

16.1 Basic Knowledge

16.1.1 Uncorrected and Corrected Visual Acuity

▶ **Uncorrected visual acuity.** This refers to the resolving power of the eye without corrective lenses. Visual acuity is determined by vision testing (see p. 3).

▶ **Corrected visual acuity.** This refers to the resolving power of the eye with an optimal correction provided by corrective lenses. Visual acuity is also determined by vision testing (see p. 3).

Both uncorrected visual acuity and corrected visual acuity provide information on how far apart two objects must be for the eye to perceive them as distinct objects (**minimum threshold resolution**). For the eye to perceive two objects as distinct, at least one unstimulated cone must lie between two stimulated cones on the retina. The cone density is greatest in the center of the retina and **central visual acuity** is highest. The interval between the cones increases toward the periphery of the retina, and both uncorrected visual acuity and corrected visual acuity decrease accordingly. Cone spacing and physical effects such as diffraction and optical aberrations limit the average minimum threshold resolution, the **minimum visual angle** to one minute of arc, that is about 1/60 degree (▶ Fig. 16.1). The theoretical minimum threshold resolution at the fovea is determined by the cone diameter of approximately 2 μm. This diameter corresponds to a "**minimum visual angle**" of about 0.5 minute of arc (ca. 0.5/60 degree), equal to a visual acuity (vision) of 2.0.

16.1.2 Refraction: Emmetropia and Ametropia

Refraction is defined as the ratio of the refractive power of the lens and cornea (the refractive media) to the axial length of the globe. Emmetropia is distinguished from ametropia.

▶ **Emmetropia (normal sight).** The ratio of the axial length of the eye to the refractive power of the cornea and lens is such that parallel light rays that enter the eye therefore meet at a focal point *on* the retina (▶ Fig. 16. 2, and see ▶ Fig. 16.6a) and not *anterior* or *posterior* to it, as is the case in ametropia.

▶ **Ametropia (refractive error).** There is a mismatch between the axial length of the eye and the refractive power of the lens and cornea. The ametropia is either **axial**, which is common, or **refractive**, which is less frequently encountered. The most common disorders are nearsightedness, farsightedness, and astigmatism.

Very few people have refraction of exactly ±0.0 diopters. Approximately 55% of persons between the ages of 20 and 30 years have refraction between +1 and −1 diopters.

> **Note** ⓘ
> Emmetropia is not necessarily identical to good visual acuity. The eye may have other disorders that reduce visual acuity, such as atrophy of the optic nerve or amblyopia.

The refractive power of an optical lens system is specified in *diopters*, which are the international unit of measure. Refractive power is calculated

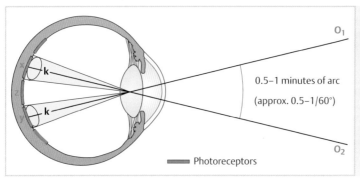

Fig. 16.1 Resolution of the eye (minimum threshold resolution). Two points (O_1 and O_2) can only be perceived as distinct if at least one unstimulated cone (z) lies between two stimulated cones (x and y) on the retina. Due to optical aberrations and diffraction, a punctiform object is reproduced as a circle (k). This results in a maximum resolution of the eye of 0.5 to 1 minute of arc or 0.5/60 to 1/60 degree. The drawing is not to scale.

O_1

0.5–1 minutes of arc

(approx. 0.5–1/60°)

O_2

▬ Photoreceptors

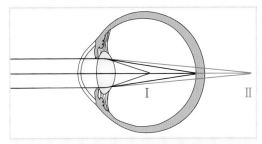

Fig. 16.2 Focal point in emmetropia and ametropia. Parallel rays of light entering the eye from an optically infinite distance meet at a focal point on the retina in emmetropia (black lines). In hyperopia, this focal point (II) lies posterior to the retina (green lines). In myopia (I), it lies anterior to the retina (red lines).

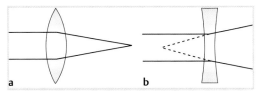

Fig. 16.3 Refraction of light rays traveling through converging and diverging lenses. (a) The converging lens (biconvex) concentrates incident light rays at a focal point behind the lens. (b) A diverging lens (biconcave) ensures that the light rays do not meet at all. The light rays appear to originate at a virtual focal point in front of the lens.

Table 16.1 Important refractive index (n) values of the various tissues of the eye. Source: Krause 1985

Eye tissue	Refractive index n
Cornea	1.376
Aqueous humor	1.336
Lens at the poles	1.385
Lens at the core	1.406
Vitreous body	1.336

according to the laws of geometric optics. According to **Snell's law**, the refraction of the incident light ray is determined by the angle of incidence and difference in the refractive indices *n* of the two media (▶ Table 16.1).

The maximum **total refractive power of an emmetropic eye** is 63 diopters with an axial length of the globe measuring 23.5 mm. The cornea accounts for 43 diopters and the lens for 10–20 diopters, depending on accommodation. However, the refractive power of the eye is not simply the sum of these two values. The optic media that surround the eye's lens system and the distance between the lens and cornea render the total system more complex.

> **Note**
> The refractive power D (specified in diopters) of an optical system is the reciprocal of the focal length of a lens f (specified in meters). This yields the equation: $D = 1/f$.

▶ **Example.** Where a lens focuses parallel incident light rays 0.5 m *behind* the lens, the refractive power is $1/(0.5\,\text{m}) = +2$ diopters. This is a converging lens. Where the *virtual* focal point is 0.5 m *in front of* the lens, the refractive power is $1/(-0.5\,\text{m}) = -2$ diopters. This is a diverging lens (▶ Fig. 16.3).

16.1.3 Accommodation

The refractive power of the eye described in the previous section is not a constant value. The eye's refractive power must alter to allow visualization of both near and distant objects with sharp contours. This accommodation is made possible by the *elasticity of the lens.*

▶ **Accommodation mechanisms.** Accommodation involves the lens, zonule fibers, and ciliary muscle.
- **Lens.** The soluble proteins of the lens are surrounded by a thin elastic capsule. The curvature of the posterior capsule of the lens is greater than its anterior curvature, with a posterior radius of 6.0 mm as opposed to an anterior radius of 10.0 mm. The *intrinsic elasticity of the lens capsule* tends to make the lens assume a spherical shape. However, in the unaccommodated state this is prevented by the pull of the zonule fibers. The elasticity of the inner tissue of the lens progressively decreases with age due to deposits of insoluble proteins.
- **Zonule fibers.** The radiating zonule fibers insert into the equator of the lens and connect it to the ciliary body. They hold the lens securely in position and transmit the pull of the ciliary muscle to the lens.
- **Ciliary muscle.** Contraction of the ring-shaped ciliary muscle decreases the tension in the zonule fibers. The lens can then approach the spherical shape (with a radius of curvature of 5.3 mm) that its physical configuration and chemical composition would otherwise dictate. This change in the curvature of the lens is especially pronounced in its anterior surface. The deformation *increases the refractive power;* the focus of the eye shifts to the near field (▶ Fig. 16.4), and close objects take

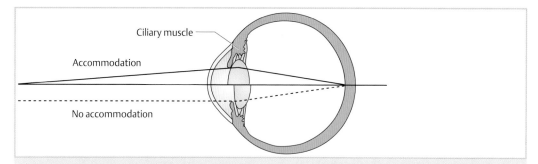

Fig. 16.4 Morphological changes in accommodation. *Top half:* In accommodation, the lens becomes increasingly globular. The curvature of the anterior surface in particular increases. The ciliary muscle is shifted slightly anteriorly, and the anterior chamber becomes shallower. Objects in the near field (continuous line) are represented on the retina with sharp contours. *Bottom half:* With the ciliary body relaxed, parallel incident light rays (dotted line) are focused on the retina. Distant objects are represented on the retina with sharp contours.

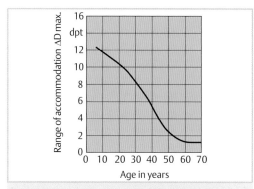

Fig. 16.5 Range of accommodation in diopters as a function of age. When the range of accommodation falls below 3 diopters, a previous emmetropic patient will require eyeglasses for reading (after Goersch 1987.)

Note
When the ciliary muscle is *at rest*, the zonule fibers are under tension and the eye focuses on distant objects.

Accommodation is regulated by a *control loop*. The control variable is the sharpness of the retinal image. The system presumably uses the color dispersion of the retinal image to determine the direction in which accommodation should be corrected.

▶ **Range of accommodation.** This specifies the *maximum increase in refractive power that is possible* by accommodation in diopters (▶ Fig.16.5). In mathematical terms, the range of accommodation is obtained by subtracting near-point refractive power from far-point refractive power. The **near point** (punctum proximum) is the shortest distance that allows focused vision; the **far point** (punctum remotum) describes the farthest point that is still discernible in focus. The near and far points define the range of accommodation; its specific location in space is a function of the refractive power of the eye.

▶ **Example.** In one patient, the near point lies at 0.1 m and the far point at 1 m. This patient's range of accommodation is then 10 diopters − 1 diopter = 9 diopters.

In an emmetropic eye, the far point is at optical infinity (▶ Fig. 16.6a). However, accommodation can also bring near-field objects into focus (▶ Fig. 16.6b). The elasticity of the lens decreases with increasing age, and the range of accommodation decreases accordingly (see ▶ Fig. 16.5). **Presbyopia** (physiologic loss of accommodation in advancing age) begins when the *range of accommodation falls*

on sharp contours. As *the ciliary muscle relaxes,* the tension on the lens increases and the lens flattens. The resulting *decrease in refractive power* shifts the focus of the eye into the distance (▶ Fig. 16.4), and distant objects take on sharp contours.

The ciliary muscle is innervated by the short ciliary nerves, postganglionic parasympathetic fibers of the oculomotor nerve. Parasympatholytics such as atropine, scopolamine, and cyclopentolate inhibit the function of the ciliary muscle and therefore prevent accommodation. Referred to as *cycloplegics,* these medications also cause *mydriasis* by inhibiting the sphincter pupillae. *Parasympathomimetics* such as pilocarpine cause the ciliary muscle and sphincter pupillae to contract, producing *miosis.*

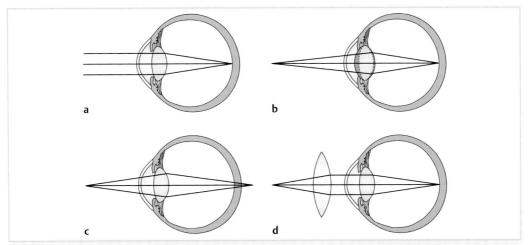

Fig. 16.6 Refraction in the emmetropic eye. (a) Parallel light rays entering the eye from optical infinity are focused on the retina in an *unaccommodated eye*. **(b)** Accommodation focuses the light rays from a close object on the retina, and the object is visualized with sharp contours. **(c)** When accommodation is insufficient, as in advanced age, close objects appear blurred. **(d)** A converging lens is required to correct insufficient accommodation for near vision in advancing age.

below 3 diopters. The gradual loss of accommodation causes the near point to recede; the patient's arms become "too short for reading." Depending on age and limitation of accommodation, presbyopia can be compensated for with converging lenses of 0.5 to 3 diopters (see ▶ Fig. 16.6c, d).

16.1.4 Adaptation to Differences in Light Intensity

Like a camera, the eye's aperture and lens system also automatically adapts to differences in light intensity to avoid "overexposure." This adjustment is effected by two mechanisms.

1. **The iris acts as an aperture to control the amount of light entering the eye**. This regulation takes about 1 second and can change the light intensity on the retina over a range of about a power of ten.
2. **The sensitivity of the retina changes** to adapt to differences in light intensity. The sensitivity of the retina to light is a function of the *concentration of photopigment in the photoreceptors* and of the *neuronal activity of the retinal cells*. The change in neuronal activity is a rapid process that takes only a few milliseconds and can alter the light sensitivity of the retina over a range of three powers of ten. The change in the concentration of photopigment takes several minutes but can cover a wide range of retinal light sensitivity, as much as eight powers of ten.

16.2 Examination Methods

Visual acuity, see Chapter 1.4.

16.2.1 Refraction Testing

Refraction testing means measuring the *additional refractive power* required to produce a sharp image on the retina. Subjective and objective methods are used. Subjective methods require information from the patient.

▶ **Subjective refraction testing.** This consists of successively placing various combinations of lenses before the patient's eye until the maximum visual acuity is reached (see Chapter 1.4).

▶ **Objective refraction testing.** Objective testing is unavoidable when the patient is unable to provide subjective information (for example, with infants) or when this information is unreliable. This method also greatly accelerates subjective refractive testing.

▶ **Retinoscopy (shadow testing).** The retina is illuminated through the pupil. The examiner observes the optical phenomena in the patient's pupil while moving the light source (▶ Fig. 16.7). A lens with a power of +2 diopters is held into the light path.

▶ **Refractometry.** The measuring principle is based on ophthalmoscopic observation of a test image projected onto the patient's retina. The distance between the test figure and the eye is changed until the image appears in focus on the retina. Refraction can then be calculated from the measured values. An alternative to changing of the distance is to place various lenses in the path of the light beam.

▶ **Automated refractometry.** The method measures refraction automatically with the aid of light-sensitive detectors and a computer until a focused image appears on the retina. These systems operate with infrared light.

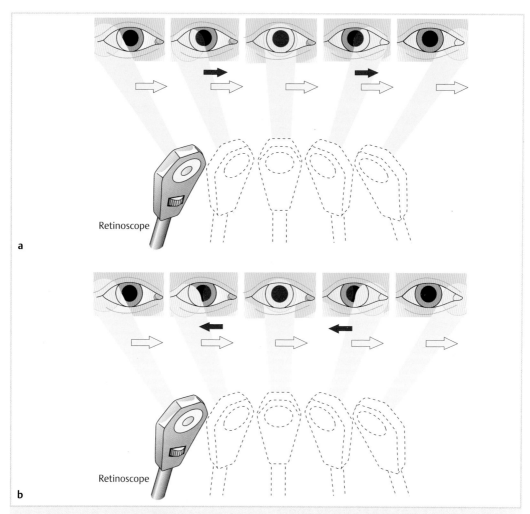

Fig. 16.7 Objective measurement of refractive power with a retinoscope. With the retinoscope, the examiner moves a light source (a beam of yellow light) across the pupil (dark spot) at a distance of about 50 cm from the patient. This produces a light reflex (red spot) in the patient's eye. It is important to note how this light reflex (red spot) behaves as the light source in the retinoscope is moved. There are two possibilities. **(a) Concurrent movement.** The light reflex in the pupil (red spot) moves in the same direction (red arrows) as the light source of the retinoscope (yellow arrows). This means that the far point of the eye is *behind* the light source. **(b) Countermovement.** The light reflex in the pupil moves in the *opposite* direction (red arrows) to the light source of the retinoscope (yellow arrows). This means that the far point of the eye lies *between* the eye and the light source. The examiner places appropriate lenses in front of the patient's eyes (plus lenses for concurrent movement and minus lenses for countermovement) until no further movement of the light reflex is observed. The movement of the retinoscope will then only elicit a brief flicker (**neutral point**). This method is used to determine the proper lens power to correct the refractive error.

Table 16.2 Overview of the major refractive anomalies

Refractive anomaly	Focal point of parallel incident light rays	Causes	Vision	Possible complications	Optical correction
Myopia (nearsightedness)	Anterior to the retina	• Eyeball too long (axial myopia) • Excessive refractive power (refractive myopia)	• Very good near vision • Poor distance vision	• Increased risk of retinal detachment	Diverging lenses (minus or concave lenses)
Hyperopia (farsightedness)	Posterior to the retina	• Eyeball too short (axial hyperopia) • Insufficient refractive power (refractive hyperopia)	• Poor near vision. • Accommodation usually permits normal distance vision (in young patients and in slight to moderate hyperopia)	• Disposition to acute angle closure glaucoma (shallow anterior chamber). Caution is advised with diagnostic and therapeutic mydriasis • Esotropia	Converging lenses (plus or convex lenses)
Astigmatism	Lack of a focal point	• Anomalies in the curvature of the normally spherical surfaces of the refractive media (cornea and lens)	• Patients see everything distorted	• Risk of refractive amblyopia	Cylindrical lenses; eyeglass correction is only possible where astigmatism is regular

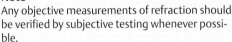

Note
Any objective measurements of refraction should be verified by subjective testing whenever possible.

16.2.2 Testing the Potential Resolving Power of the Retina in the Presence of Opacified Ocular Media

Special examination methods are indicated in the presence of opacification of the ocular media of the eye (such as a cataract) to determine the potential visual acuity of the retina. This permits the ophthalmologist to estimate whether optimizing the refractive media with techniques such as cataract surgery or corneal transplantation would achieve the desired improvement.

▶ **Laser interference visual acuity testing.** Lasers are used to project interference strips of varying widths onto the retina. The patient must specify the direction in which these increasing narrower strips are aligned. This examination can no longer be performed where there is severe opacification of the optic media such as in a mature cataract. The

preliminary examination then consists of evaluating the pattern of the transilluminated retinal vasculature (see p. 193).

16.3 Refractive Anomalies

For a summary of the most important refraction defects, see ▶ Table 16.2.

16.3.1 Myopia (Shortsightedness)

Definition
A discrepancy between the refractive power and axial length of the eye such that parallel incident light rays converge at a *focal point anterior to the retina* (▶ Fig. 16.8a).

▶ **Epidemiology.** Aside from age-related functional disorders of the eye, no change occurs as frequently as myopia. An average of 23 epidemiological examinations in 19 countries, the frequency in youths is 35%. In some developed nations (Far East), the frequency is as high as 80 to 90%. Approximately 25% of persons between the ages of 20 and 30 years have refraction less than −1 diopter.

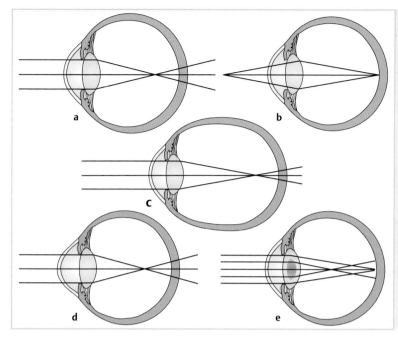

Fig. 16.8 Refraction in myopia. (a) The focal point of parallel light rays entering the eye lies anterior to the retina. (b) Only close objects from which the light rays diverge until they enter the eye are focused on the retina and appear sharply defined. The far point is a finite distance from the eye. (c) Axial myopia: normal refractive power in an excessively long globe. (d) Refractive myopia: excessive refractive power in a normal-length globe. (e) Nuclear cataract with a secondary focal point (the patient sees double).

▶ **Etiology.** The etiology of myopia is not clear. Familial patterns of increased incidence suggest the influence of genetic factors.

▶ **Pathophysiology.** Whereas parallel incident light rays converge at a focal point on the retina in emmetropic eyes, they converge at a focal point *anterior to* the retina in myopic eyes (▶ Fig. 16.8a). This means that *no sharply defined images* appear on the retina when the patient *gazes into the distance.* The myopic eye can only produce *sharply defined images* of *close objects* from which the light rays diverge until they enter the eye (▶ Fig. 16.8b). The far point moves closer; in myopia of −1 diopter it lies at a distance of 1 m.

> **Note**
> In myopia, the far point (distance from the eye = A) can be calculated using the formula: A (m) = $1/D$, where D is myopia in diopters.

Possible causes include an *excessively long globe* with normal refractive power (**axial myopia**; ▶ Fig. 16.8c) and, less frequently, *excessive refractive power* in a normal-length globe (**refractive myopia**; ▶ Fig. 16.8d).

> **Note**
> A difference in globe length of 1 mm with respect to a normal eye corresponds to a difference of about 3 diopters in refractive power.

▶ **Special forms of refractive myopia**
- Myopic sclerosis of the nucleus of the lens (*cataract*) in advanced age (see p. 106). This causes a secondary focal point to develop, which can lead to monocular diplopia (double vision) (▶ Fig. 16.8e).
- Keratoconus (see p. 72): increase in the refractive power of the cornea.
- Spherophakia: spherically shaped lens.

▶ **Forms of myopia:** Forms of myopia include the following:
- **Simple myopia** (school-age myopia): Onset is at the age of 10 to 12 years. Usually the myopia does not progress after the age of 20 years. Refraction rarely exceeds 6 diopters. However, a *benign progressive myopia* also exists, which stabilizes only after the age of 30 years.
- **Pathologic myopia.** This disorder is largely hereditary and progresses continuously, independently of external influences.

▶ **Symptoms and diagnostic considerations.** The diagnosis is made on the basis of a typical clinical

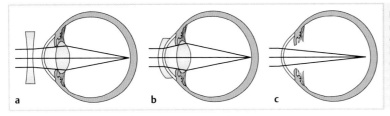

Fig. 16.9 Correction of myopia. (a) Correction with diverging lenses (minus lenses). **(b)** Correction with a contact lens. **(c)** Correction by removing the lens to reduce the refractive power of the eye.

picture and refraction testing. Myopic patients have very good near vision. When gazing into the distance, they squint in an attempt to improve their uncorrected visual acuity by further narrowing the optic aperture of the pupil. The term "myopia" comes from this squinting; the Greek word *myein* means to squint or close the eyes. *Older* myopic patients can read without corrective lenses by holding the reading material at about the distance of the far point.

The typical **morphological changes** occurring in myopia are referred to as **myopia syndrome**. Progressive myopia in particular is characterized by *thinning of the sclera,* a so-called staphyloma posticum verum (see p. 96). The *elongation of the globe* causes a *shift in the axes of the eye.* In addition, enlargement of the globe can lead to a unilateral or bilateral pseudoexophthalmos. This also simulates esotropia. The *anterior chamber* is deep. *Atrophy of the ciliary muscle* is present as it is hardly used. The volume of the vitreous body is too small for the large eye, and it may collapse prematurely. This results in *vitreous opacifications* that the patient perceives as floaters.

For morphological changes of the fundus (myopic maculopathy) see Chapter 12.4.6.

The **risk of retinal detachment** is increased in myopia. However, it *does not* increase in proportion to the severity of the myopia.

Note
Because of the increased risk of retinal detachment, patients with myopia should be examined particularly thoroughly for prodromal signs of retinal detachment, such as equatorial degeneration or retinal tears. Therefore, examination of the fundus with the pupil dilated is indicated both when the first pair of eyeglasses is prescribed and at regular intervals thereafter.

Glaucoma is more difficult to diagnose in patients with myopia. Measurements of intraocular pressure obtained with a Schiøtz tonometer (see p. 147) will be lower than normal due to the decreased rigidity of the sclera.

Note
Applanation tonometry (see p. 147) yields the most accurate values in patients with myopia because the rigidity of the sclera only slightly influences results.

The **optic cup** is also difficult to evaluate in patients with myopia because the optic nerve enters the eye obliquely. This also makes glaucoma more difficult to diagnose.

▶ **Treatment.** The excessive refractive power of the refractive media must be reduced. This is achieved through the use of **diverging lenses** (minus or concave lenses; ▶ Fig. 16.9a). These lenses cause parallel incident light rays to diverge behind the lens. The divergent rays converge at a virtual focal point in front of the lens. The refractive power (D) is negative (hence the term "minus lens") and is equal to $1/f$, where f is the focal length in meters. Previously, *biconcave* or *planoconcave* lens blanks were used in the manufacture of corrective lenses. However, these entailed a number of optical disadvantages. Today lenses are manufactured in a *positive meniscus shape* to reduce lens aberrations.

Correction with contact lenses (see p. 289) offers optical advantages (▶ Fig. 16.9b). The reduction in the size of the image is less than with eyeglass correction. Aberrations are also reduced. These advantages are clinically relevant with myopia exceeding 3 diopters.

Note
The closer the "minus lens" is to the eye, the weaker its refractive power must be to achieve the desired optic effect.

Minus lenses to be used to correct myopia should be no stronger than absolutely necessary. Although accommodation could compensate for an overcorrection, patients usually do not tolerate this well. Accommodative asthenopia (rapid ocular fatigue) results from the excessive stress caused by chronic contraction of the atrophic ciliary muscle.

Note
Myopic patients have "lazy" accommodation due to atrophy of the ciliary muscle. A very slight undercorrection is often better tolerated than a perfectly sharp image with minimal overcorrection.

In certain special cases, **removal of the crystalline lens** (▸ Fig. 16.9c) can be performed to reduce the refractive power of the myopic eye. However, this operation is associated with an increased risk of retinal detachment. There is also the possibility of implanting an **anterior chamber intraocular lens** (diverging lens) anterior to the natural lens to reduce refractive power. For additional surgical options see Chapter 5.7.2.

Popular health books describe exercises that can allegedly treat refractive errors such as nearsightedness without eyeglasses or contact lenses. Such exercises cannot influence the sharpness of the retinal image; they can only seemingly improve uncorrected visual acuity by training the patient to make better use of additional visual information. However, after puberty no late sequelae of chronically uncorrected vision are to be expected.

16.3.2 Hyperopia (Farsightedness)

Definition
In hyperopia, there is a discrepancy between the refractive power and axial length of the eye such that parallel incident light rays converge at a *focal point posterior to the retina* (▸ Fig. 16.10a).

▸ **Epidemiology.** Approximately 20% of persons between the ages of 20 and 30 years have refraction exceeding +1 diopter. Most newborns exhibit slight hyperopia (*newborn hyperopia*). This decreases during the first few years of life. In advanced age, refraction tends to shift toward the myopic side due to sclerosing of the nucleus of the lens.

▸ **Etiology.** The mechanisms that coordinate the development of the eyeball so as to produce optic media of a given refractive power are not yet fully understood.

▸ **Pathophysiology.** In farsighted patients, the virtual *far point* of the eye lies *posterior to the retina* (▸ Fig. 16.10b). Only convergent incident light rays can be focused on the retina (▸ Fig. 16.10b). This is due either to an *excessively short globe* with normal refractive power (**axial hyperopia**; ▸ Fig. 16.10d)

or, less frequently, to *insufficient refractive power* in a normal-length globe (**refractive hyperopia**; ▸ Fig. 16.10e). Axial hyperopia is usually congenital and is characterized by a shallow anterior chamber with a thick sclera and well developed ciliary muscle.

Note
Hyperopic eyes are predisposed to acute angle closure glaucoma because of their shallow anterior chamber. This can be provoked by diagnostic and therapeutic mydriasis.

▸ **Special forms of refractive hyperopia**
• Absence of the lens (aphakia) due to dislocation.
• Postoperative aphakia following cataract surgery without placement of an intraocular lens (see ▸ Fig. 16.10f).

To bring the focal point onto the retina, a farsighted person *must accommodate even when gazing into the distance* (▸ Fig. 16.10c). *Close objects remain blurred* because the eye is unable to accommodate any further in near vision. As accommodation is linked to convergence, this process can result in *esotropia* (accommodative esotropia or accommodative convergent strabismus, see ▸ Fig. 17.6).

▸ **Symptoms.** In young patients, accommodation can compensate for slight to moderate hyperopia. However, this leads to chronic overuse of the ciliary muscle. Reading in particular can cause **asthenopic symptoms** such as eye pain or headache, burning sensation in the eyes, blepharoconjunctivitis, blurred vision, and rapid fatigue. **Esotropia** can also occur, as was mentioned above. As accommodation decreases with advancing age, near vision becomes increasingly difficult. For this reason, hyperopic persons tend to become presbyopic early.

▸ **Diagnostic considerations.** Ophthalmoscopic examination of the fundus may reveal a slightly blurred **optic disc** that may be **elevated** (hyperopic pseudoneuritis). However, this is not associated with any functional impairment such as visual field defects, loss of visual acuity, or color vision defects. The retina is too large for the small eye, which leads to **tortuous retinal vascular structures**. Transitions to abnormal forms of axial shortening, such as in microphthalmos, are not well defined.

The ciliary muscle is chronically under tension in slight or moderate hyperopia to compensate for

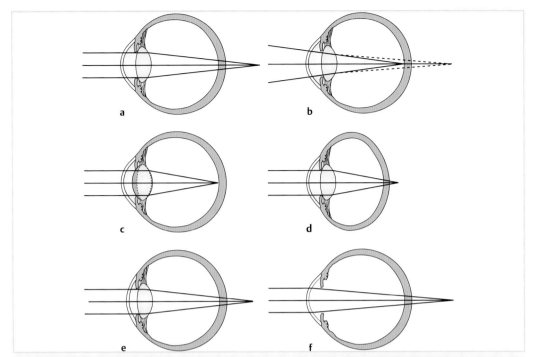

Fig. 16.10 Refraction in hyperopia. (a) The focal point of parallel light rays entering the eye lies posterior to the retina. **(b)** Divergent light rays are focused on the retina. The virtual far point lies posterior to the eye (dashed line). **(c)** To bring the focal point onto the retina, a farsighted person has to accommodate even when gazing into the distance. **(d)** Axial hyperopia. The refractive power is normal, but the globe is too short (more common). **(e)** Refractive hyperopia. The globe has a normal length, but the refractive power is insufficient (less common). **(f)** A special form of refractive hyperopia is aphakia (absence of the lens).

the hyperopia. This overuse of the ciliary muscle leads to a condition of residual accommodation in which the muscle is unable to relax even after the hyperopia has been corrected with plus lenses. This residual or **latent hyperopia** may be overlooked if refraction testing is performed without first completely paralyzing the ciliary body with cycloplegic agents such as cyclopentolate or atropine. The full extent of hyperopia includes both this residual hyperopia and clinically manifest hyperopia.

Note

In the presence of asthenopic symptoms of uncertain origin, refraction testing under cycloplegia is indicated to rule out latent hyperopia.

▶ **Treatment.** The insufficient refractive power must be augmented with **converging lenses** (plus or convex lenses; ▶ Fig. 16.11a). A watch-and-wait approach is indicated with asymptomatic young patients with slight hyperopia. Spherical plus lenses converge parallel incident light rays at a focal point behind the lens. The refractive power (D) in plus lenses is positive. It is equal to $1/f$, where f is the focal length in meters. Previously, *biconvex* or *planoconvex* lens blanks were used in the manufacture of corrective lenses. However, these entailed a number of optical disadvantages. The optical aberrations of the *positive meniscus* lenses used today are comparatively slight.

The clinician should determine the *total degree of hyperopia present* (see Diagnostic considerations) prior to prescribing corrective lenses. The second step is to prescribe the **strongest plus lens** that the patient can tolerate without compromising visual acuity. Care should be taken to avoid overcorrection. This will compensate for the manifest component of the hyperopia. If the patient wears these corrective lenses permanently, then with time it will also become possible to correct the latent component (see Diagnostic considerations). This is because the permanent tension in the ciliary body is no longer necessary.

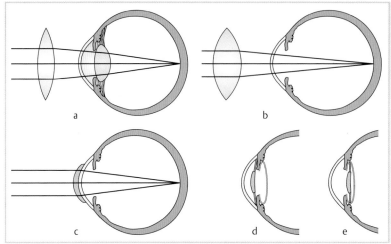

Fig. 16.11 Correction of hyperopia. (a) Correction with converging lenses (plus lenses). **(b)** Correction of aphakia with a cataract lens. **(c)** Contact lens. **(d)** Anterior chamber intraocular lens. **(e)** Posterior chamber intraocular lens.

Note

Prior to any correction of hyperopia, refraction testing should be performed after administering cycloplegics to the patient. The correction is then made with the strongest plus lens that the patient can subjectively tolerate without compromising visual acuity.

In contrast, refraction testing to **correct aphakia** *does not require cycloplegia.* Here, too, *plus lenses* are required to correct the hyperopia. The closer the plus lens is to the retina, the stronger its refractive power must be to converge incident light at a point on the retina. For this reason, a cataract lens (▶ Fig. 16.11b) has a refractive power of about 12 diopters, a contact lens (▶ Fig. 16.11c) about 14 diopters, an anterior chamber intraocular lens (▶ Fig. 16.11d) about 20 diopters, and a posterior chamber lens about 23 diopters (▶ Fig. 16.11e).

16.3.3 Astigmatism

Definition

Astigmatism is derived from the Greek word *stigma* (point) and literally means lack of a focal point. The disorder is characterized by a curvature anomaly of the refractive media such that parallel incident light rays do not converge at a point but are drawn apart to form a line.

▶ **Epidemiology.** Forty-two percent of humans have astigmatism greater than or equal to 0.5 diopters. In approximately 20%, this astigmatism is greater than 1 diopter and requires optical correction.

▶ **Pathophysiology.** The refractive media of the astigmatic eye are not spherical, but *refract differently along one meridian and along the meridian perpendicular to it* (▶ Fig. 16.12). Any amount of astigmatism at the axis orientation introduces a Sturm conoid into the image system. This produces two focal points. A *punctiform object* is therefore represented as a sharply defined *line segment* at the focal point of the first meridian, but also appears as a sharply defined line segment rotated 90° at the focal point of the second meridian. Midway between these two focal points is what is known as the "*circle of least confusion.*" This refers to the location at which the image is equally distorted in every direction—i.e., the location with the least loss of image definition. The aggregate system lacks a focal point.

The combined astigmatic components of all of the refractive media comprise the **total astigmatism** of the eye. These media include:
- Anterior surface of the cornea.
- Posterior surface of the cornea.
- Anterior surface of the lens.
- Posterior surface of the lens.

Rarely, nonspherical curvature of the retina may also contribute to astigmatism.

▶ **Classification and causes.** Astigmatism can be classified as follows:
- **External astigmatism.** Astigmatism of the anterior surface of the cornea.
- **Internal astigmatism.** The sum of the astigmatic components of the other media.

Note
The degree of astigmatism and its axis can change during life.

Astigmatism can also be classified *according to the location of the meridian of greater refraction:*
- **With-the-rule astigmatism** (most common form). The meridian with the greater refractive power is vertical—i.e., between 70° and 110°.
- **Against-the-rule astigmatism.** The meridian with the greater refractive power is horizontal—i.e., between 160° and 20°.
- **Oblique astigmatism.** The meridian with the greater refractive power is oblique—i.e., between 20° and 70° or between 110° and 160°.

The discussion up to this point has proceeded from the assumption that the anomaly is a **regular astigmatism** involving only two meridians approximately perpendicular to each other (see ▶ Fig. 16.12). This is presumably caused by excessive eyelid tension that leads to astigmatic changes in the surface of the cornea.

The condition above should be distinguished from **irregular astigmatism** (▶ Fig. 16.13a,b). Here, the curvature and the refractive power of the refractive media are *completely irregular* (▶ Fig. 16.13a). There are multiple focal points, a situation that produces a completely blurred image on the retina. This condition may be caused by the following diseases:
- Corneal ulcerations with resulting scarring of the cornea.

- Penetrating corneal trauma.
- Advanced keratoconus (see p. 72).
- Cataract.
- Lenticonus (see p. 104).

▶ **Symptoms.** Patients with astigmatism see everything distorted, both near and far. Attempts to compensate for the refractive error by accommodation can lead to asthenopic symptoms such as a burning sensation in the eyes or headache.

▶ **Diagnostic considerations.** The **keratoscope** (Placido disk) permits *gross estimation* of astigmatism. The examiner evaluates the mirror images of the rings on the patient's cornea. In *regular astigmatism*, the rings are *oval*; in *irregular astigmatism*, they are *irregularly distorted*. Computerized corneal topography (**video keratoscopy**) or cross-sectional imaging of anterior and posterior corneal surfaces (Scheimpflug principle) can be used to obtain an image of the distribution of refractive values over the entire cornea (see ▶ Fig. 5.4). A **Helmholtz** or **Javal ophthalmometer** can be used to *measure the central corneal curvature*, which determines the refractive power of the cornea (▶ Fig. 16.14).

▶ **Treatment.** Early correction is crucial. Untreated astigmatism in children will eventually lead to uncorrectable refractive amblyopia because a sharp image is not projected on the retina.

▶ **Treatment of regular astigmatism.** The purpose of the correction is to bring the "focal lines" of two

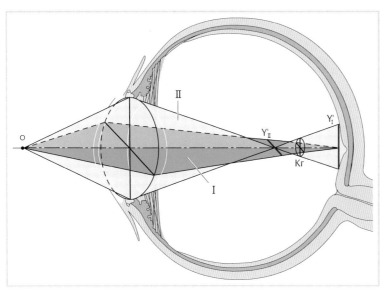

Fig. 16.12 Image formation with an astigmatic cornea (Sturm conoid). The two main meridians (I and II) are perpendicular to each other. A punctiform object (o) is represented as a line segment Y'_{II} and Y'_I at the focal points of the two meridians. Midway between these two focal points is the "circle of least confusion" (Kr), the location with the least loss of image definition.

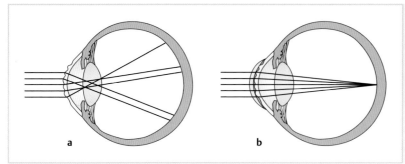

Fig. 16.13 Irregular corneal astigmatism. (a) Curvature and refractive power of the refractive media are totally irregular, resulting in multiple focal points. (b) Correction of irregular corneal astigmatism with a rigid contact lens.

main meridians together at one focal point. This requires a lens that *refracts in only one plane*. **Cylinder lenses** are required for this application (▶ Fig. 16.15a). Once the two "focal lines" have been converged into a focal point, **additional spherical lenses** can be used to shift this focal point onto the retina if necessary (= eyeglass correction with so-called spherocylindrical combination lenses).

▶ **Treatment of irregular astigmatism.** This form *cannot* be corrected with eyeglasses. *External astigmatism* can be managed with a rigid contact lens (see ▶ Fig. 16.13b), keratoplasty (see p. 88), or surgical correction of the refractive error (see p. 90). Irregular *internal astigmatism* is usually lens-related. In this case, removal of the lens with implantation of an intraocular lens is indicated.

> **Note**
> Only regular astigmatism can be corrected with eyeglasses.

16.3.4 Anisometropia

Definition
In anisometropia, there is a difference in refractive power between the two eyes.

▶ **Epidemiology.** Anisometropia of at least 4 diopters is present in less than 1% of the population.

▶ **Etiology.** The reason for the varying development of the two eyes is not clear. This primarily congenital disease is known to exhibit a familial pattern of increased incidence.

▶ **Pathophysiology.** In anisometropia, there is a difference in refractive power between the two eyes. This refractive difference can be corrected

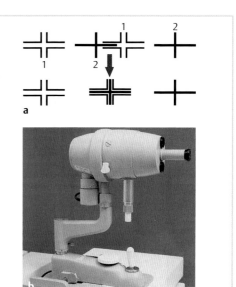

Fig. 16.14 Diagnosis of corneal astigmatism with an ophthalmometer. (a) The diagram shows the corneal reflex images (outline cross, 1; solid cross, 2) of the Zeiss ophthalmometer (so-called "Zeiss Bomb", see b). (b) These images are projected onto the cornea; the distance between them will vary depending on the curvature of the cornea. The examiner has to align the images by changing their angle of projection. After aligning them, the examiner reads the axis of the main meridian, the corneal curvature in millimeters, and the appropriate refractive power in diopters on a scale in the device. This measurement is performed in both main meridians. The difference yields the astigmatism. In irregular astigmatism, the images are distorted, and often a measurement cannot be obtained.

separately for each eye with different lenses as long as it *lies below 4 diopters*. Where the difference in refraction is greater than or equal to 4 diopters, the size difference of the two retinal images becomes too great for the brain to fuse the two images into one. Known as **aniseikonia**, this condition jeopardizes binocular vision because it can lead to devel-

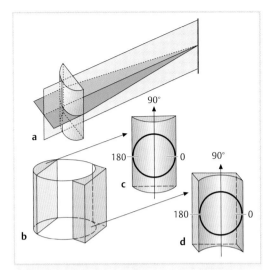

Fig. 16.15 Correction of regular astigmatism with cylinder lenses. **(a)** Cylinder lenses refract light only in the plane perpendicular to the axis of the cylinder. The axis of the cylinder defines the nonrefracting plane. **(b–d)** Cylinder lenses can be manufactured as plus cylinders (**c**) or minus cylinders (**d**).

opment of amblyopia (*anisometropic amblyopia*). The aniseikonia, or differing size of the retinal images, as well as depending on the degree of refractive anomaly also depends significantly on the **type of correction**. The closer to the site of the refraction deficit the correction is made, the less the retinal image changes in size. Correction with *intraocular lenses* results in almost no difference in image size. Contact lenses produce a slight and *usually irrelevant difference in image size*. However, *eyeglass correction* resulting in a difference of *more than 4 diopters* leads to *intolerable aniseikonia* (see ▶ Table 7.4).

▶ **Symptoms.** Anisometropia is usually congenital and *often asymptomatic*. Children are not aware that their vision is abnormal. However, there is a tendency toward strabismus as binocular functions may remain underdeveloped. Where the correction of the anisometropia results in unacceptable aniseikonia, patients will report unpleasant visual sensations of *double vision*.

▶ **Diagnostic considerations.** Anisometropia is usually diagnosed during routine examinations. The diagnosis is made on the basis of refraction testing.

▶ **Treatment.** The refractive error should be corrected. Anisometropia exceeding 4 diopters cannot be corrected with **eyeglasses** because of the clinically relevant aniseikonia. **Contact lenses** and, in rare cases, surgical treatment are indicated (see p. 90). Patients with unilateral aphakia or who do not tolerate contact lenses will require implantation of an **intraocular lens**.

Note
Correction of unilateral aphakia with unilateral glasses is usually contraindicated because it results in aniseikonia of approximately 25%.

16.4 Impaired Accommodation

16.4.1 Accommodation Spasm

Definition
An accommodation spasm is defined as inadequate, protracted contraction of the ciliary muscle.

▶ **Etiology.** Accommodation spasms are *rare*. They may occur as *functional impairment* or they may occur *iatrogenically* when treating young patients with parasympathomimetic agents (miotic agents). The functional impairments are frequently attributable to heightened sensitivity of the accommodation center, which especially in children (often girls) can be psychogenic. *Rarely* the spasm is due to *organic* causes. In these cases, it is most often attributable to irritation in the region of the oculomotor nuclei (from cerebral pressure or cerebral disorders) or to change in the ciliary muscle such as in an ocular contusion.

▶ **Symptoms.** Patients complain of deep eye pain and blurred distance vision (lenticular myopia).

▶ **Diagnostic considerations and differential diagnosis.** The diagnosis is made on the basis of presenting symptoms and refraction testing, including measurement of the range of accommodation. This is done with an accommodometer, which determines the difference in refractive power between the near point and far point. A *differential diagnosis* should exclude latent hyperopia. In children, this will frequently be associated with accommodative esotropia and accommodative pupil narrowing.

▶ **Treatment.** This depends on the underlying disorder. Cycloplegic therapy with agents such as tropicamide or cyclopentolate may be attempted in the presence of recurrent accommodation spasms.

▶ **Prognosis.** Iatrogenic spasms are completely reversible by discontinuing the parasympathomimetic agents. The prognosis is also good for patients with functional causes. Spasms due to organic causes require treatment of the underlying disorder but once treatment is initiated the prognosis is usually good.

16.4.2 Accommodation Palsy

> **Definition**
> Failure of accommodation due to palsy of the ciliary muscle.

▶ **Etiology.** This *rare* disorder is primarily due to one of the following causes:
- **Iatrogenic drug-induced palsy** due to parasympatholytic agents such as atropine, cyclopentolate scopolamine, homatropine, and tropicamide.
- **Peripheral causes.** Oculomotor palsy, lesions of the ciliary ganglion, or the ciliary muscle.
- **Systemic causes.** Damage to the accommodation center in diphtheria, diabetes mellitus, chronic alcoholism, meningitis, cerebral stroke, multiple sclerosis, syphilis, lead or ergotamine poisoning, medications such as isoniazid or piperazine, and tumors.

▶ **Symptoms.** The failure of accommodation leads to blurred near vision and may be associated with mydriasis where the sphincter pupillae muscle is also involved. The clinical syndromes listed below exhibit a specific constellation of clinical symptoms and therefore warrant further discussion.
- **Postdiphtheria accommodation palsy.** This transitory palsy is a toxic reaction and occurs *without* pupillary dysfunction approximately 4 weeks after infection. Sometimes it is associated with palsy of the soft palate and/or impaired motor function in the lower extremities.
- **Accommodation palsy in botulism.** This is also a toxic palsy. It *does* involve the pupil, producing *mydriasis,* and can be the first symptom of botulism. It is associated with speech, swallowing, and ocular muscle dysfunction accompanied by double vision.
- **Tonic pupillary contraction** is associated with tonic accommodation. See additional information on tonic pupil in Chapter 9.4.2.

- **Sympathetic ophthalmia** (see p. 132) is characterized by a decrease in the range of accommodation, even in the unaffected eye.

> **Note**
> Measurement of the range of accommodation is indicated whenever sympathetic ophthalmia is suspected.

▶ **Diagnostic considerations.** In addition to measuring the range of accommodation with an accommodometer, the examiner should inquire about other ocular and general symptoms.

▶ **Treatment.** Treatment depends on the underlying disorder.

▶ **Prognosis.** The clinical course of **tonic pupillary contraction** is chronic and results in irreversible loss of accommodation. The **toxic accommodation palsies** are reversible once the underlying disorder is controlled.

16.5 Correction of Refractive Errors

16.5.1 Eyeglass Lenses

Monofocal Lenses

There are two basic types:
- **Spherical lenses** refract light equally along every axis.
- **Toric lenses** (known as cylindrical lenses) refract light only along one axis. Spherical and toric lenses can be combined where indicated.

The **refractive power of the lenses** is measured manually or automatically with an optical interferometer. The measured refraction is specified as *spherocylindrical combination.* By convention, the specified axis of the cylindrical lens is perpendicular to its axis of refraction (see ▶ Fig. 16.15b, c). The orientation of this axis with respect to the eye is specified on a standardized form (▶ Fig. 16.16).

▶ **Example.** +4.00 diopters −2.00 diopters/90° means that the lens represents a combination of converging lens (+4 diopters) and cylindrical lens (−2 diopters) with its axis at 90°. Opticians often use plus cylinders. The spectacle lens would then be described as 2.00 diopters + 2.00 diopters/180°.

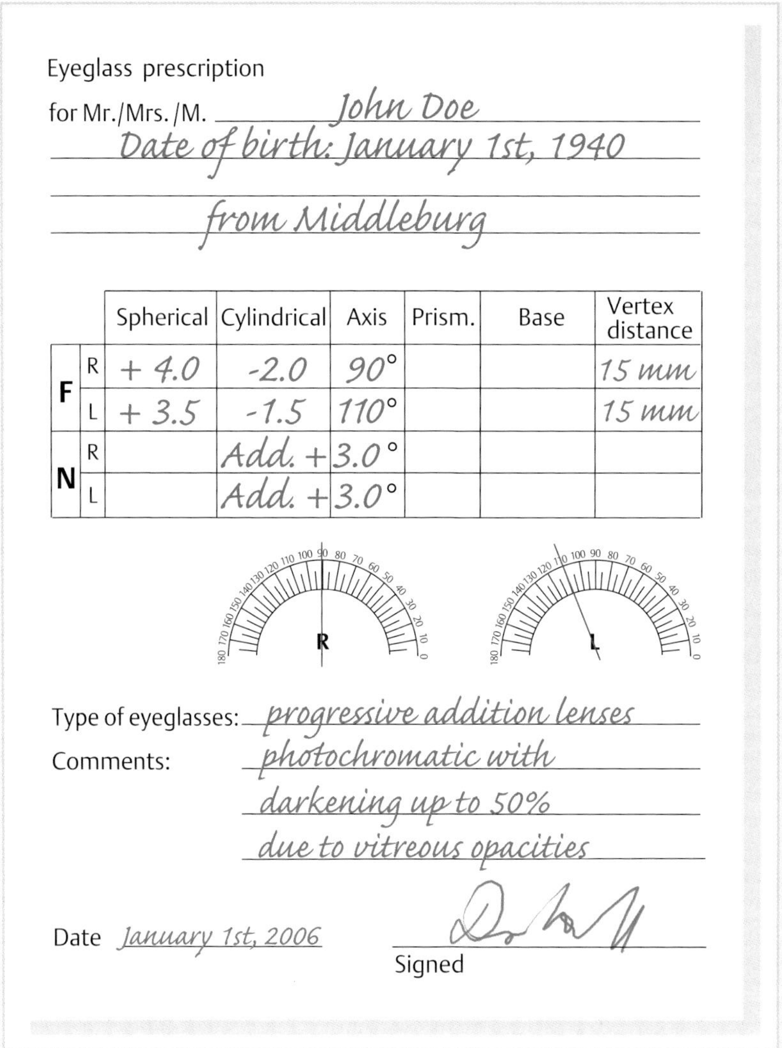

Eyeglass prescription

for Mr./Mrs./M. _____ *John Doe* _____

_____ *Date of birth: January 1st, 1940* _____

_____

_____ *from Middleburg* _____

		Spherical	Cylindrical	Axis	Prism.	Base	Vertex distance
F	R	+ 4.0	-2.0	90°			15 mm
	L	+ 3.5	-1.5	110°			15 mm
N	R		Add. +3.0°				
	L		Add. +3.0°				

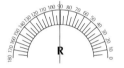 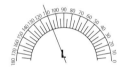

Type of eyeglasses: *progressive addition lenses*

Comments: *photochromatic with darkening up to 50% due to vitreous opacities*

Date *January 1st, 2006*

Signed

Fig. 16.16 Eyeglass prescription. The refraction values have been entered. The cylindrical axis has also been entered (red line). The diagram specifies the position of the cylindrical axis with respect to the eye. On the standard form, the perpendicular cylindrical axis (red line) represents 90°.

Note

Eyeglass lenses exhibit typical characteristics when moved back and forth a few inches in front of one's eye. Objects viewed through minus lenses appear to move in the same direction as the lens; objects viewed through plus lenses move in the opposite direction. A cylindrical lens produces image distortions when turned.

Multifocal Lenses

Multifocal lenses differ from the monofocal lenses of uniform refractive power discussed in the previ-ous section in that different areas of the lens have different refractive powers. These lenses are best understood as *combinations of two or more lenses in a single lens.*

▶ **Bifocals.** The *upper and middle portion of the lens* is ground for the *distance correction;* the lower portion is ground for the *near-field correction* (▶ Fig. 16.17). Patients are able to view distant objects in focus and read using *one pair* of eyeglasses, eliminating the need to constantly change glasses. The gaze is lowered and converged to read. This portion of the lens contains the near-field correction. This near-field correction can be placed in a different part of the lens for special applications.

▶ **Trifocals.** These lenses include a *third refractive correction* between the distance and near-field portions. This intermediate portion *sharply images the intermediate field between distance vision and reading range* without any need for accommodation (▶ Fig. 16.17).

▶ **Progressive addition lenses.** These lenses were developed to *minimize abrupt image changes* when the gaze moves through the different correction zones of the lens while *maintaining a sharp focus at every distance* (▶ Fig. 16.17).

These eyeglasses also offer cosmetic advantages. They produce *well-focused images in the central region* but have a *high degree of peripheral astigmatism*. However, many patients learn to tolerate this peripheral distortion.

Note
Presbyopic patients tolerate progressive addition lenses better when they still have only slight presbyopia and have not previously worn bifocals.

Special Lenses

The following types of lens have been developed for special applications:

▶ **Plastic lenses.** These lenses reduce the weight of eyeglasses where severe ametropia must be corrected. Another advantage is that these lenses are largely shatterproof, which is why they are preferred for children. However, they are easily scratched.

▶ **Absorption lenses.** These lenses are indicated in patients with *increased sensitivity to glare*.

Note
Operating motor vehicles in twilight or at night with eyeglasses that absorb more than 20% of incident light is dangerous because of the resulting reduction in visual acuity.

▶ **Photochromatic lenses.** These lenses darken in response to the intensity of ultraviolet light. The lenses become darker at low temperatures than at high temperatures; they lighten more slowly at low temperatures and more rapidly at high temperatures. Light attenuation ranges between 15 and 50% in some lenses and between 30 and 65% in others.

Note
Photochromatic lenses pose problems for patients operating motor vehicles. The lenses darken only slightly in a warm car with the windows closed, due to the lack of ultraviolet light. Dark lenses lighten too slowly when the car enters a tunnel.

▶ **Anti-reflective coated lenses.** Extremely thin coatings of magnesium fluoride can be applied to lenses to reduce surface reflection on the front and back of the lens.

Subjective Refraction Testing for Eyeglasses

While the patient looks at vision charts, the examiner places various combinations of lenses in front of the patient's eye. The patient reports which of two lenses produces the sharper image. The better of the two is then compared with the next lens.

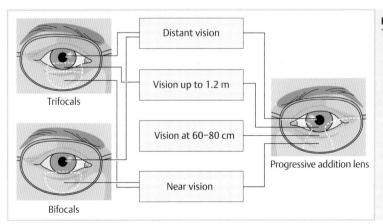

Fig. 16.17 Multifocal lenses. Trifocals, bifocals, progressives.

This incremental method identifies the optimal correction. It is expedient to use the patient's objective refraction as the starting point for subjective testing. Refraction testing is performed either with a series of **test lenses** from a case or with a Phoroptor, which contains many lenses that can be automatically or manually placed before the patient's eye. The examination proceeds in three stages:

- **Monocular testing.** The optimal refraction for achieving best visual acuity is determined *separately for each eye.* The weakest possible minus lens is used in *myopic patients,* and the strongest possible plus lens in *hyperopic patients.* The red–green chromatic aberration test can be used for fine refraction. In this test, the patient compares optotypes on green and red backgrounds. Fine adjustment of refraction permits precise shifting of the focal point of the light on the retina. Optotypes on both red and green backgrounds then appear equally sharply defined.
- **Binocular testing.** The objective of this stage is to achieve a *balance* between both eyes.
- **Near point testing.** The final stage of the examination determines the patient's *near visual acuity,* and, if necessary, the *presbyopic addition.* Allowance is made for the patient's preferred reading and working position.

The values determined by this examination are entered in the eyeglass prescription (see ▶ Fig. 16.16). The **vertex distance** at which refraction was performed is an important additional parameter for the optician. This is the *distance between the back surface of the test lens and the anterior surface of the cornea.* If the manufactured eyeglasses have a different vertex distance, then the strength of the lenses should be altered accordingly. This is because the optical effect of eyeglass lenses varies according to the distance from the eye.

Before the lenses are fitted into the frame, the **distance between the pupils** must be measured to ensure that the lenses are properly centered. The *center of the lens* should be *in front of the pupil.* The prismatic effects of eccentric lenses might otherwise cause asthenopic symptoms such as headache or a burning sensation in the eyes.

Note

To facilitate early detection of glaucoma, intraocular pressure should be measured in any patient over the age of 40 years presenting for refraction testing for eyeglasses.

16.5.2 Contact Lenses

Advantages and Characteristics of Contact Lenses

Contact lenses are in immediate contact with the cornea. Although they are foreign bodies, most patients adapt to properly fitted contact lenses. Contact lenses differ from eyeglasses in that they correct the refractive error closer to the location of its origin. For this reason, the *quality of the optical image viewed through contact lenses is higher than that viewed through eyeglasses.* Contact lenses have significantly less influence on the size of the retinal image than does correction with eyeglasses. Lenses do not cloud up in rainy weather or steam, and peripheral distortion is minimized. The cosmetic disadvantage of thick eyeglasses in *severe ametropia* is also eliminated. *Severe anisometropia (see p. 284)* requires correction with contact lenses for optical reasons—i.e., to minimize aniseikonia.

Contact lenses are defined by the following **characteristics:**
- Diameter of the contact lens.
- Radius of curvature of the posterior surface.
- Geometry of the posterior surface—i.e., spherical, aspherical, complex curvature, or toric.
- Refractive power.
- Material.
- Oxygen permeability of the material (Dk value).

The cornea requires oxygen from the precorneal tear film. To ensure this supply, *contact lens materials must be oxygen permeable.* This becomes all the more important the less the contact lens moves and permits circulation of tear fluid. Contact lenses can be made of *rigid* or *flexible* materials.

Rigid (Hard) Contact Lenses

These contact lenses have a stable, nearly unchanging shape. Patients *take some time to become used to them* and should therefore wear them often. The goal is to achieve the best possible intimacy of fit between the posterior surface of the lens and the anterior surface of the cornea (▶ Fig. 16.18). This allows the contact lens to float on the precorneal tear film. Every time the patient blinks, the lens is displaced superiorly and then returns to its central position. This permits circulation of the tear film.

Previously, polymethylmethacrylate (PMMA) was used as a material. However, this is practically impermeable to oxygen. The lenses were fitted in small diameters with a very shallow curvature; the central area maintained contact with the cornea while the periphery projected. This allowed

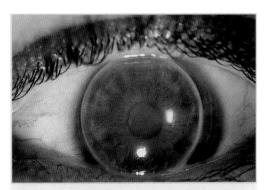

Fig. 16.18 Fitting of a rigid contact lens. There is a tear film between the anterior surface of the cornea and the posterior surface of the lens (visualized by green fluorescein dye).

excellent tear film circulation, and patients were able to wear the lenses for surprisingly long periods. Today, highly oxygen-permeable materials such as silicone copolymers are available. This eliminates the time limit for *daily wearing*. These lenses may also remain in the eye overnight in special cases, such as in aphakic patients with poor coordination (*prolonged wearing*).

Rigid contact lenses can be manufactured as *spherical lenses and toric lenses*. **Spherical** contact lenses can almost completely compensate for **corneal astigmatism of less than 2.5 diopters**. This is possible because the space between the posterior surface of the spherical contact lens and the anterior surface of the astigmatic cornea is filled with tear fluid that forms a "*tear lens*." Tear fluid has nearly the same refractive index as the cornea. **More severe corneal astigmatism** or **internal astigmatism** requires correction with **toric** contact lenses. Rigid contact lenses can even correct severe **keratoconus**.

Soft Contact Lenses

The material of the soft contact lens, such as hydrogel, is soft and pliable. Patients find these lenses *significantly more comfortable*. The *oxygen permeability* of the material depends on its water content, which may range from 36 to 85%. The higher the water content, the better the oxygen permeability. However, it is typically *lower* than that of *rigid lenses*. The material is more permeable to foreign substances, which can accumulate in it. At 12.5 to 16 mm, flexible lenses are larger in diameter than rigid lenses. Flexible lenses are often supported by the limbus. The lens is often displaced only a few tenths of a millimeter when the patient blinks. This *greatly reduces the circulation of tear film under the*

lenses. This limits the *maximum daily period* that patients are able to wear them and requires that they be removed at night to allow regeneration of the cornea. Deviation from this principle is only possible in exceptional cases under the strict supervision of a physician.

As the lenses are almost completely in contact with the surface of the cornea, *corneal astigmatism cannot be corrected with spherical soft lenses*. This requires toric soft lenses.

Special Lenses

The following types of special lens are available for specific situations:

▶ **Therapeutic contact lenses.** In the presence of **corneal erosion,** soft ultrathin (0.05 mm) contact lenses act as a bandage and thereby accelerate reepithelialization of the cornea. They also reduce pain. Soft contact lenses may also be used in patients receiving topical medication as they store medication and only release it very slowly.

▶ **Corneal shields.** These are collagen devices that resemble contact lenses. These shields are gradually broken down by the collagenase in the tear film. They are used as **bandages** and **substrates for topical medication** in the treatment of anterior disorders, such as erosion or ulcer.

▶ **Iris print lenses.** These colored contact lenses with a clear central pupil are used in patients with **aniridia** and **albinism.** They produce good cosmetic results, reduce glare, and can correct a refractive error where indicated.

▶ **Bifocal contact lenses.** These lenses were developed to allow the use of contact lenses in presbyopic patients. As in eyeglasses, a *near-field correction* is ground into the lens. This near-field portion is always located at the bottom of the lens because the lens is heavier there. When the patient gazes downward to read, the immobile lower eyelid pushes this near-field portion superiorly where it aligns with the pupil and becomes optically effective. Another possibility is *diffraction* (bending of light rays as opposed to refraction) through concentric rings on the posterior surface of the contact lens. This produces two images, a distant refractive image and a near-field diffractive image. The patient chooses the image that is important at the moment. It is also possible to correct one eye for distance vision and the fellow eye for near vision (*monocular vision*).

Disadvantages of Contact Lenses

Contact lenses exert mechanical and metabolic influences on the cornea. They therefore require the *constant supervision of an ophthalmologist.*

▶ **Mechanical influences on the cornea.** These can lead to *transient changes in refraction.* "Spectacle blur" can result when eyeglasses suddenly no longer provide the proper correction after removal of the lens. Contact lenses require careful *daily cleaning* and disinfection. This is more difficult, time-consuming, and more expensive than eyeglass care and is particular important with soft lenses.

▶ **Metabolic influences on the cornea.** The macromolecular mesh of material absorbs proteins, protein breakdown products, low molecular-weight substances such as medications and disinfectants, and bacteria and fungi. Serious complications can occur if care of the contact lenses is inadequate (see p. 75). With their threshold oxygen permeability, soft contact lenses interfere with corneal metabolism. Contact lenses are less suitable for patients with symptoms of keratoconjunctivitis sicca (see p. 82).

Contact Lens Complications

Complications have been observed primarily in patients wearing *soft* contact lenses. They include the following:

▶ **Infectious keratitis, Chapter 5.4.** Corneal infiltrations and ulcers caused by bacteria, fungi, and protozoans.

Note
Acanthamoeba keratitis is a serious complication affecting wearers of soft contact lenses and often requires penetrating keratoplasty.

▶ **Giant papillary conjunctivitis.** This is an allergic reaction of the palpebral conjunctiva of the upper eyelid to denatured proteins. It results in proliferative "cobblestone" conjunctival lesions. For details see Chapter 5.5.4.

▶ **Severe chronic conjunctivitis.** This usually makes it impossible to continue wearing contact lenses.

16.5.3 Prisms

Prisms can change the direction of parallel light rays. The optical strength of a prism is specified in *prism diopters.* Prism lenses can be combined with spherical and toric lenses. When prescribing eyeglasses, the ophthalmologist specifies the strength and the position of the base of the prism. Prism lenses are used to correct heterophoria (latent strabismus) and ocular muscle palsies, and in preparation for surgery to correct strabismus.

Note
A 1-diopter prism deflects a ray of light 1 cm at a distance of 1 m from the base of the prism.

16.5.4 Magnifying Vision Aids

The **reduction in central corrected visual acuity** as a result of destruction of the fovea with a central scotoma requires magnifying vision aids. However, magnification is always associated with a *reduction in the size of the visual field.* As a result, these vision aids require patience, adaptation, motivation, and dexterity. Cooperation between ophthalmologist and optician is often helpful. The following **systems** are available in order of magnification:

▶ **Increased near-field corrections.** The stronger the near-field correction, the shorter the reading distance. Magnification (V) is a function of the refractive power of the near-field correction (D) and is determined by the equation $V = D/4$.

▶ **Example.** Eyeglasses with a 10-diopter near-field correction magnify the image 2½ times. However, the object must be brought to within 10 cm of the eye.

▶ **Magnifying glasses.** Magnifying glasses are available in various strengths, with or without illumination.

▶ **Monocular and binocular loupes, telescopes, and prism loupes.** An optical magnifying system is mounted on one or both eyeglass lenses. The optical system functions on the principle of Galilean or Keplerian optics.

▶ **Closed-circuit TV magnifier.** This device displays text at up to 45-power magnification.

16.6 Aberrations of Lenses and Eyeglasses

Optical lens systems (eyeglasses or lenses) always have minor aberrations. These aberrations are not material flaws, rather they are due to the laws of physics. Expensive optical systems can reduce these aberrations by using many different lenses in a specific order.

16.6.1 Chromatic Aberration (Dispersion)

This means that the **refractive power of the lens varies according to the wavelength of the light.**

Light consists of a blend of various wavelengths. Light with a *short wavelength* such as blue is refracted more than light with a *long wavelength* such as red (▶ Fig. 16.19). This is why monochromatic light (light of a single wavelength) produces a sharper image on the retina.

> **Note**
> Chromatic aberration is the basis of the red–green test used for fine refraction testing (see p. 275).

16.6.2 Spherical Aberration

This means that the **refractive power of the lens varies according to the location at which the light ray strikes the lens.**

The further peripherally the light ray strikes the lens, the more it will be refracted (▶ Fig. 16.20). The iris intercepts a large share of these peripheral light rays. A narrow pupil will intercept a particularly large share of peripheral light rays, which improves the *depth of field.* Conversely, *depth of field is significantly poorer* when the pupil is dilated.

> **Note**
> Modern intraocular lenses are fabricated so as to minimize spherical aberration. Patients may report being able to see better when looking through a disk with a pinhole (a stenopeic aperture) than without it. This usually is a sign of an uncompensated refractive error in the eye.

16.6.3 Astigmatic Aberration

A punctiform object **viewed through a spherical lens** appears as a line.

If one looks through a lens obliquely to its optical axis, it will act as a *prism* (▶ Fig. 16.21a). A prism refracts a light ray toward its base (▶ Fig. 16.21b). In addition to this, the light is split into its component spectral colors (dispersion). Light with a *short wavelength* (blue) is refracted more than light with a *long wavelength* (red). Astigmatic aberration is an undesired side effect that is present whenever one looks through a lens at an oblique angle.

This phenomenon should be distinguished from *astigmatic or toric lenses* (see p. 286), which correct for astigmatism of the eye when the patient looks through them *along the optical axis.*

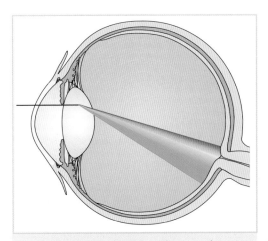

Fig. 16.19 Chromatic aberration. Chromatic aberration splits white light into its component spectral colors. Red is refracted least, and blue is refracted most.

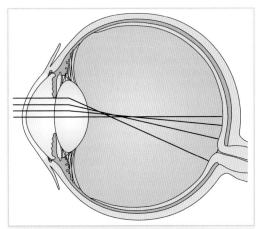

Fig. 16.20 Spherical aberration. Due to spherical aberration, the refraction of light rays increases the further peripherally they strike the lens.

16.6.4 Distortion

This refers to the curved appearance of straight lines as seen through the periphery of a lens. Distortion also renders the image seen through the periphery of a lens more blurred than the image seen through the center of the lens.

Note

Because of these physiologically and optically determined image defects, the optical resolution capacity is limited to approximately 0.5/60–1/60 degree. The spatial distribution of the retinal photoreceptors corresponds fairly accurately to this resolution capacity. Thus a significantly finer retinal structure would have no purpose.

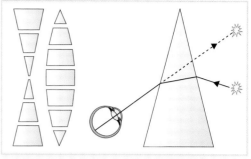

Fig. 16.21 Astigmatic aberration. (a) Lenses can be regarded as consisting of a large number of prisms, which explains many of the optical phenomena of lenses, such as dispersion. **(b)** A prism refracts a light ray toward its base twice (solid line). It appears to the observer that the object is shifted toward the apex of the prism (dashed line).

17 Ocular Motility and Strabismus

Joachim Esser, Doris Recker, and Gerhard K. Lang

Definition

Strabismus is defined as deviation of an eye's visual axis from its normal position, in which the visual axes of both eyes point at the fixated object.

Strabismus can be manifest or latent. If one visual axis always deviates, the strabismus is manifest (heterotropia). If the deviation only occurs from time to time (e.g., due to fatigue) or only under certain conditions (e.g., if one eye is covered), the strabismus is called latent (heterophoria).

There are **two major types of manifest strabismus, or heterotropia.**

1. Concomitant strabismus (from the Latin *comitare*, "accompany"). The deviating eye *accompanies* the leading eye in every direction of movement. The angle of deviation (i.e., the angle between the fixating and the deviating visual axes) remains the same in all directions of gaze.

2. Paralytic strabismus (Chapter 17.5). The causes of this can be neurogenic paralysis of the extraocular muscles or myogenic changes (e.g., myasthenia, Graves's disease, entrapment of one or more eye muscles). All these forms have in common that the angle of deviation is different in various directions of gaze. This is often offset by compensatory head positions.

▶ **Epidemiology.** The incidence of strabismus is about 5 to 7%. Concomitant strabismus is generally congenital or noticeable within the first few years of life, whereas paralytic strabismus is usually acquired.

17.1 Basic Knowledge

▶ **Neurophysiology of eye movements.** In principle, the two eyeballs can only move simultaneously ("yoked function"). In parallel movement of the gaze (**versions:** horizontal, vertical and/or cyclorotatory) one pair of eye muscles is always synergistically activated (e.g., if looking to the left: the left lateral rectus muscle and the right medial rectus muscle). In alternation between distant and near objects, opposing eye movements (vergences) are necessary. In *convergence* (fixation of a near object), both medial rectus muscles are activated and both eyeballs are turned toward the nose. In *divergence*, on the other hand, both lateral rectus muscles are activated and the eyeballs are turned outward. The concepts convergence and divergence are also used for pathologic malpositions of the eyeballs (e.g., inward strabismus = convergent strabismus).

Vergences can be initiated voluntarily or as a reflex. Voluntary rapid eye movements (**saccades**) have the purpose of imaging an object that was first noticed in the periphery of the visual field in the fovea. They are initiated in the premotor cortex (▶ Fig. 17.1). In contrast, **ocular pursuit** movements are not initiated voluntarily but are reflex movements toward an object of fixation. They serve to keep the foveal line of sight of each eye pointed at a moving object as well as to maintain retinal stabilization of the visual surroundings during the subject's head movements. They are relatively slow since they have a longer reflex arc (closed-loop reflex with negative feedback): detection of object movement by the retina → occipital cortex → pontomesencephalic gaze centers (generated by the archicerebellum) → oculomotor nuclei → eye muscles. Another form of reflex eye movement is triggered by the **vestibulo-ocular** reflex (VOR): this open-loop reflex (head movement → vestibular nuclei → pontomesencephalic gaze centers with generation by the archicerebellum → oculomotor nuclei → eye muscles) is more rapid than that of the ocular pursuit reflex and serves to stabilize the gaze during head movements (e.g., reading while walking: less possible with archicerebellar lesions).

One can easily demonstrate the differing speeds of the two reflex eye movements on oneself: look at a small object with a large amount of detail (lettering on a pencil) and shake your head with increasing speed. Even at high shaking frequencies, you can see the object clearly. Now keep your head still and let the object swing back and forth. The object will become blurred even at a low swing frequency.

The pontomesencephalic gaze centers (▶ Fig. 17.1) are organized in relation to direction of movement: for horizontal version PPRF (right PPRF for gaze to the right, left for gaze to the left), for vertical version: riMLF. The convergence center lies close to the riMLF.

The oculomotor nuclei lie close to the pontomesencephalic gaze centers. Thus, the nucleus of the oculomotor nerve (innervated eye muscles: ▶ Table 17.1 and see ▶ Fig. 17.2) lies close to the vertical

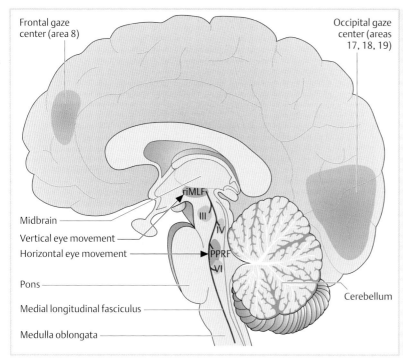

Occipital gaze
center (areas
17, 18, 19)

riMLF

III

Midbrain

IV

Vertical eye movement

Horizontal eye movement

PPRF

VI

Pons

Cerebellum

Medial longitudinal fasciculus

Medulla oblongata

Fig. 17.1 Position of the oculomotor nuclei and gaze centers. The oculomotor nerve (cranial nerve [CN] III) innervates all eye muscles with the exception of the superior oblique muscle (trochlear nerve, CN IV) and the lateral rectus muscle (abducens nerve, CN VI). The rostral interstitial nucleus of the medial longitudinal fascicle (riMLF) is responsible for vertical eye movements and rapid phases of nystagmus, i.e., quivering eyes; the paramedian pontine reticular formation (PPRF) is responsible for horizontal eye movements.

gaze center (riMLF) and the abducens nucleus lies close to the horizontal gaze center (PPHR) (▶ Fig. 17.1). There is a noticeable anatomical peculiarity here: for a lateral gaze, the right PPRF generates the contraction of the ipsilateral lateral rectus muscle (through the nearby right abducens nucleus). But at the same time, innervation of the left medial rectus muscle is required. The connection between PPRF and the more rostral oculomotor nucleus runs through the medial longitudinal fascicle (▶ Fig. 17.1) which is susceptible to damage, especially in demyelinating diseases (such as disseminated encephalomyelitis).

▶ **Anatomy of the extraocular muscles.** The movements of the eyeballs are produced by the following extraocular muscles (▶ Fig. 17.2):
- The **four rectus muscles:** the superior, inferior, medial, and lateral rectus muscles.
- The **two oblique muscles:** the superior and inferior oblique muscles.

All of these muscles originate at the tendinous ring except for the inferior oblique muscle, which has its origin near the nasolacrimal canal. The *rectus muscles* envelop the globe posteriorly, and their respective tendons insert ventral to the eyeball equator on the sclera. The *oblique muscles* insert into the temporal globe posterior to the equator. The inser-

tion of the muscles determines the direction of their pull (▶ Table 17.1).

The ligaments on which the globe is "hung" keep the globe in place within the orbit and allow it to move freely, like a ball bearing. Stability is ensured by a tendinous ring connected to the periorbita by close-fitting ligaments. Free mobility is ensured by the following anatomical structure: **Tenon's capsule** is the anterior border between the orbital fat and the sclera. The ocular muscles are embedded in **Tenon's capsule** (which provides good contractility) and perforate it to reach the sclera. On contraction they are constrained in their course by these openings in the capsule, so-called "pulleys," and not displaced to the side.

▶ **Direction of pull of the extraocular muscles.** The **horizontal ocular muscles** pull the eye in only *one* direction: The lateral rectus pulls the eye outward (*abduction*); the medial rectus pulls it inward (*adduction*). **All other extraocular muscles** have a *secondary direction of pull* in addition to the primary one. Depending on the path of the muscle, where it inserts on the globe (see ▶ Fig. 17.2), and the direction of gaze, these muscles may elevate or depress the eye, adduct or abduct it, or rotate it medially (intorsion) or laterally (extorsion). The secondary direction of pull becomes most effective when the direction of gaze is not straight ahead.

For instance, when the eyeball is in the adducted position, the depressing action of the superior oblique muscle comes to the fore and when the eyeball is in the abducted position, the internal rotation function comes to the fore.

▶ Table 17.1 shows the primary and secondary actions of the six extraocular muscles. Knowledge of these actions is important to understanding paralytic strabismus.

Note
All extraocular muscles except for the superior oblique and lateral rectus are supplied by the oculomotor nerve.

▶ **Physiology of binocular vision.** Strictly speaking, we "see" with the brain. The eyes are merely

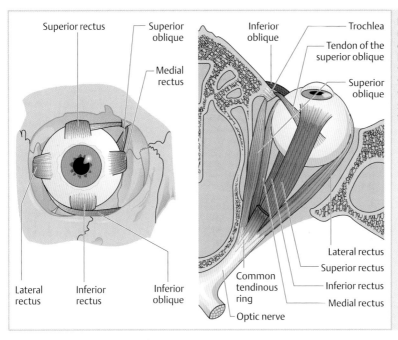

Fig. 17.2 (a, b) Extraocular muscles of the right eye. The two oblique ocular muscles insert on the temporal aspect posterior to the equator. The four rectus muscles insert on the superior, inferior, nasal, and temporal sclera.

Table 17.1 Function of the extraocular muscles with the gaze directed straight ahead

Muscle	Primary action	Secondary action	Example (right eye)	Nerve supply
Lateral rectus	Abduction	None		Abducens nerve
Medial rectus	Adduction	None		Oculomotor nerve

Table 17.1 Function of the extraocular muscles with the gaze directed straight ahead (continued)

Muscle	Primary action	Secondary action	Example (right eye)	Nerve supply
Superior rectus	Elevation	Intorsion and adduction	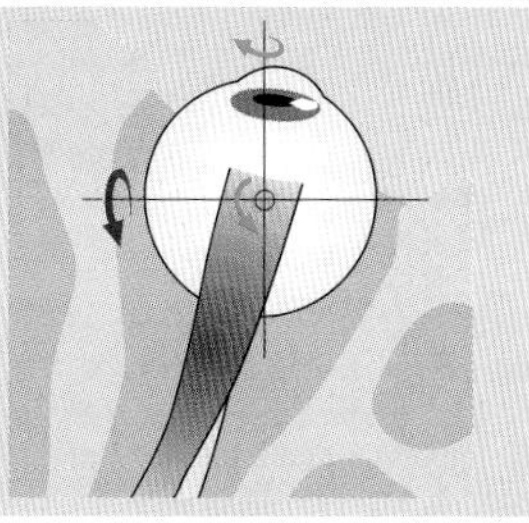	Oculomotor nerve
Inferior rectus	Depression	Extorsion and adduction	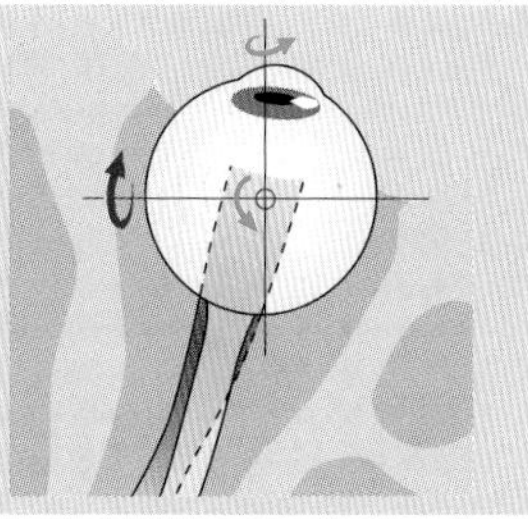	Oculomotor nerve
Superior oblique	Intorsion	Depression and abduction	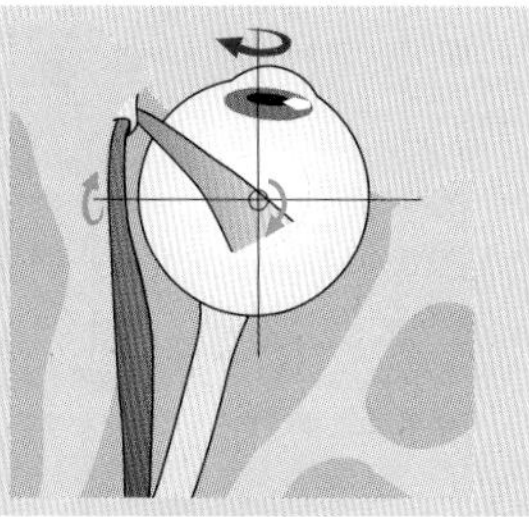	Trochlear nerve
Inferior oblique	Extorsion	Elevation and abduction	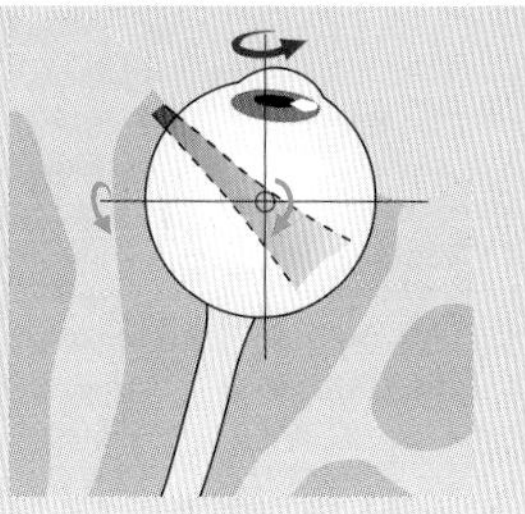	Oculomotor nerve

the organs of sensory reception. Their images are stored by coding the stimuli received by the retina. The optic nerve and visual pathway transmit this information in coded form to the visual cortex (sensory system). The motor system (see p. 296) described above directs both eyes to a fixated object so that the same or very similar objects are imaged on both retinas. The brain can then process this information into **binocular visual perception**. A person has no subjective awareness of this interplay between sensory and motor systems.

There are **three distinct levels of quality of binocular vision:**

▶ **Simultaneous vision.** The retinas of the two eyes perceive two images *simultaneously*. In normal binocular vision, both eyes have the *same point* of fixation, which lands on the fovea centralis in each eye. The image of an object always lands on *identical* areas of the retina, referred to as *corresponding points on the retina*. Objects lying on an imaginary circle known as the *geometric horopter* (▶ Fig. 17.3a) are projected to these points on the retina. A different horopter will apply for any given fixation distance. The images of both retinas are therefore identical in normal binocular vision. This phenomenon can be examined by presenting different

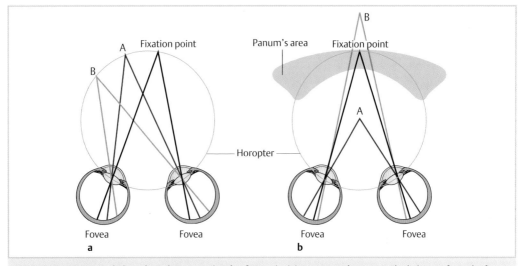

Fig. 17.3 Geometric and physiologic horopters (circle of vision). (a) Geometric horopter. The light rays from the fixation point strike the fovea centralis in both eyes in normal simultaneous vision. Objects A and B on the geometric horopter are therefore projected to corresponding points on the retina. **(b) Physiologic horopter.** In a narrow range in front of and behind the horopter (Panum's area), two retinal images can blend into a three-dimensional image. Points A and B, which lie outside Panum's area, are perceived as double.

images to each retina; normally both images will be perceived. This is known as *physiologic diplopia.*

Note
Physiologic diplopia can be demonstrated by placing two vertical pencils in a line slightly higher than the subject's visual axis, with the second pencil approximately twice as far from the subject as the first. When the subject focuses on one pencil, the other will appear double. If one of the pencils is fixated while the other one is moved toward the fixated pencil, the double image suddenly disappears and both pencils are perceived stereoscopically. The second pencil "ducked" into the Panum area as a result of the movement (see ▶ Fig. 17.3b).

▶ **Fusion.** Only when the two retinas convey the same visual impression—i.e., transmit identical images to the brain—will the two retinal images blend into *a single perception.* Impaired fusion can result in double vision (horror fusionis or diplopia).

▶ **Stereoscopic vision (perception of depth).** This is the highest level of quality of binocular vision and is possible only when several conditions are met. For objects to be projected to corresponding or identical points on the retina, they must lie on the

same geometric horopter. Objects lying in front of or behind this circle will not be projected to corresponding points but to *noncorresponding or disparate points* on the retina. The result is that these objects are perceived as double images (diplopia). However, objects within a narrow range in front of and behind the horopter are fused into a *single image.* This area is referred to as *Panum's area.* The brain processes noncorresponding retinal images within Panum's area into a single three-dimensional visual perception and does not interpret them as double images (▶ Fig. 17.3b).

17.2 Concomitant Strabismus

Definition
Concomitant strabismus differs from paralytic strabismus in that the angle of deviation remains the same in every direction of gaze. The angle of deviation (i.e., the angle between the fixating and the deviating visual axis) is the same in all directions of gaze. This form of strabismus occurs as unilateral right/left strabismus (only one eye deviates) and alternating strabismus (alternating eyes deviate).

▶ **Epidemiology.** Concomitant strabismus occurs almost exclusively in children. Approximately 5 to

7% of children are affected. In 60 to 70% of cases, the disorder initially manifests itself within the first 2 years of life.

▶ **Etiology.** Both sensorimotor coordination and binocular vision are very unstable during the first few years of life. *Impairments of the sensory or motor systems or central processing of visual perceptions* that occur during this time can disturb the coordination between the eyes and lead to strabismus. However, the causes of concomitant strabismus are often unclear. The following causes have been identified to date:

- **Genetic factors.** Approximately 60% of children with strabismus have a family history of increased incidence.
- **Uncorrected refractive errors** are partially responsible for the occurrence of strabismus. Children with *hyperopia* tend to have *esotropia*. This is because convergence (simultaneous inward movement of both eyes while focusing on a nearby object), accommodation (focusing on an object), and near miosis (pupillary constriction) are coupled (near reflex). Children with hyperopia have to accommodate *without converging* when gazing into the distance to compensate for their refractive error. However, accommodation always triggers a convergence impulse that can cause esotropia, especially when there is insufficient fusion. If in addition hyperopia is markedly greater on one side (anisohyperopia), there is often a convergent squint: through accommodation (which can only occur symmetrically on both sides), the hyperopia is only compensated to the level of the less hyperopic eye. The more hyperopic eye thus always sees a blurred image. Unilateral astigmatism also leads to blurred retinal imaging in one eye.
- **Unilateral visual impairment.** Severe myopia, corneal scarring, lens opacities (cataract), aniseikonia (unequal image size at the retinas), macular changes, and retinal disorders can cause secondary strabismus. *Retinal causes* include retinoblastoma, Coats's disease, retinopathy of prematurity, retinal detachment, or central retinal scarring in congenital toxoplasmosis.

Note

⚠

Any initial examination of a patient with strabismus must invariably include examination of the fundus of both eyes under mydriasis in addition to examination of the anterior segments of the eye.

- **Other possible causes** of concomitant strabismus include:
  - Perinatal lesions such as preterm birth and asphyxia.
  - Cerebral trauma and encephalitis.

▶ **Pathophysiology.** Deviation of the visual axis of the deviating eye causes objects to be projected to noncorresponding points on the retina. In adults, this would lead to the perception of double images. But two mechanisms have developed in children, in the early years of life, to prevent double images:

▶ **Suppression.** A central inhibiting mechanism suppresses the visual stimuli from the deviating eye. There are two different types of suppression:

- As a fixation point scotoma. The object fixated by the dominant eye is not seen by the deviating eye (double image is avoided). *Example:* In convergent strabismus, a nasal location on the retina is suppressed.
- As a central scotoma: The image projected on the fovea of the deviating eye is suppressed (confusion is avoided).

▶ **Anomalous retinal correspondence.** In small-angle strabismus (usually <5°, microstrabismus) a location outside the fixation point scotoma can take over the macular function of the fixation point ("pseudomacula"). This even permits coarse stereoscopic vision. This mechanism only functions when both eyes are used. After the fixating eye is covered, the previously deviating eye fixates centrally again (foveola). In addition, there is a form of microstrabismus in which the deviating eye does not fixate with the foveola, even with monocular vision. For details, see Determining the Type of Fixation (see p. 306) and/or Treatment and Avoidance of Strabismic Amblyopia (see p. 306).

▶ **Amblyopia secondary to suppression.** A disadvantage of the evolutionary advantage gained through suppression (or anomalous retinal correspondence) is the fact that the inhibitory mechanisms lead to delayed development of visual acuity in the inhibited eye so that visual development in this eye is weak (amblyopia), especially in children below the age of 6 years. The prospects for successful treatment decrease with age, and amblyopia may become irreversible beyond the age of 6 to 8 years. Amblyopia only occurs in unilateral strabismus. In alternating strabismus, fixation or deviation alternates between both eyes so that both eyes "learn" to see. Causes of amblyopia other than strabismus are possible (▶ Table 17.2).

Note
Strabismus occurring before the age of 6 years will frequently lead to amblyopia. Early examination and treatment by an ophthalmologist are crucial.

17.2.1 Forms of Concomitant Strabismus

These essentially include the following forms:
- **Esotropia.** Inward deviation of the visual axis.
- **Exotropia.** Outward deviation of the visual axis.
- **Hypertropia and hypotropia.** Ocular deviation with one eye higher or lower than the other.
- **Cyclotropia.** This refers to the rotation of one eye around its visual axis. An isolated form of strabismus (i.e., one that does not occur in combination with paralytic strabismus), this disorder is extremely rare and therefore will not be discussed in greater detail.

Esotropia

▶ **Epidemiology.** Esotropia is one of the most commonly encountered forms of strabismus.

▶ **Symptoms and diagnostic considerations.** There are three forms of esotropia:
1. **Congenital or infantile esotropia.** Strabismus is *present at birth* or develops *within the first 6 months of life.* This form is characterized by a large angle of convergent deviation (▶ Fig. 17.4a, b), lack of binocular vision, latent nystagmus (involuntary oscillation of the eyeballs that only occurs or becomes more pronounced when one eye is covered), intermittent torticollis, and additional hypertropia (see p. 304), primary oblique muscle dysfunction and dissociated vertical deviation. Another motility disorder that occurs in infantile strabismus syndrome is the A or V pattern deviation:
   - *"A pattern deviation"* refers to an inward angle of deviation that increases in upgaze and decreases in downgaze.
   - *"V pattern deviation"* refers to an inward angle of deviation that decreases in upgaze and increases in downgaze.
2. **Acquired strabismus.** Two forms are distinguished:
   - Strabismus begins *at the age of incomplete sensory development*—i.e., between the ages of 1 and 3 years. Usually the disorder manifests itself at the age of 2 years and leads to sensory adaptation syndromes in the form of *unilateral* strabismus. Amblyopia is usually already present, and correspondence is primarily anomalous.
   - Strabismus becomes manifest *between the ages of 3 and 7 years.* This form of *acute late strabismus with normal sensory development* is encountered far less frequently than other forms. As binocular vision is already well

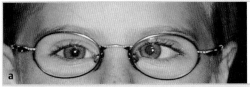
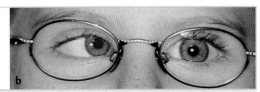

Fig. 17.4 **Alternating esotropia.** This 5-year-old girl has had alternating esotropia since birth with additional slight vertical deviation and a large angle of deviation both distant and near. Before she entered school she underwent strabismus surgery on her left eye. For details, see Surgery in infantile strabismus syndrome (p. 307) and ▶ Fig. 17.12a, b. In this form of strabismus, the eyes take the lead alternately: **(a)** Eye position when fixating an object on the right. **(b)** Eye position when fixating an object on the left.

Table 17.2 Forms of amblyopia

Forms of amblyopia	Cause	Treatment
Amblyopia with strabismus	Suppression of the deviating eye	Occlusion therapy (see p. 307)
Deprivation amblyopia	Organic disease, such as ptosis or cataract	Early surgery and occlusion therapy in applicable cases
Refractive amblyopia	Different refractive errors	Correction with eyeglasses or contact lenses and occlusion therapy in applicable cases
Bilateral amblyopia	Nystagmus (see p. 316), astigmatism, late correction of refractive errors	None

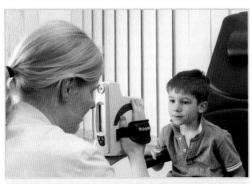

Fig. 17.5 Determination of refraction in a child, using a hand-held refractometer.

developed, affected children cannot immediately suppress the visual images of the deviating eye. As a result, they suffer from *sudden* double vision at the onset of strabismus, which they attempt to suppress by closing one eye. *Immediate* treatment is indicated to preserve binocular vision. This consists of the following steps: Objective examination of refraction (see p. 275) with cycloplegia with atropine or cyclopentolate is performed (often higher, asymmetrical hyperopia). In infants, objective examination of refraction is performed with a skiascope (see Chapter 16.2.2, ▶ Fig. 16.7) or alternatively with a portable hand-held refractometer suitable for children, equipped with light reflex and acoustic signal (▶ Fig. 17.5). After the required eyeglass correction is determined (corresponding to the objective refractometry), the measured angle of deviation is offset with the appropriate prismatic correction. If the angle of deviation cannot be relaxed in a few weeks with eyeglasses or if the eyes are in a state of emmetropia, surgery on the extraocular muscles is indicated.

Note

Binocular vision is well developed in late strabismus with normal sensory development. Surgery within 3–6 months will allow the patient to maintain or regain stereoscopic vision.

3. **Microstrabismus.** This is defined as unilateral esotropia with a usually *minimal cosmetic effect*—i.e., an angle of deviation of 5° or less. As a result, microstrabismus is often diagnosed too late—i.e., only at the age of 4 to 6 years. By that time the resulting amblyopia in the deviating eye may be severe. Another sequela of microstrabismus is anomalous retinal corre-

spondence (see p. 301). Binocular vision is partially preserved despite anomalous retinal correspondence and amblyopia (Bagolini test positive, coarse stereoscopic vision). The microstrabismus is untreatable. For this reason, treatment is limited to occlusion therapy to correct the amblyopia.

Accommodative Esotropia

Bilateral hyperopia leads to blurred projection on the retina. As a result, the near reflex (accommodation, convergence, and miosis) is activated. If a fusion disorder is present, strong demands made of the near reflex (accommodation) lead to a permanent convergence position that can be decreased by plus lenses. Two types of accommodative esotropia can be distinguished:

1. **Accommodative strabismus**: Convergent strabismus disappears for distant and near fixation after correction of hyperopia (distance glasses), since the constant triggering of the near reflex (and the resulting convergent squint elicited even by gazing into the distance) no longer occurs.

2. **Convergence excess esotropia**: Esotropia is markedly greater in near than in distant focus. A pathologically increased near reflex causes excessive increase of the convergent angle of deviation. This condition usually affects children of school age. If a near correction of +3.0 diopters is prescribed (in addition to the necessary distance correction), the difference between the large near angle of deviation and the small (or nonexistent) distant angle of deviation disappears, since the near reflex is no longer needed. Two forms are distinguished:

- In the **more frequent** form, the accommodation amplitude is normal (**normaccommodative** or **hyperkinetic convergence excess**). Treatment consists of bifocal glasses with a large near section (dividing line at the level of the pupils), since the young patient must be forced to use the near portion of the glasses. This is the only way, in this case, to prevent undesirable accommodation. As the near reflex is gradually attenuated, especially during puberty, the near portion of the glasses can usually be made weaker (or removed entirely). It is useful to check annually whether the near portion can be made weaker (▶ Fig. 17.6). A large basic angle of deviation (distance angle of deviation measured through the distance part, near angle of deviation measured through the near portion of the glasses) can be eliminated by eye muscle surgery.

- In rare **hypoaccommodative convergence excess** the outstanding aspect is hypoaccommodation, which can also occur in isolation (with convergence excess). In this form, the amplitude of accommodation is pathologically decreased. This can also be caused by trauma. This can also cause asthenopic complaints in young patients (e.g., headaches, blurred near vision, and occasionally reading and writing weakness). Treatment consists of bifocal glasses with a small near portion (similar to the prescription for presbyopia [loss of ability to focus with aging], since the patient will use it actively and will not need to be "forced" to use it by a particularly large near portion. Varifocal glasses are also well accepted. Eye muscle surgery is not required since, in any case, the bifocals are worn constantly.

Exotropia

Exotropia (divergent strabismus) is less common than esotropia. Exotropia less frequently leads to amblyopia because the strabismus is often alternating. Occasionally what is known as "panorama vision" will occur, in which case the patient has an expanded binocular field of vision. The following forms are distinguished:

- **Intermittent exotropia.** This is the *most common form* of divergent strabismus. In many cases of intermittent exotropia, an angle of deviation is present only when the patient gazes into the distance; the patient has normal binocular vision in near fixation (▶ Fig. 17.7a, b). The image from the deviating eye is suppressed in the deviation phase.
- **Secondary exotropia** occurs with reduced visual acuity in one eye resulting from disease or trauma.
- **Consecutive exotropia** occurs after esotropia surgery (after recession of the medial rectus muscle).

Vertical Deviations (Hypertropia and Hypotropia)

The most frequently occurring forms of vertical deviation are the V and A patterns (strabismus sursoadductorius and deorsoadductorius) that typically occur in early childhood strabismus (see p. 302) and dissociated vertical deviation.

- Strabismus sursoadductorius is characterized by *upward vertical* deviation of the adducting eye during *horizontal* eye movements. This is often associated with a V-pattern.

Fig. 17.6 Accommodative convergence excess. A 7-year-old girl with a convergent squint and bifocal glasses. When fixating a distant point through the distance portion of the glasses (a) and fixating a near point through the near portion (in each case, in addition, +3.0 diopters) (b), there is a slight convergent squint (+3°). With near fixation through the distance portion of the glasses, there is a convergent squint of +15° (c).

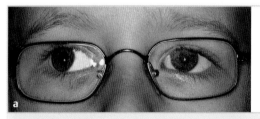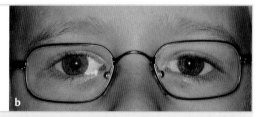

Fig. 17.7 Intermittent right divergent strabismus. This 5-year-old boy has had intermittent divergent strabismus in his right eye since the age of 2 years. In order to maintain the visual acuity of the deviating eye at 100%, the nondeviating left eye is covered with a patch for 3 hours a day. Strabismus surgery was performed before the boy started school. **(a)** In a distant gaze, the right eye deviates. **(b)** There is no deviation in a near gaze.

- Strabismus deorsoadductorius is a vertical downward deviation of the adducted eye in a lateral version and is combined with an A-pattern (see p. 304).
- Dissociated vertical deviation is *alternating upward deviation of the eyes.* The respective non-fixating eye or the eye occluded in the cover test will be elevated.

17.2.2 Diagnosis of Concomitant Strabismus

Evaluating Ocular Alignment with a Focused Light

This is a fundamental examination and is usually the first one performed by the ophthalmologist in patients with suspected concomitant strabismus. The examiner holds the light beneath and close to his or her own eyes and observes the light reflexes on the patient's corneas (*Hirschberg's method*) in near fixation at a distance of 30 cm. Normally these reflexes are symmetrical. Strabismus is associated with an asymmetrical corneal reflex (▶ Fig. 17.7).

Diagnosis of Unilateral and Alternating Strabismus (Unilateral Cover Test)

The unilateral cover test can confirm the presence of manifest strabismus more precisely than Hirschberg's corneal reflex test (see above). The subject is asked to fixate a point. The examiner first covers the right eye and observes whether the left eye moves. Then bilateral fixation is permitted again and then the left eye is covered and the right eye is observed. Manifest strabismus is present if an eye movement is observed ("adjustment movement"). It is also possible to distinguish between manifest monolateral and alternating strabismus.

- In unilateral strabismus, the *same eye always deviates.* When the deviating eye is covered, the uncovered eye (the leading, nondeviating eye) remains focused on the point of fixation and no adjustment movement is observed. When the nondeviating eye is covered, the uncovered deviating eye has to take the lead. To do so, it will first make a visible adjustment. If there is an outward adjustment, the eye is esotropic (▶ Fig. 17.8a–c); if the movement is inward, it is exotropic.
- In alternating strabismus, *both eyes* will *alternately* fixate: covering the right eye will trigger left fixation and covering the left side will then trigger right fixation.

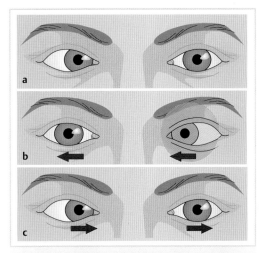

Fig. 17.8 Response of the deviating eye to a unilateral cover test. (a) Unilateral esotropia of the right eye. **(b)** Unilateral cover test. When the leading left eye is covered, the deviating right eye adjusts with a movement from medial to lateral and then takes the lead. The covered left eye deviates. **(c)** When the leading left eye is uncovered again, the right eye reverts to its deviation. The leading left eye is realigned with the fixation point.

Measuring the Angle of Deviation (Prism Cover Test)

Exact measurement of the angle of deviation is crucial to prescribing the proper prism correction to compensate for the angle of deviation and to the corrective surgery. A measurement error may lead to undercorrection or overcorrection of the angle of deviation during the operation.

The angle of deviation is measured with a **cover test with the use of prism lenses of various refractive powers**. The patient fixates on a certain point with the *leading eye* at a distance of 5 m (distant) or 30 cm (near). The examiner places prism lenses of different refractive power before the patient's deviant eye until no further adjustment movement is observed.

Prism bars simplify the examination. These bars contain a series of prisms of progressively increasing strength arranged one above the other.

Note
The angle of deviation can be measured in centimeters per meter [cm/m] (previously prism diopters) or degrees. One prism diopter refracts light rays approximately half a degree, so that two prism diopters correspond to 1 degree.

Determining the Type of Fixation

This examination is used to ascertain *which part of the retina of the deviating eye* the image of the fixated point falls on. The examiner observes the fundus (Chapter 12.2) with a direct ophthalmoscope. At the same time, the ophthalmoscope projects a small star onto the retina and the patient is asked to fixate it:

- In **central fixation**, the image of the star falls on the fovea centralis (▶ Fig. 17.9[1]).
- In **eccentric fixation**, the image of the star falls on an area of the retina outside the fovea (▶ Fig. 17.9 [2–6]). Usually this point lies between the fovea and the optic disc.

Aside from the type of fixation, one can also estimate potential *visual acuity*. The greater the distance between where the point of fixation lies and the fovea, the lower the resolving power of the retina and the poorer visual acuity will be. Initial treatment consists of occlusion therapy to shift an eccentric point of fixation onto the fovea centralis.

Testing Binocular Vision

▶ **Bagolini test.** This test uses flat lenses with fine parallel striations. The striations spread light from a point source into a strip. The lenses are mounted in the examination eyeglasses in such a manner that the strips of light form a diagonal cross in patients with intact binocular vision. The patient is asked to describe the pattern of the strips of light while looking at the point source. Children can also demonstrate the light strips with hand movements through space. Patients who describe a cross have normal simultaneous vision. Patients who see only one diagonal strip of light are suppressing the image received by the respective fellow eye.

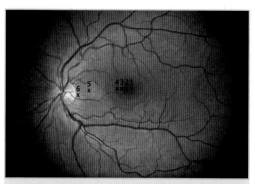

Fig. 17.9 Ophthalmoscopic testing of fixation: 1, foveal fixation; 2, parafoveal fixation; 3, macular fixation; 4, paramacular fixation; 5 and 6, parapapillar fixation.

▶ **Lang's test.** This test can be used to determine depth perception (stereopsis) in infants. A card depicts various objects that the child only sees if it can perceive depth.

Diagnosis of Infantile Strabismic Amblyopia (Preferential Looking Test)

The preferential looking test can be used for early evaluation of visual acuity beginning at the age of 4–6 months (▶ Fig. 17.10). In this way, defects of the entire visual system can be revealed. Since the onset of strabismus most often occurs in infants and young children, an associated visual impairment (strabismic amblyopia) can be recognized and treated early, thus preventing permanent visual impairment.

17.2.3 Treatment of Concomitant Strabismus

▶ **Treatment of concomitant strabismus in children.** Treatment is generally long-term. The duration of treatment may extend from the first months of life to about the age of 10 years. The whole course of treatment (after ruling out other diseases, such as retinal diseases) can be divided into **three phases with corresponding interim goals**:

1. The ophthalmologist determines whether the cause of the strabismus can be treated with **eyeglasses**. The hyperopia frequently present in esotropia should always be corrected in this way.
2. If the strabismus cannot be fully aligned with eyeglasses, the next step in treatment (parallel to prescribing eyeglasses) is to minimize the risk of amblyopia by **occlusion therapy**.
3. Once the occlusion therapy has produced sufficient visual acuity in both eyes, the alignment of one or both eyes is corrected by **surgery**. The alignment correction is required for normal binocular vision and has the added benefit of esthetic improvement.

▶ **Treatment of concomitant strabismus in adults.** A functional improvement in binocular vision can usually no longer be achieved. However, esthetic improvement with surgery is indicated to avoid or reduce psychological suffering.

Eyeglass Prescription

Where the strabismus is due to a cause that can be treated with eyeglasses, then eyeglasses can elimi-

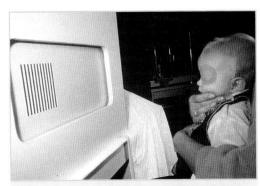

Fig. 17.10 Diagnosis of strabismus in children with the Teller acuity card. The Teller acuity card is located in a viewing case behind which the examiner sits. An observation pinhole in the middle of the card allows the examiner to see upon which half of the card the infant fixates. The cards are successively replaced with cards that have increasingly narrow black and white stripe patterns, so that with increasing spatial frequency of stripes the patterns increasingly resemble the background gray. The examiner tests up to which stripe pattern density a preferred gaze direction can still be observed.

nate at least the accommodative component of the disorder (see p. 303). Often residual strabismus requiring further treatment will remain despite eyeglass correction.

Treatment and Avoidance of Strabismic Amblyopia

Strict occlusion therapy by eye patching or eyeglass occlusion is the most effective method of avoiding or treating strabismic amblyopia. *Primarily the leading eye* is patched.

▶ **Eye patching.** The most effective method for avoiding strabismic amblyopia or treating it is strict occlusion treatment with a skin adhesive bandage. The leading eye is covered (▶ Fig. 17.11). If the skin does not tolerate the bandage, a possible alternative is to cover the eyeglass lens of the leading eye with an opaque film. Eyeglass occlusion entails the risk that the child might attempt to circumvent the occlusion of the good eye by looking over the rim of the eyeglasses with the leading eye. This would compromise the effectiveness of occlusion therapy, whose purpose is to train the amblyopic eye.

▶ **Procedure.** In amblyopia, the occlusion period must be selected case by case, such that visual acuity increases (regular vision check!). There are established rules for this, but flexibility is necessary in individual cases: The leading eye is occluded for several hours at a time in **mild amblyopia**, and

for several days at a time in **severe amblyopia** *depending on the patient's age.* For example, the nondeviating eye in a *4-year-old patient* with severe amblyopia is patched for *4 days* while the deviating eye is left uncovered. Both eyes are then left uncovered for 1 day. This is important in order to prevent the better eye from losing visual acuity. This treatment cycle is repeated beginning on the following day.

> **Note**
> Amblyopia must be treated in early childhood. The earlier therapy is initiated, the sooner amblyopia can be eliminated. Often, the treatment must be continued until the child is of school age.

▶ **Treatment goal.** The goal of treatment in infantile strabismus is to achieve *alternating strabismus* with *full visual acuity* and *central fixation* in both eyes. But even after this goal has been achieved, there can be a decline in vision after cessation of occlusion therapy, requiring resumption of the therapy ("maintenance occlusion"). Binocular vision is less important in this setting. It is not normally developed anyway in patients who develop strabismus at an early age and cannot be further improved.

Surgery

▶ **Surgery in infantile strabismus syndrome.** Surgery should be postponed until after amblyopia has been successfully treated (see p. 306). In contrast to treatment for amblyopia, strabismus surgery is not subject to time pressure. It is advisable to wait since exact preoperative measurement of the angle of deviation and adequate aftercare (e.g., regular

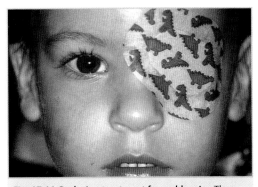

Fig. 17.11 Occlusion treatment for amblyopia. The leading eye is patched for several hours or days at a time to improve visual acuity in the deviating amblyopic eye.

and exact monitoring of visual acuity with tests that require the patient's cooperation) are not assured in patients who are too young (under 4 years of age). Surgical correction in a very young patient prior to successful treatment of amblyopia involves a risk that a decrease in visual acuity in one eye may go unnoticed after the strabismus has been corrected. However, the child should undergo surgery prior to entering school so as to avoid the social stigma of strabismus. In such a case, surgery achieves only a *cosmetic correction of strabismus* (▶ Fig. 17.12).

▶ **Surgery in late strabismus with normal sensory development.** In this case, surgery should be performed as early as possible because the primary goal is to preserve binocular vision, in contrast to infantile strabismus syndrome.

▶ **Procedure.** The position of the eyes in forward gaze is altered with an operative procedure. **Esotropia** is corrected by a combined procedure involving a medial rectus recession and a lateral rectus resection (or tucking). The medial rectus is released because its pull is "too strong" (see ▶ Fig. 17.2), whereas the lateral rectus is shortened to increase its pull. The degree of correction depends on the angle of deviation. **Strabismus sursoadductorius** is treated by recession of the inferior oblique muscle, and **strabismus deorsoadductorius** is treated by recession of the superior oblique muscle. **Exotropia** is corrected by a lateral rectus recession in combination with a medial rectus resection (or tucking).

17.3 Heterophoria

Definition

- If both eyes are parallel and remain so when one eye is covered, this is called orthophoria. However, many people have a latent strabismus that they constantly correct with a fusion reflex. This fusion reflex keeps the eyes parallel in order to avoid double vision and enable three-dimensional vision. When the fusion reflex is interrupted, the eyes resume their inborn strabismic position ("resting position"). This tendency to strabismus is called heterophoria. Asthenopic problems (such as headache, burning eyes, rapid tiring) are very rare in heterophoria. When these problems do occur, the condition is called pathophoria. The state in which there are no problems is called normophoria.

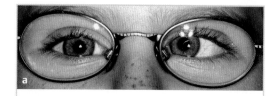
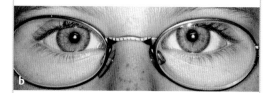
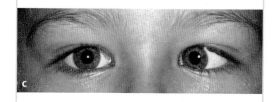
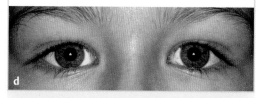

Fig. 17.12 Operation in infantile strabismus. This 5-year-old girl with alternating esotropia (see ▶ Fig. 17.4a,b) was operated on before starting school. **(a)** Condition before the operation: alternating convergent strabismus. Patient's preferred eye position: right fixation, angle of deviation before the operation F: +17° – N: +19°. **(b)** Condition after strabismus surgery on the left eye: recession of the internal rectus muscle 5.0 mm, external rectus myectomy 6.0 mm, angle of deviation after surgery: F: +2° – N: +3°. **(c,d)** In this 6-year-old boy, the unilateral esotropia in the left eye was operated on. Because of preexistent strabismic amblyopia in the left eye, a three-year amblyopia therapy was carried out. In addition, the right eye was occluded daily as appropriate for his age (see ▶ Fig. 17.11) Before the strabismus operation, the left eye had full visual acuity. **(c)** Convergent strabismus in the left eye. Right fixation, angle of deviation before the operation: F: +14° – N: +14°. **(d)** Condition after strabismus operation on the left eye: recession of the internal rectus muscle 4.0 mm, external rectus muscle myectomy 4.0 mm, angle of deviation after surgery: F: +1° – N: + 3°.

The following forms are distinguished, analogously to manifest strabismus:
- **Esophoria.** Latent inward deviation of the visual axis.
- **Exophoria.** Latent outward deviation of the visual axis.
- **Hyperphoria.** Latent upward deviation of one eye.
- **Hypophoria.** Latent downward deviation of one eye.
- **Cyclophoria.** Latent rotation of one eye around its visual axis.

▶ **Epidemiology.** This disorder occurs in 70 to 80% of the population. The incidence increases with age.

▶ **Etiology and symptoms.** Heterophoria does not manifest itself as long as image fusion is unimpaired. Where fusion is impaired as a result of alcohol consumption, stress, fatigue, concussion, or emotional distress, the muscular imbalance can cause intermittent or occasionally permanent strabismus.

▶ **Diagnostic considerations.** Heterophoria is diagnosed by the **uncover test**. This test simulates the special conditions under which heterophoria becomes manifest (decreased image fusion such as can occur due to extreme fatigue or consumption of alcohol) and eliminates the *impetus to fuse images*. In contrast to the cover test (see p. 305), the uncover test focuses on the *response of the previously covered eye immediately after being uncovered*. Once uncovered, the eye makes a visible adjustment to permit fusion and recover binocular vision. The size of the latent angle of deviation is measured by the alternating prism cover test. The eyes are covered alternately, without an interval of binocular vision. As in the unilateral cover test (see p. 305), prismatic lenses of various strengths are set before one eye until no further adjustment movement is observed.

▶ **Treatment.** Heterophoria requires treatment only in symptomatic cases. In pathophoria, a **strabismus operation** offers a possibility of a permanent solution.

17.4 Pseudostrabismus

A broad dorsum of the nose with epicanthal folds through which the nasal aspect of the palpebral fissure appears shortened can often simulate strabismus in small children (▶ Fig. 17.13). The child's eyes appear esotropic especially when gazing to the side. Testing with a focused light (see p. 305) will

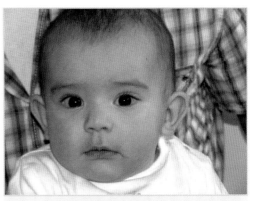

Fig. 17.13 **Pseudostrabismus caused by epicanthus.** In this child, esotropia is simulated by a broad dorsum of the nose. The corneal reflexes, however, demonstrate parallel visual axes. The epicanthus disappears in the first years of life after the dorsum of the nose develops.

reveal that the corneal reflexes are symmetrical, and there will be no eye adjustments in the cover test (see p. 305). Usually the epicanthal folds will spontaneously disappear during the first few years of life as the dorsum of the nose develops.

17.5 Ophthalmoplegia and Paralytic Strabismus

Definition
Ophthalmoplegia can affect one or more ocular muscles at the same time. The condition may be neurogenic, myogenic, or mechanically caused. Neurogenic paralysis may be partial (paresis, more common) or complete (paralysis, less common). If the cause of neurogenic paralysis is located in the area of the oculomotor nuclei or the peripheral cranial nerves (III, IV, or VI), the result is paretic strabismus; if it lies above the oculomotor nuclei, the result is gaze palsy. Internuclear ophthalmoplegia is in an intermediate position: the lesion is localized between the nuclei of cranial nerves III and VI (see p. 297).
- **Paralytic strabismus.** Strabismus due to an isolated limitation of motility in one or more eye muscles. The angle of deviation does not remain constant in every direction of gaze, as in concomitant strabismus (see p. 300), but increases in the direction of pull of the paralyzed muscle. This is referred to as an *incomitant* angle of deviation.
- **Gaze palsy.** Impairment or failure of coordinated eye movements, i.e., the coordinated eye movements of both eyes.

17.5.1 Etiology and Forms of Ocular Motility Disorders

Two forms are distinguished.

- **Congenital ocular motility disorders** may be due to the following causes:
  - Prenatal encephalitis.
  - Aplasia of the ocular muscles.
  - Birth trauma.
- **Acquired ocular motility disorders** may be due to the following causes:
  - Diabetes mellitus.
  - Multiple sclerosis.
  - Tumors (intracranial, intraorbital).
  - Arteriosclerosis.
  - Central ischemia (apoplexy).
  - AIDS.
  - Trauma and other causes.

17.5.2 Forms of Eye Movement Disorders

Neurogenic ocular motility disturbances are distinguished according to the location of the lesion (▶ Table 17.3).

- *Lesions of the nerves supplying the ocular muscles.* This condition is referred to as an *infranuclear* ocular motility disorder; for details of the commonest type of paralysis see p. 313. The following nerves may be affected See ▶ Table 17.1):
  - Oculomotor nerve lesions are rare and cause paralysis of several muscles.
  - Trochlear nerve lesions are common and cause paralysis of the superior oblique.
  - Abducens nerve lesions are common and cause paralysis of the lateral rectus.
- *Lesions of the ocular muscle nuclei.* This condition is referred to as a *nuclear* ocular motility disorder (see ▶ Fig. 17.1).
- *Lesions of the gaze centers.* This condition is referred to as a *supranuclear* ocular motility disorder (see gaze centers, ▶ Fig. 17.1). It very often causes gaze palsy.
- Also possible is a disorder or *lesion in the fiber tract connection* (fasciculus longitudinalis medialis) between the nuclei of cranial nerves III and VI (internuclear ocular motility disorder) (see ▶ Table 17.2 and ▶ Fig. 17.14).

▶ **Myogenic ocular motility disorders.** A heterogeneous group of primary myogenic ocular motility disorders in which muscle stretch is impaired or there are changes in muscular metabolism (e.g., chronic progressive external ophthalmoplegia or acute myositis) by which muscle contractility is limited.

- Impairment of ocular muscle stretching.
  - Graves's disease (see p. 262) is the most common cause of myogenic ocular motility disorders. Sometimes significant motility disorders caused by fibrotic changes in eye muscles (most frequently the inferior rectus and medial rectus muscles) that lead to a decrease in elasticity of these muscles.
  - Orbital wall fractures (e.g., blowout fracture): entrapment of eye muscles (rare!) or their sheaths (frequent!) in the fracture gap. Because the orbital floor is thin, stretching of the inferior rectus muscle is most likely to be impeded (restricted vertical movement of the upward gaze!).
  - Hematomas or swelling of the orbits or facial bones (e.g., orbital abscess, orbital tumor).
- Restriction of eye muscle contractility:
  - *Ocular myasthenia gravis* is a disorder of neuromuscular transmission characterized by the presence of acetylcholine receptor antibodies. Typical symptoms of ocular myasthenia gravis include fluctuating weakness that is clearly attributable to any one cranial nerve. The weakness typically increases in severity during the course of the day with fatigue.
  - *Chronic progressive external ophthalmoplegia (CPEO)* is usually a bilateral, gradually progressive paralysis of one or more extraocular muscles.
  - *Ocular myositis* is inflammation of one or more extraocular muscles. The pathogenesis is uncertain. Ocular motility is often limited not so much in the direction of pull of the inflamed muscle as in the opposite direction. While there is paresis of the muscle, it is characterized primarily by insufficient ductility. Often additional symptoms are present, such as pain during eye movement.

17.5.3 Symptoms of Ocular Motility Disorders

▶ **Strabismus.** Paralysis of one or more ocular muscles can cause its respective antagonist to dominate. This results in a typical strabismus that allows which muscle is paralyzed to be determined—see Chapter 17.5.5. This is readily done especially in abducens or trochlear nerve palsy as the abducens nerve and the trochlear nerve each supply only one extraocular muscle (see ▶ Table 17.1).

Example: abducens nerve palsy (▶ Fig. 17.15). A lesion of the abducens nerve paralyzes the lateral rectus so that the eye can no longer be *abducted*. Since the tensile force of the lateral rectus muscle is

Table 17.3 Classification of neurogenic ophthalmoplegia according to the location of the lesion (see ▶ Fig.17.1)

Ocular motility disorder	Causes	Location of lesion	Effects

Infranuclear ocular motility disorder	• In younger patients:
	  ○ Trauma
	  ○ Multiple sclerosis
	  ○ Infectious disease
	  ○ Brain tumors
	• In older patients:
	  ○ Vascular disease
	  ○ Diabetes
	  ○ Hypertension
	  ○ Arteriosclerosis
		• Lesion in one of the nerves supplying the ocular muscles:
		  ○ Oculomotor nerve
		  ○ Trochlear nerve
		  ○ Abducens nerve
			Palsy of one or several extraocular muscles of one or both eyes resulting in strabismus or limited eye motility

Nuclear ocular motility disorder	• Multiple sclerosis • Myasthenia gravis • Meningoencephalitis • Syphilis • AIDS	Lesion of the ocular muscle nucleus	Palsy of the extraocular muscles of both eyes in varying degrees of severity
Supranuclear ocular motility disorder			
• Horizontal gaze palsy	• Diabetes • Apoplexy • Tumor • Encephalitis • Vascular insult • Multiple sclerosis	Lesion in the paramedian pontine reticular formation (PPRF; see ▶ Fig. 17.1)	• All conjugate eye movements on the side of the lesion are impaired • Peripheral facial paresis is often also present • Both eyes are affected
• Vertical gaze palsy (Parinaud's syndrome)	• Midbrain infarctions • Tumors of the quadrigeminal region such as pineal gland tumors and germinomas	Lesion in the medial longitudinal fasciculus (MLF; see Fig. ▶ 17.1)	• Isolated upward or downward gaze palsy • Combined upward and downward gaze palsy • Moderately wide pupils • Impaired accommodation • Convergence nystagmus
Internuclear ocular motility disorder (INO)	• Younger patients with bilateral INO: multiple sclerosis • Older patients with unilateral INO: brain stem infarction	Lesion in the medial longitudinal fasciculus (MLF; see Fig. ▶ 17.1)	• Medial nerve palsy or impaired adduction in one eye in side gaze with intact near reflex convergence (see ▶ Fig. 17.14) • Jerk nystagmus in the abducted eye

lacking even with a forward gaze, inward strabismus results.

▶ **Incomitant angle of deviation.** It is typical of paretic strabismus that the angle of deviation varies in size depending on whether the paralyzed eye or nonparalyzed eye is fixating:
• A *primary angle of deviation* is the angle of deviation when fixating with the normal eye.
• A *secondary angle of deviation* is the angle of deviation when fixating with the paralyzed eye. *Explanation:* The secondary angle of deviation is always larger than the primary angle. This is because both the paralyzed muscle and its synergist in the fellow eye receive increased impulses when the paralyzed eye fixates. For

example, when the right eye fixates in right abducens nerve palsy, the left medial rectus will receive increased impulses. This increases the angle of deviation.

▶ **Gaze palsy.** If synergistically acting muscles of both eyes are paralyzed, the gaze is paralyzed.

For example, *vertical gaze palsy or Parinaud's syndrome*, which occurs in the presence of a pineal gland tumor, involves a lesion of the rostral interstitial nucleus of the medial longitudinal fasciculus (see ▶ Fig. 17.1).

▶ **Double vision.** Loss of binocular coordination between the two eyes due to ophthalmoplegia leads to double vision. Normal vision can be

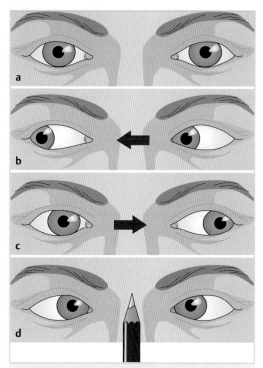

Fig. 17.14 Right internuclear ophthalmoplegia. (a) Parallel visual axes. (b) Normal right gaze. (c) In left gaze, the right eye cannot be adducted, because the medial longitudinal fasciculus is interrupted. (d) Convergence is preserved in both eyes.

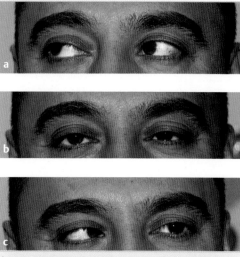

Fig. 17.15 Left abducens nerve palsy. (a) In a gaze to the right, the parallel position persists without diplopia. (b) In a forward gaze, the left eye deviates inward and diplopia is experienced. (c) In a gaze to the left, the inward deviation increases, as well as the distance between the double images.

expected in patients with only moderate paresis. As the onset of paresis is usually sudden, double vision is the typical symptom that induces patients to consult a physician. Some patients learn to suppress one of the two images within a few hours, days, or weeks. Other patients suffer from persistent double vision. Children usually learn to suppress the image more quickly than adults.

▶ **Causes.** Double vision occurs when the image of the fixated object only falls on the fovea in one eye while falling on a point on the peripheral retina in the fellow eye. As a result, the object is perceived in two different directions and therefore seen double (▶ Fig. 17.16). The double image of the deviating eye is usually somewhat out of focus as the resolving power of the peripheral retina is limited. Despite this, the patient cannot tell which is real and which is a virtual image and has difficulty in reaching to grasp an object.

In ophthalmoplegia the *distance between the double images* is greatest in the original direction of pull of the affected muscle.

Example: trochlear nerve palsy (▶ Fig.17.17). The superior oblique supplied by the trochlear nerve is primarily an intorter and depressor in adduction (see ▶ Table 17.1); it is also an abductor when the gaze is directed straight ahead.

Therefore, the limited motility and upward deviation of the affected eye is most apparent in depression (as when reading). The distance between the double images is greatest and the diplopia most irritating in this direction of gaze, which is the main direction of pull of the paralyzed superior oblique.

▶ **Compensatory head posture.** The patient can avoid diplopia only by attempting to avoid using the paralyzed muscle. This is done by assuming a typical compensatory head posture in which the gaze lies within the binocular visual field; the patient tilts the head and turns it toward the shoulder opposite the paralyzed eye.

The *Bielschowsky head tilt test* uses this posture to confirm the diagnosis of trochlear or fourth cranial nerve palsy (▶ Fig. 17.18). In this test, the examiner tilts the patient's head toward the side of the paralyzed eye. If the patient then fixates with the normal eye, the paralyzed eye will deviate upward. When the patient's head is tilted toward the normal side, there will be no vertical deviation (see Chapter 17.5.5 for further diagnostic procedures).

▶ **Ocular torticollis.** The compensatory head posture in trochlear nerve palsy is the most pronounced and typical of all cranial nerve palsies. *Congenital* trochlear nerve palsy can lead to what is known as ocular torticollis.

17.5.4 Ocular Muscle Paralysis Caused by Cranial Nerve Damage

Since paralyses caused by cranial nerve damage are the most frequent ones, they will be treated here in greater detail than other disorders of ocular motility. Diagnosis of an ocular muscle paralysis must always be followed by further diagnostic investigation (often by a neurologist), for instance in order to rule out a tumor or a specific underlying disease such as diabetes mellitus.

▶ **Abducens nerve palsy**
▶ **Causes.** The main causes of this relatively common palsy include vascular disease (diabetes mellitus, hypertension, or arteriosclerosis) and intracerebral tumors. Often a tumor will cause increased cerebrospinal fluid pressure, which particularly affects the abducens nerve because of its long course along the base of the skull. In *children*, these transient isolated abducens nerve palsies can occur in infectious diseases, febrile disorders, or secondary to inoculations.

▶ **Effects.** The lateral rectus is paralyzed, causing its antagonist, the medial rectus, to dominate. Abduction is impaired or absent altogether, and the affected eye remains medially rotated (see ▶ Fig. 17.15). Horizontal homonymous (uncrossed) diplopia is present (see ▶ Fig. 17.16). The images are farthest apart in abduction.
　Example: right abducens nerve palsy:
- Compensatory head posture with right tilt.
- Esotropia when the gaze is directed straight ahead.
- Largest angle of deviation and distance between images in right gaze.
- No angle of deviation or diplopia in left gaze.

▶ **Trochlear nerve palsy**
▶ **Causes.** The commonest cause is trauma (often bilateral); less common causes include vascular disease (diabetes mellitus, hypertension, and arteriosclerosis). Trochlear nerve palsy is a relatively common phenomenon.

▶ **Effects.** The superior oblique is primarily an intorter and a depressor in adduction. This results in upward vertical deviation of the paralyzed eye in adduction and vertical strabismus (see ▶ Fig. 17.17). Patients experience vertical diplopia; the images are farthest apart in depression and intorsion (e.g., while reading or walking up or down

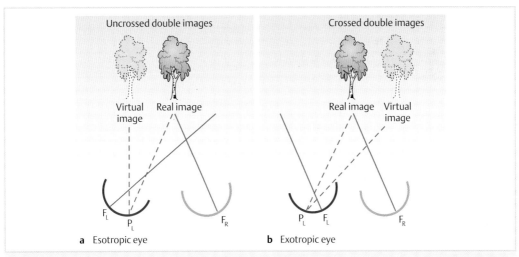

Fig. 17.16 Crossed and uncrossed diplopia. (a) Convergent position of the left eye (L) with uncrossed images. The right eye (R) is the leading eye, and the left eye is esotropic. The visual image falling on the fovea in the leading eye falls on the nasal retina next to the fovea (P_L) in the esotropic eye and is perceived in space in a temporal location. The object is seen as two uncrossed or homonymous images. **(b)** Divergent positon of the left eye (L) with crossed images. The right eye (R) is the leading eye, and the left eye is exotropic. The visual image falling on the fovea in the leading eye falls on the temporal retina next to the fovea (P_L) in the exotropic eye and is perceived in space in a nasal location. The object is seen as two crossed or heteronymous images.

stairs). Compensatory head posture is discussed in the section on symptoms (see p. 312). Diplopia is absent in elevation.

▶ **Oculomotor nerve palsy**

▶ **Causes.** The causes oculomotor nerve palsy are mainly diseases of the vascular system, e.g., aneurysms and other vascular processes.

▶ **Effects**

- Complete oculomotor nerve palsy. *Every intraocular and almost every extraocular muscle* is affected, with loss of both accommodation and pupillary light reaction. The failure of the parasympathetic fibers in the oculomotor nerve produces mydriasis. Ptosis is present because the levator palpebrae is also paralyzed. The paralyzed eye deviates in extorsion and depression as the function of the lateral rectus and superior oblique is preserved. Patients do not experience diplopia because the ptotic eyelid covers the pupil.

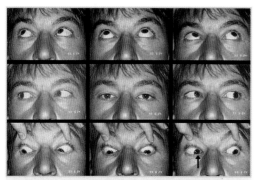

Fig. 17.17 Right trochlear nerve palsy. Vertical deviation of the right eye in left downward gaze (arrow).

- Partial oculomotor nerve palsy:
  - External oculomotor nerve palsy (isolated paralysis of the *extraocular* muscles supplied by the oculomotor nerve; see ▶ Table 17.1) is characterized by deviation in extorsion and depression. If the ptotic eyelid does not cover the pupil, the patient will experience diplopia.
  - Internal oculomotor nerve palsy is isolated paralysis of the *intraocular* muscles supplied by the oculomotor nerve. This is characterized by loss of accommodation (due to paralysis of the ciliary muscle) and mydriasis (due to paralysis of the sphincter pupillae). Patients do not experience diplopia as there is no strabismic deviation (see also Tonic Pupil and Adie's syndrome in Chapter 9.4.2).

17.5.5 Diagnosis of Ocular Motility Disorders

▶ **Examination of the nine diagnostic positions of gaze** (see ▶ Table 17.1). The patient is asked to follow the movements of the examiner's finger or a pencil with his or her eyes only. The six cardinal directions of gaze (right, upper right, lower right, left, upper left, lower left) provide the most information; upward and downward movements are performed with several muscles and therefore do not allow precise identification of the action of a specific muscle. Immobility of one eye when the patient attempts a certain movement suggests involvement of the muscle responsible for that movement.

▶ **Bielschowsky head tilt test.** This test is performed only where trochlear nerve palsy is suspected (see Symptoms in Chapter 17.5.3).

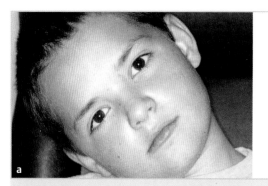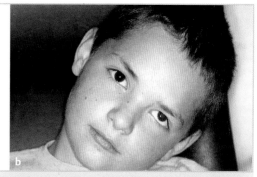

Fig. 17.18 Bielschowsky head tilt test (trochlear paresis left). (a) When the 8-year-old patient tilts his head to the right (toward the normal side), the left eye does not deviate upward when the normal right eye fixates. **(b)** When the patient tilts his head to the left (toward the side of the paralyzed muscle), the left eye deviates upward when the normal right eye fixates.

▶ **Measuring the angle of deviation.** Measuring this angle in the nine diagnostic directions of gaze provides information about the severity of the palsy, which is important for surgical correction. This is done using a Harms tangent table (▶ Fig. 17.19). In addition to the vertical and horizontal graduations of Maddox's cross, the Harms table also has diagonals. These diagonals permit the examiner to measure the angle of deviation even in patients with a compensatory head tilt, such as can occur in trochlear nerve palsy.

17.5.6 Differential Diagnosis

▶ Table 17.4 shows the most important differences between paralytic strabismus and concomitant strabismus.

17.5.7 Treatment of Ophthalmoplegia and Myogenic Motility Disorders

▶ **Surgery.** Surgery for paralytic strabismus should be postponed for at least 1 year to allow for possible spontaneous remission. Preoperative diagnostic studies to determine the exact cause are indicated to permit treatment of a possible underlying disorder, such as diabetes mellitus. In myogenic disorders as well, an attempt should first be made to treat the underlying disease (Graves's disease, myasthenia, etc.).

If double images are disturbing, it is possible to cover the paralyzed eye with a patch until the operation or to cover the eyeglass lens over the affected eye with Fresnel press-on prisms that will correct the angle of deviation and thus eliminate the double images, at least with a forward gaze. With

extreme strabismus, correction with Fresnel prisms is not possible.

If surgery is indicated, care must be taken to correctly *gauge the angle of deviation.* The goal of surgery is to eliminate diplopia in the normal visual field—i.e., with head erect, in both near and distance vision. It is usually not possible to surgically eliminate diplopia in the *whole* field of vision.

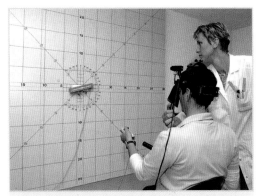

Fig. 17.19 Measuring the angle of deviation with the Harms tangent table. The patient sits at a distance of 2.5 meters from the table and fixates on the light in the center. The examiner evaluates the nine diagnostic positions of gaze. The grid provides the coordinates for measuring the horizontal and vertical deviations, and the diagonals are used to measure the angle of deviation at a head tilt of 45° (Bielschowsky head tilt test in trochlear nerve palsy). A small projector with positioning cross hairs mounted on the patient's forehead permits the examiner to determine the patient's head tilt with a relatively high degree of precision. The tilt of the image (paralytic strabismus often leads to image tilting) can also be measured with the Harms tangent table. To do so, the fixation light in the center of the table is spread into a band of light.

Table 17.4 Differential diagnosis between concomitant strabismus and paralytic strabismus

Differential criterion	Concomitant strabismus	Paralytic strabismus
Onset	At an early age, initially only periodically	At any age, sudden onset
Cause	Hereditary, uncorrected refractive error, perinatal injury	Disease of or injury to ocular muscles, supplying nerves, or nuclei
Diplopia	None; image suppressed (except in late strabismus with normal sensory development)	Diplopia is present
Compensatory head posture	Rare	Frequent
Depth perception	Not present	Only present when the patient assumes compensatory head posture (see Chapter 17.5.3)
Visual acuity	Unilaterally reduced visual acuity possible	No change in visual acuity
Angle of deviation	Constant in every direction of gaze	Variable, increasing in the direction of pull of the paralyzed muscle

▶ **Procedure.** The treatment of choice in paretic strabismus and myogenic disorders with limited contraction (e.g. myasthenia) is resection of the affected muscle(s). In pronounced paresis and paralysis, adjacent ocular muscles can be partly or entirely transposed to the insertion of the paralyzed muscles. In myogenic restriction of motility with (entrapment) or loss of elasticity (Graves's disease), recession of the affected muscles is the therapy of choice.

> **Note**
> Ocular muscle surgery for ophthalmoplegia is possible only after a 1-year regeneration period.

17.6 Nystagmus

> **Definition**
> • Nystagmus refers to bilateral involuntary rhythmic oscillation of the eyes, which can be jerky or pendular (jerk nystagmus and pendular nystagmus).

The various forms of nystagmus are listed in ▶ Table 17.5.

▶ **Treatment.** If nystagmus can be reduced by convergence, prisms with an outward-facing base may be prescribed. With good binocular vision, a convergence impulse can be released by ocular muscle surgery ("artificial divergence operation"). This calms the nystagmus. If nystagmus is inhibited in a specific gaze direction (and a compensatory head posture is assumed), both eyeballs can be surgically moved into parallel alignment (Kestenbaum's operation). This does not decrease the nystagmus, but in the best case its relative "resting position" is shifted to the forward gaze position so that at least the patient no longer assumes a compensatory head posture when looking straight ahead.

Table 17.5 Forms of nystagmus

Forms	Onset	Characteristics	Type of nystagmus
Ocular nystagmus	Congenital or acquired in early childhood	• Occurs in organic disorders of both eyes, such as albinism, cataract, color blindness, vitreous opacification, or macular scarring • Significant visual impairment • Secondary strabismus may also be present	• Pendular nystagmus
Congenital nystagmus	Congenital or acquired in early childhood (at the age of 3 months)	• Nystagmus is not curbed by fixation • Oscillation is usually horizontal • Intensity varies with the direction of gaze (compensatory head position) usually less in near fixation than in distance fixation	• Usually pendular nystagmus
Latent nystagmus	Congenital or acquired in early childhood	• Always associated with congenital strabismus • Manifested only by spontaneously uncovering one eye when fixation changes • Direction of oscillation changes when fixation changes	• Right oscillating nystagmus in right fixation • Left oscillating nystagmus in left fixation • Nystagmus occurs as jerk nystagmus
Fixation nystagmus	Acquired	• Occurs in disorders of the brainstem or cerebellum due to vascular insults, multiple sclerosis, trauma, or tumors	• Jerky form of oscillation

Chapter 18

Ocular Trauma

18 Ocular Trauma

Gerhard K. Lang

18.1 General Introductory Remarks

Eye injuries occur more often in combination with other injuries (in cases of polytrauma) than in isolation. Life-threatening injuries should always be treated before ophthalmologic treatment is started.

Definition
Life takes priority over vision. Eye injuries should be treated in patients who have been fully examined and stabilized.

18.2 Examination Methods

The incidence of ocular injuries is still high despite improved safety regulations in recent years, such as the mandatory use of seat belts and protective eyewear for persons operating high-speed rotating machinery. It is therefore important that every general practitioner and member of healthcare staff should be able to recognize an ocular injury and provide initial treatment. The patient should then be referred to an ophthalmologist, who should be solely responsible for evaluation of the injury and definitive treatment. The following diagnostic options are available to determine the nature of the injury more precisely.

▶ **Patient history.** Obtaining a thorough history will provide important information about the cause of the injury.

- Work with a hammer and chisel nearly always suggests an intraocular foreign body.
- Cutting and grinding work suggests corneal foreign bodies.
- Welding and flame-cutting work suggests ultraviolet keratoconjunctivitis.

Note
The examiner should always ascertain whether the patient has adequate tetanus immunization.

▶ **Inspection (gross morphological examination).** Ocular injuries frequently cause pain, photophobia, and blepharospasm. A few drops of topical anesthetic are recommended to allow the injured eye to be examined at rest with minimal pain to the patient. The cornea and conjunctiva are then examined for signs of trauma using a focused light, preferably one combined with a magnifying loupe (see ▶ Fig. 1.7 for examination technique). The eyelids can be everted to inspect the tarsal surface and conjunctival fornix. A foreign body can then be removed immediately.

▶ **Ophthalmoscopy.** Examination with a focused light or ophthalmoscope will allow gross evaluation of deeper intraocular structures, such as whether a vitreous or retinal hemorrhage is present. Vitreous hemorrhage can be identified by the lack of red reflex on retroillumination. Care should be taken to avoid unnecessary manipulation of the eye in an obviously severe open-globe injury (characterized by a soft globe, pupil displaced toward the penetration site, prolapsed iris, and intraocular bleeding in the anterior chamber and vitreous body). Such manipulation might otherwise cause further damage, such as extrusion of intraocular contents.

Note
To properly estimate the urgency of treating palpebral and ocular trauma, it is particularly important to differentiate between open-globe injuries (see p. 326) and closed-globe injuries (see p. 325). Open-globe injuries have highest priority due to the risk of losing the eye.

18.3 Classification of Ocular Injuries by Mechanism of Injury

- **Mechanical injuries**
  - Eyelid injuries.
  - Injuries to the lacrimal system.
  - Conjunctival laceration.
  - Foreign body in the cornea and conjunctiva.
  - Corneal erosion.
  - Nonpenetrating injury (blunt trauma to the globe).
  - Injury to the floor of the orbit (blow-out fracture).
  - Penetrating injury (open-globe injury).
  - Impalement injury to the orbit.
- **Chemical injuries**

- **Injuries due to physical agents**
  - Burns.
  - Radiation injuries (ionizing radiation).
  - Ultraviolet keratoconjunctivitis.
- **Indirect ocular trauma.** Transient traumatic retinal angiopathy (Purtscher's retinopathy).

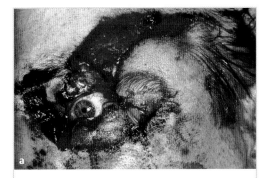

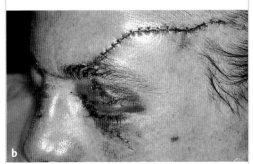

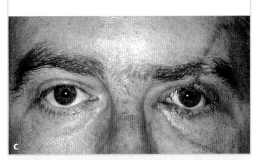

Fig 18.1 Laceration of the upper and lower eyelids with avulsion of the lacrimal system. **(a)** The injury has exposed the cornea. The patient is unable to close the eye, and the cornea and conjunctiva can no longer be moistened. During transport to the hospital, the first responder *must* create a moist environment (a gauze sponge dipped in saline solution) to prevent desiccation **(b)** Postoperative findings. **(c)** The findings 2 months postoperatively after the wound had been treated with placement of a plastic stent (see also ▶ Fig. 18.3 for surgical technique).

18.4 Mechanical Injuries

18.4.1 Eyelid Injury

▶ **Etiology.** Eyelid injuries can occur in practically every facial injury. The following types warrant special mention:

- Eyelid lacerations with involvement of the eyelid margin.
- Avulsions of the eyelid in the medial canthus with avulsion of the lacrimal canaliculus.

▶ **Clinical picture.** The highly vascularized and loosely textured tissue of the eyelids causes them to bleed profusely when injured. Hematoma and swelling will be severe (▶ Fig. 18.1). *Abrasions* usually involve only the superficial layers of the skin, whereas *punctures*, *cuts*, and all *eyelid avulsions due to blunt trauma* (such as a fist) frequently involve all layers. Bite wounds (such as dog bites) are often accompanied by injuries to the lacrimal system.

▶ **Treatment.** Surgical repair of eyelid injuries, especially lacerations with involvement of the eyelid margin, should be performed with care. The wound should be closed in layers and the edges properly approximated to ensure a smooth margin without tension to avoid later complications, such as cicatricial ectropion (▶ Fig. 18.2). Lid swellings are best treated by cold compresses (ice-pack).

18.4.2 Injuries to the Lacrimal System

▶ **Etiology.** Lacerations and tears in the medial canthus (such as dog bites or glass splinters) can divide the **lacrimal duct**. Obliteration of the **punctum**

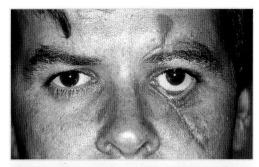

Fig. 18.2 Cicatricial ectropion in the left lower eyelid after incorrect repair. Failure to close the wound in layers without creating tension in the wound results in a scar that pulls the lower eyelid downward.

and **lacrimal canaliculus** is usually the result of a burn or chemical injury (see p. 328). Injury to the **lacrimal sac** or **lacrimal gland** usually occurs in conjunction with severe craniofacial trauma (such as a kick from a horse or a traffic accident). Dacryocystitis is a common sequela, which often can only be treated by surgery (dacryocystorhinostomy, see ▶ Fig. 3.10)

▶ **Clinical picture.** For **dacryocystitis** see Chapter 3.3, Disorders of the Lower Lacrimal System. ▶ Fig. 18.3a shows avulsion of the lower lacrimal system (avulsions in the medial canthus).

▶ **Treatment.** Lacrimal system injuries are repaired under an operating microscope. A ring-shaped silicone stent is advanced into the canaliculus using a special probe (▶ Fig. 18.3b,c). The silicone stent remains in situ for 3 to 4 months and is then removed.

> **Note**
> Surgical repair of eyelid and lacrimal system injuries must be performed by an ophthalmologist.

18.4.3 Conjunctival Laceration

▶ **Epidemiology.** Due to its exposed position, thinness, and mobility, the conjunctiva is susceptible to lacerations, which are usually associated with subconjunctival hemorrhage.

▶ **Etiology.** Conjunctival lacerations most commonly occur as a result of penetrating wounds (such as from bending over a spiked-leaf palm plant or from a branch that snaps back onto the eye).

▶ **Symptoms and diagnostic considerations.** The patient experiences a foreign-body sensation. Usually this will be rather mild. Examination will reveal circumscribed conjunctival reddening or subconjunctival hemorrhage in the injured area. Occasionally only application of fluorescein dye to the injury will reveal the size of the conjunctival gap.

▶ **Treatment.** Minor conjunctival injuries do not require treatment as the conjunctiva heals quickly. Larger lacerations with mobile edges are closed with absorbable sutures.

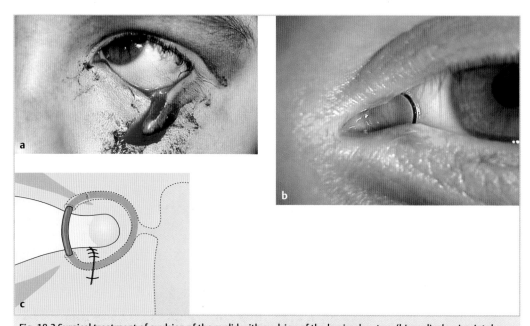

Fig. 18.3 Surgical treatment of avulsion of the eyelid with avulsion of the lacrimal system (bicanalicular ring intubation). (a) The findings before treatment of the wound. **(b)** Appearance after wound care. **(c)** Appearance after wound care (schematic).

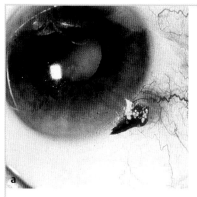
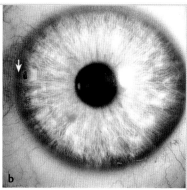
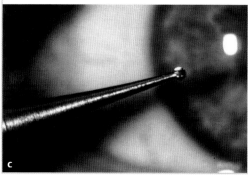

Fig. 18.4 Corneal and conjunctival foreign bodies and the reamer used to remove them. **(a)** A conjunctival foreign body (a grain kernel that has become caught) on the limbus of the cornea, with conjunctival injection. **(b)** A foreign body that has burned its way into the cornea. When the patient was using a grinder without protective eyewear the previous day, a splinter flew into the eye (arrow), which now exhibits a slight halo of visible infiltration. The conjunctival and ciliary injection at the site of the foreign body should be noted (see also ▶ Fig. 4.6). **(c)** The drill used to ream out the defect created by the foreign body.

Note
The possibility of a perforating injury should always be considered in conjunctival injuries. When the wound is treated, the physician should inspect the underlying sclera after application of topical anesthetic.

18.4.4 Corneal and Conjunctival Foreign Bodies

▶ **Epidemiology.** Foreign bodies on the cornea and conjunctiva are the commonest ocular emergency encountered by general practitioners and ophthalmologists.

▶ **Etiology.** Airborne foreign bodies and metal splinters from grinding or cutting disks in particular often become lodged in the conjunctiva or cornea or burn their way into the tissue.

▶ **Symptoms and diagnostic considerations.** The patient experiences a foreign-body sensation with every blink of the eye. This is accompanied by epiphora (tearing) and blepharospasm. Depending

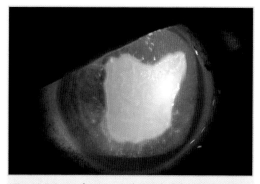

Fig. 18.5 Corneal erosion. The epithelial defect in the cornea is readily visible when the eye is examined with blue light after administration of fluorescein sodium dye.

on the time elapsed since the injury—i.e., after a few hours or several days—conjunctival or ciliary injection will be present (▶ Fig. 18.4a,b). The foreign bodies on the conjunctiva or cornea are themselves often so small that they are visible only under loupe magnification. There may be visible infiltration or a ring of rust. Where there is *no* visible foreign body but fluorescein dye reveals vertical corneal striations, the foreign body will be attached to the tarsus (see ▶ Fig. 5.15).

Note

A foreign-body sensation with every blink of the eye accompanied by epiphora, blepharospasm, and vertical striations on the surface of the cornea are typical signs of a subtarsal foreign body.

▶ **Treatment**

▶ **Corneal and conjunctival foreign bodies.** The foreign body is prised out of its bed with a fine needle or cannula. The defect created by the foreign body will often be contaminated with rust or infiltrated with leukocytes. This defect is carefully reamed out with a drill (▶ Fig. 18.4c) and treated with an antibiotic eye ointment and bandaged if necessary.

▶ **Subtarsal foreign bodies.** Everting the upper and lower eyelids will usually reveal the foreign body, which may then be removed with a moist cotton swab. An antibiotic eye bandage is placed until the patient is completely free of symptoms.

18.4.5 Corneal Erosion

▶ **Etiology.** This disorder follows initial **trauma** to the surface cornea, such as from the fingernail of a child carried in the parent's arms, a spiked-leaf palm plant, or a branch that snaps back onto the eye. Properly treated, this epithelial defect usually heals within a short time—i.e., 24 to 48 hours depending on the size of the defect. However, *occasionally* the epithelial cells do not properly adhere to Bowman's layer so that the epithelium repeatedly ruptures at the site of the initial injury even after weeks and months. This characteristically

Table 18.1 Overview of possible injuries resulting from blunt trauma to the globe

Description of injury	Definition	Sequelae	Treatment
Iridodialysis	Avulsion of the root of the iris	• Loss of pupillary roundness • Increased glare • Optical impairment results if there is a large gap at the palpebral fissure leading to a "double pupil"	Suture of the base of the iris is indicated for severe injuries (patient has two pupils due to severe avulsion; see ▶ Fig. 18.6). Other cases do not require treatment
Traumatic aniridia	Total avulsion of the iris	Patient suffers from increased glare	• Sunglasses • Where a simultaneous cataract is present, a black prosthetic lens with an optical aperture the size of the pupil is inserted during cataract surgery
Recession of the angle	Widening of the angle of the anterior chamber	Late sequela: secondary glaucoma	See Chapter 10
Cyclodialysis	Avulsion of the ciliary body from the sclera	• Intraocular hypotonia with choroidal folds and optic disc edema • Visual impairment	The ciliary body must be reattached with sutures to prevent phthisis bulbi (shrinkage of the eyeball)
Subluxation of the lens	Avulsion of the zonule fibers	• Dislocation of the lens and iridodonesis • Decreased visual acuity	Removal of the lens and implantation of a prosthetic lens; see Chapter 7.5
Vitreous detachment	Separation of the base of the vitreous body	Patient sees floaters (see Chapter 11)	See Chapter 11.3
Oradialysis	Avulsion of the peripheral retina (ora serrata)	Retinal detachment resulting in flashes of light, shadows, and blindness	Retinal surgery; see ▶ Fig. 12.27
Sphincter tear	Tear in the sphincter pupillae with elongation of the iris	Traumatic mydriasis or impaired pupillary function may be present	Sunglasses are indicated. Otherwise, no treatment is possible; if cataract surgery is necessary, pupil constriction by means of iris constriction suture is possible

Table 18.1 Overview of possible injuries resulting from blunt trauma to the globe (continued)

Description of injury	Definition	Sequelae	Treatment
Contusion rosette	Traumatic lens opacity (traumatic cataract)	• Rosette-shaped subcapsular opacity on the anterior surface of the lens, which with time migrates into the deeper cortex due to the apposition of lens fibers yet otherwise remains unchanged • Patient suffers from gradually increasing loss of visual acuity	Opacity in the optical center is routinely an indication for surgery (for details of surgery see Chapter 7, ► Fig. 7.19)
Berlin's edema	Retinal and macular edema at the posterior pole of the globe (contrecoup location) possibly associated with bleeding	Loss of visual acuity	Watch-and-wait approach is advised until swelling recedes
Choroidal ruptures	Crescentic concentric choroidal tears around the head of the optic nerve	Tears that extend through the macula can result in decreased visual acuity	No treatment is possible. Watch-and-wait approach is advised until scarring develops
Traumatic retino-choroido-pathy	Choroidal and retinal atrophy due to avulsion or impingement of the short posterior ciliary arteries	Loss of visual acuity	No treatment is possible
Avulsion of the globe	Traumatic avulsion of the globe out of the orbit, frequently associated with avulsion of the optic nerve (see next row)	Immediate blindness	Enucleation
Avulsion of the optic nerve	Avulsion of the entire optic nerve at its point of entry into the globe	Immediate blindness	The separation of the nerve fibers is irreversible
Injury to the optic nerve	Possible injuries include: • Hematoma of the optic nerve sheath • Optic nerve contusion • Fracture of the optic nerve canal	Atrophy of the optic nerve with loss of visual acuity and visual field defects	No treatment is possible
Retrobulbar hematoma	Injury to retrobulbar vascular structures	• Orbital bleeding • Eyelid hematoma • Exophthalmos	• Wait for blood to be absorbed • Surgery is indicated only when the central retinal artery is occluded by pressure
Hyphema	Bleeding into the anterior cavity	Patient has blurred vision	• Patient should assume an upright posture to allow blood to settle. This will restore vision • Hyphema will resolve spontaneously
Vitreous hemorrhage	Bleeding into the vitreous chamber	• Identified by the lack of red reflex on retroillumination during ophthalmoscopy • Loss of visual acuity	Wait for spontaneous recession (always keep in mind retinal detachment with bleeding from a torn retina)
Orbital fracture (blow-out fracture)	Fracture of the floor of the orbit with displacement into the maxillary sinus	• Diplopia in the affected eye • Elevation or depression deficit	• Patient should refrain from blowing his or her nose if paranasal sinuses are involved (crepitus upon palpation) • Surgical repair of the orbital floor and release of impinged orbital contents

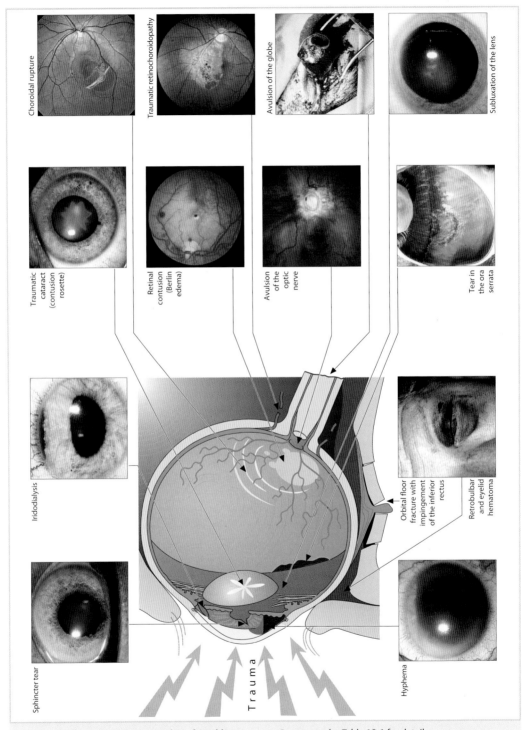

Choroidal rupture

Traumatic retinochoroidopathy

Avulsion of the globe

Subluxation of the lens

Traumatic cataract (contusion rosette)

Retinal contusion (Berlin edema)

Avulsion of the optic nerve

Tear in the ora serrata

Iridodialysis

Orbital floor fracture with impingement of the inferior rectus

Retrobulbar and eyelid hematoma

Sphincter tear

Trauma

Hyphema

Fig. 18.6 Possible ocular injuries resulting from blunt trauma. See text and ▸ Table 18.1 for details.

occurs in the morning when the patient wakes up and suddenly opens his or her eyes. This **recurring erosion** often creates severe emotional stress for the patient.

▶ **Symptoms and diagnostic considerations.** Immediately after the injury, the patient experiences a severe foreign-body sensation associated with tearing. Because there is actually a defect in the *surface* of the cornea, the patient has the subjective sensation of a foreign body *within* the eye. The epithelial defect causes severe pain, which immediately elicits a blepharospasm. Additional symptoms associated with corneal erosion include immediate eyelid swelling and conjunctival injection. Fluorescein sodium dye will readily reveal the corneal defect when the eye is examined through a blue light (▶ Fig. 18.5).

▶ **Treatment.** Application of a dressing with antibiotic ointment or treatment of the eye with a therapeutic contact lens and additional antibiotic eye drops.

Note
Treatment of recurrent corneal erosion often requires hospitalization. Bilateral bandages are placed to ensure that the eyes are completely immobilized. Photorefractive keratectomy (PRK) and corneal anterior stromal micropuncture are additional treatment options.

18.4.6 Blunt Ocular Trauma (Ocular Contusion)

▶ **Epidemiology and etiology.** Ocular contusions resulting from blunt trauma such as from a fist, ball, champagne cork, or stone, or a fall onto the eye, are very common. Less common, but no less severe, is trauma caused by animals, for example a blow from a cow's horn. Significant deformation of the globe can result where the diameter of the blunt object is less than that of the bony structures of the orbit.

▶ **Clinical picture and diagnostic considerations.** Deformation exerts significant traction on intraocular structures and can cause them to tear. Often there will be blood in the anterior chamber, which will initially prevent the examiner from evaluating the more posterior intraocular structures.

Note
Do not administer medications that act on the pupil as there is a risk of irreversible mydriasis from a sphincter tear, and pupillary movements increase the risk of subsequent bleeding. The posterior intraocular structures should only be thoroughly examined in mydriasis to determine the extent of injury after a week to 10 days.

Common injuries are listed in ▶ Table 18.1 and ▶ Fig. 18.6.
Late sequelae of blunt ocular trauma include:

- Secondary glaucoma.
- Retinal detachment.
- Cataract.

Note
Late sequelae of blunt ocular trauma may occur years after the injury.

▶ **Treatment.** Treatment involves immobilizing the eye initially, to allow intraocular blood to settle. See ▶ Table 18.1 for details.

Note
Subsequent bleeding 3 to 4 days after the injury is common.

18.4.7 Blow-Out Fracture

▶ **Etiology.** Blow-out fractures of the orbit result from blunt trauma. Blunt objects of small diameter, such as a fist, tennis ball, or baseball, can compress the contents of the orbit so severely that the orbital wall fractures. This fracture usually occurs where the bone is thinnest, *along the paper-thin floor of the orbit over the maxillary sinus*. The ring-shaped bony orbital rim usually remains intact. The fracture can result in protrusion and impingement of orbital fat and the inferior rectus and its sheaths in the fracture gap. Where the *medial ethmoid wall* fractures instead of the orbital floor, emphysema in the eyelids will result.

▶ **Symptoms and diagnostic considerations.** The more severe the contusion, the more severe the intraocular injuries and resulting visual impairment will be. Impingement of the inferior rectus can result in **diplopia**, especially in upward gaze. Initially, the diplopia may go unnoticed when the eye is still swollen shut. A large bone defect may result in displacement of larger portions of the contents of the orbital cavity. The eye may recede into the orbit (**enophthalmos**) and the **palpebral fissure may narrow**. Injury to the infraorbital nerve, which runs along the floor of the orbit, may result. This can cause **hypesthesia of the facial skin**.

Crepitus upon palpation during examination of the eyelid swelling is a sign of emphysema due to collapse of the ethmoidal air cells. The crepitus is caused by air entering the orbit from the paranasal sinuses. The patient should refrain from blowing his or her nose for the next 4 to 5 days to avoid forcing air or germs into the orbit. Radiographs should be obtained and an ear, nose, and throat specialist consulted to help determine the **exact location of the fracture.** CT studies are more precise and may be indicated to evaluate difficult cases.

In rare cases of extreme orbital trauma and usually complete bursting of the eyeball (fall onto bicycle handlebars, eye injury by fireworks rocket), there can be fractures of the more stable orbital roof.

> **Note**
> Tissue displaced into the maxillary sinus will resemble a hanging drop of water in the CT image.

▶ **Treatment.** Surgery to restore normal anatomy and the integrity of the orbit should be performed within 10 days. This minimizes the risk of irreversible damage from scarring of the impinged inferior rectus. Where treatment is prompt, the prognosis is good (see Chapter 15.8, Orbital Surgery).

> **Note**
> Tetanus prophylaxis and treatment with antibiotics are crucial.

18.4.8 Open-Globe Injuries

▶ **Etiology.** Together with severe chemical injuries, open-globe injuries are the most devastating forms of ocular trauma. They are caused by sharp objects that penetrate the cornea and sclera. A distinction is made between penetration with and without an intraocular foreign body. However, even blunt trauma can cause an open-globe injury in an eye weakened by previous surgery or injury where extremely high-energy forces are involved

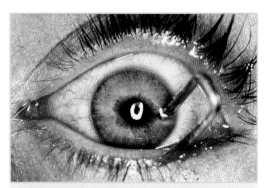

Fig. 18.7 Penetrating injury. An open-globe injury by a staple, involving the cornea, iris, lens, sclera, and retina.

(such as falling onto a stick or a blow from a squash ball).

▶ **Clinical picture and diagnostic considerations.** Penetrating injuries cover the entire spectrum of clinical syndromes. Symptoms can range from massive penetration of the cornea and sclera (▶ Fig. 18.7) with loss of the anterior chamber to tiny, nearly invisible injuries that close spontaneously. The latter may include a fine penetrating wound or the entry wound of a foreign body. Depending on the severity of the injury, the patient's visual acuity may be severely compromised or not influenced at all.

One of the most common sequelae is a **traumatic cataract**. The rupture in the lens capsule allows aqueous humor to penetrate, causing the lens to swell. This results in lens opacification of varying severity. Large defects will lead to total opacification of the lens within hours or a few days. Smaller defects that close spontaneously often cause a circumscribed opacity. Typically, penetration results in a rosette-shaped anterior or posterior subcapsular opacity.

Depending on the severity of the injury, the following **diagnostic signs** will be present in an open-globe injury:

• The anterior chamber will be shallow or absent.
• The pupil will be displaced toward the penetration site.
• Swelling of the lens will be present (traumatic cataract).
• There will be bleeding in the anterior chamber and vitreous cavity.
• Hypotonia of the globe will be present.

The rupture of the lens capsule and vitreous hemorrhage often render examination difficult as they

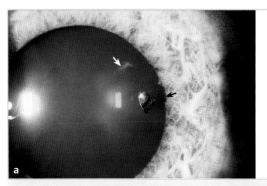
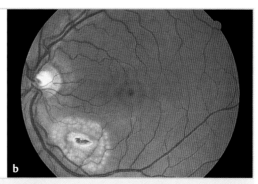

Fig. 18.8 Intraocular foreign body sustained while working with a hammer and chisel. (a) An iron splinter has caught in the lens; the cornea closed spontaneously immediately after the injury (white arrow). A sphincter injury is also present (black arrow). (b) The iron splinter has entered through the sclera and is now lodged in the retina on the posterior wall of the globe, which it has "coagulated" (white discoloration of the surrounding retinal tissue). Focal burns are placed around the foreign body with an argon laser to fix the retina before a vitrectomy is performed to remove the foreign body.

prevent direct inspection. These cases, as well as tentative diagnosis of an intraocular foreign body (see p. 318), based on information in the medical history, require one or both of the following diagnostic imaging studies:

- Radiographs in two planes to determine whether there is a foreign body in the eye.
- CT examinations, which allow precise localization of the foreign body and can also image radiolucent foreign bodies such as Plexiglas.

Note
An injury sustained while working with a hammer and chisel suggests an intraocular foreign body. The diagnosis can be confirmed by examining the fundus in mydriasis and obtaining radiographic images.

▶ **Treatment**
▶ **First aid.** Where penetrating trauma is suspected, a sterile bandage should be applied and the patient referred to an eye clinic for treatment. Tetanus immunization or prophylaxis and prophylactic antibiotic treatment are indicated as a matter of course.

▶ **Surgery.** Surgical treatment of penetrating injuries must include suturing the globe and reconstructing the anterior chamber. Any extruded intraocular tissue (such as the iris) must be removed. Intraocular foreign bodies (▶ Fig. 18.8) should be removed when the wound is repaired (i.e., by vitrectomy and extraction of the foreign body).

▶ **Late sequelae**
- **Improper reconstruction of the anterior chamber** may lead to adhesions between the iris and the angle of the anterior chamber, resulting in secondary angle closure glaucoma.
- A **retinal injury** (for example at the site of the impact of the foreign body) can lead to retinal detachment.
- Failure to remove **iron foreign bodies** can lead to ocular siderosis, which causes irreparable damage to the receptors and may manifest itself years later.
- **Copper foreign bodies** cause severe inflammatory reactions in the eye (ocular chalcosis) within a few hours. Symptoms range from uveitis and hypopyon to phthisis bulbi (shrinkage and hypotonia of the eyeball).
- **Organic foreign bodies** (such as wood) in the eye lead to fulminant endophthalmitis.

18.4.9 Impalement Injuries in the Orbit

▶ **Etiology.** Impalement injuries occur most frequently in situations such as the following:

- Children may fall on pencils held in their hands (▶ Fig. 18.9).
- Injuries may result from the actions of other persons (such as arrows or darts).
- A knife may slip while a butcher or cook is removing a bone from a cut of meat.

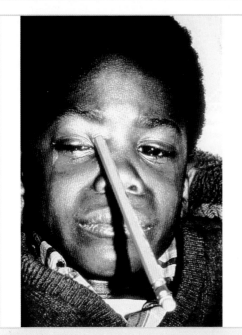

Fig. 18.9 Impalement injury in the right orbit. Orbital injury without injury to the globe following a fall on a pencil the patient was holding in his hand. (Photograph courtesy of Professor W.R. Green, MD, Baltimore, Maryland, USA.)

Often the impaling "stake" will glance off the round hard outer layer of the globe (*cornea and sclera*) and lodge in the soft tissue of the orbit.

▶ **Symptoms and diagnostic considerations.** The stake can cause displacement of the globe. Often there will be minimal bleeding in the surrounding tissue. Diagnostic studies used to ascertain possible damage to intraocular structures include ophthalmoscopy, radiography, and ultrasonography.

▶ **Treatment.** First aid treatment should leave the stake in situ. Removing the stake could cause severe bleeding and orbital hematoma. If necessary, the stake should be stabilized before the patient is transported to an eye hospital. Once the patient is in the hospital, the foreign body is removed from the orbit and the integrity of the globe is verified, depending on specific findings. Any bleeding is controlled. Prophylactic antibiotic treatment is indicated routinely to minimize the risk of orbital cellulitis (see p. 263).

18.5 Chemical Injuries

▶ **Etiology.** Chemical injuries can be caused by a variety of substances such as acids, alkalis, detergents, solvents, adhesives, and irritants such as tear gas and pepper spray. The severity can range from slight irritation of the eye to total blindness.

Note
Chemical injuries are among the most dangerous ocular injuries. First aid at the site of the accident is crucial to minimize the risk of severe sequelae such as blindness.

As a general rule, acid burns are less dangerous than alkali burns. This is because most acids do not act deeply. **Acids** differ from alkalis in that they cause immediate *coagulation necrosis* in the superficial tissue. This has the effect of preventing the acid from penetrating deeper so that the burn is effectively a self-limiting process. However, some acids penetrate deeply like alkalis and cause similarly severe injuries. Concentrated sulfuric acid (such as from an exploding car battery) draws water out of tissue and simultaneously develops intense heat that affects every layer of the eye. Hydrofluoric acid and nitric acid have a similar penetrating effect.

Alkalis differ from most acids in that they can penetrate by hydrolyzing structural proteins and dissolving cells. This is referred to as *liquefactive necrosis*. They then cause severe intraocular damage by alkalizing the aqueous humor.

▶ **Symptoms.** Epiphora, blepharospasm, and severe pain are the primary symptoms. Acid burns usually cause immediate loss of visual acuity due to the superficial necrosis. In alkali injuries, loss of visual acuity *often* manifests itself only several days later.

▶ **Clinical picture and diagnostic considerations.** Proper diagnosis of the cause and severity of the burn is crucial to treatment and prognosis.

Note
Alkali burns can appear less severe initially than acid burns, but they may lead to blindness.

Morphological findings and the resulting prognosis can vary greatly depending on the severity and duration of exposure to the caustic agent. This information is summarized in ▶ Table 18.2.

▶ **Treatment.** First aid rendered at the scene of the accident often decides the fate of the eye. The first few seconds and minutes and resolute action by persons at the scene are crucial. Immediate copious irrigation of the eye can be performed with any watery solution of neutral pH, such as tap water, mineral water, soft drinks, coffee, tea, or similar liquids. Milk should be avoided as it increases the penetration of the burn by opening the epithelial barrier. A second person must rigorously restrain the severe blepharospasm to allow effective irrigation. A topical anesthetic to relieve the blepharospasm will rarely be available at the scene of the accident. Coarse particles (such as lime particles in a lime injury) should be flushed and removed from the eye. Only after these actions have been taken should the patient be brought to an ophthalmologist or eye hospital.

▶ **Chronology of treatment of chemical injuries**
- **First aid at the scene of the accident (coworkers or family members):**
  ○ Restrain blepharospasm by rigorously holding the eyelids open.
  ○ Irrigate the eye within seconds of the injury using tap water, mineral water, soft drinks, coffee, tea, or similar liquids. Carefully remove coarse particles from the conjunctival sac.
  ○ Notify emergency services at the same time.

  ○ Transport the patient to the nearest ophthalmologist or eye clinic.
- **Treatment by the ophthalmologist or at the eye hospital:**
  ○ Administer topical anesthesia to relieve pain and neutralize blepharospasm.
  ○ With the upper and lower eyelids fully everted, carefully remove small particles such as residual lime from the superior and inferior conjunctival fornices under a microscope using a moist cotton swab.
  ○ Flush the eye with a buffer solution. Long-term irrigation using an irrigating contact lens may be indicated (the lens is connected to a cannula to irrigate the eye with a constant stream of liquid).
  ○ Initiate systemic pain therapy if indicated.
- **Additional treatment on the ward in an eye hospital.** The following therapeutic measures for severe chemical injuries are usually performed on the ward:
  ○ Continue irrigation.
  ○ Initiate topical cortisone therapy (dexamethasone 0.1% eye drops and prednisolone 1% eye drops).
  ○ Administer subconjunctival steroids.
  ○ Immobilize the pupil with atropine 1% eye drops or scopolamine 0.25% eye drops twice daily.

Table 18.2 Findings in chemical injuries of various degrees of severity

Severity of the injury	Damage to the corneal epithelium	Damage to the conjunctiva	Damage to the corneal stroma	Intraocular involvement	Prognosis
Slight	• Superficial punctate keratitis • No corneal erosion	• Conjunctival epithelium largely intact • Slight chemosis (edematous conjunctival swelling) • Limbal vessels (palisades of Vogt) filled with blood	Clear	None	Good: healing without loss of function
Moderate to severe	Moderate to total corneal erosion	• Moderate chemosis • Segmental ischemia of the limbal vessels	Slightly opacified	Slight irritation of the anterior chamber (slight amount of cellular and protein exudate in the anterior chamber)	Defect healing with functional impairment and possibly symblepharon
Severe	Total corneal erosion including erosion of the conjunctival epithelium at the limbus	• Severe chemosis • Total ischemia of the limbal vessels	All layers are opacified ("cooked fish eye"; see ▶ Fig. 18.11)	• Severe irritation of the anterior chamber • Damage to the iris, lens, ciliary body, and angle of the anterior chamber	• Poor • Defect healing with functional impairment that may include loss of the eye • Symblepharon

○ Administer anti-inflammatory agents (two oral doses of 100 mg indomethacin or diclofenac) or 50 to 200 mg systemic prednisolone.

○ Administer oral and topical vitamin C to neutralize cytotoxic radicals.

○ Administer 500 mg of oral acetazolamide (Diamox) to reduce intraocular pressure as prophylaxis against secondary glaucoma.

○ Administer hyaluronic acid for corneal care to promote re-epithelialization and stabilize the physiologic barrier.

○ Administer topical antibiotic eye drops.

○ Carry out débridement of necrotic conjunctival and corneal tissue and make radial incisions in the conjunctiva (Passow's method) to drain the subconjunctival edema.

- **Additional surgical treatment in the presence of impaired wound healing following extremely severe chemical injuries:**
  ○ A *conjunctival and limbal transplantation* (stem cell transfer) can replace lost stem cells that are important for corneal healing. This will allow reepithelialization.

  ○ Where the cornea does not heal, an amnion membrane patch is fixed onto the cornea or cyanoacrylate glue can be used to attach a *hard contact lens* (artificial epithelium) to promote healing.

  ○ Tenon's capsuloplasty (mobilization and advancement of a flap of subconjunctival tissue of Tenon's capsule to cover defects) can help eliminate conjunctival and scleral defects.

- **Surgical treatment after the eye has stabilized.**
  ○ Lysis of symblepharon (symblepharon refers to adhesions between the palpebral and bulbar conjunctiva; see also prognosis and complications) to improve the motility of the globe and eyelids.

○ Plastic surgery of the eyelids to release the globe. Defects are covered with amniotic membrane. (This should only be performed 12 to 18 months after the injury.)

○ Where there is total loss of the goblet cells, transplantation of nasal mucosa usually relieves pain (the lack of mucus is substituted by goblet cells from the nasal mucosa).

○ Penetrating keratoplasty (see p. 88) can be performed to restore vision. Because the traumatized cornea is highly vascularized (▶ Fig. 18.10), these procedures are plagued by a high incidence of graft rejection. A clear cornea can rarely be achieved in a severely burned eye even with an HLA-typed corneal graft and immunosuppressive therapy.

▶ **Prognosis and possible complications.** The degree of ischemia of the conjunctiva and the limbal vessels is an indicator of the severity of the

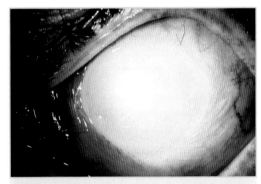

Fig. 18.11 **"Cooked fish eye" following alkali injury.** The cornea is as white as chalk and opaque. The vascular supply to the limbus (capillaries on the edge) has been obliterated.

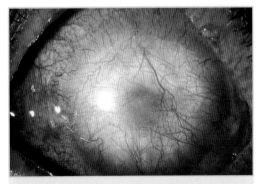

Fig. 18.10 **Lime injury.** Superficial and deep corneal vascularization is present, and the eye is dry due to loss of most of the goblet cells.

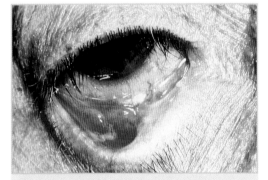

Fig. 18.12 **Symblepharon.** Moderate and severe chemical injuries can produce adhesions between the palpebral and bulbar conjunctiva.

injury and the prognosis for healing (see ▶ Table 18.2). The *greater the ischemia of the conjunctiva and limbal vessels, the more severe the burn will be.* The most severe form of chemical injury presents as a "**cooked fish eye**" (▶ Fig. 18.11), for which the prognosis is very poor—i.e., blindness is possible.

Moderate to severe chemical injuries involving the bulbar and palpebral conjunctiva can result in **symblepharon** (adhesions between the palpebral and bulbar conjunctiva; ▶ Fig.18.12). Inflammatory reactions in the anterior chamber secondary to chemical injuries can lead to **secondary glaucoma**.

18.6 Injuries Due to Physical Agents

18.6.1 Ultraviolet Keratoconjunctivitis

▶ **Etiology.** Injury from ultraviolet radiation can occur from welding without proper eye protection, from exposure to high-altitude sunlight with the eyes open without proper eye protection, or due to sunlight reflected off snow when skiing at high altitudes on a sunny day. Intense ultraviolet light can lead to ultraviolet keratoconjunctivitis within a short time (for example, just a few minutes of welding without proper eye protection). Ultraviolet radiation penetrates only slightly and therefore causes only superficial necrosis in the corneal epithelium. The exposed areas of the cornea and conjunctiva in the palpebral fissure become edematous, disintegrate, and are finally cast off.

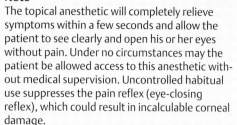

> **Note**
> Ultraviolet keratoconjunctivitis is one of the most common ocular injuries.

▶ **Symptoms and diagnostic considerations.** Symptoms typically manifest themselves after a latency period of 6–8 hours. This causes patients to seek the aid of an ophthalmologist or eye clinic in the middle of the night, complaining of "acute blindness" accompanied by pain, photophobia, epiphora, and an intolerable foreign-body sensation. Often severe blepharospasm will be present. Slit lamp examination will require administration of a topical anesthetic. This examination will reveal epithelial edema and superficial punctate keratitis or erosion in the palpebral fissure under fluorescein dye (see ▶ Fig. 18.5).

> **Note**
> The topical anesthetic will completely relieve symptoms within a few seconds and allow the patient to see clearly and open his or her eyes without pain. Under no circumstances may the patient be allowed access to this anesthetic without medical supervision. Uncontrolled habitual use suppresses the pain reflex (eye-closing reflex), which could result in incalculable corneal damage.

▶ **Treatment.** The "blinded" patient should be instructed that the symptoms will resolve completely under treatment with antibiotic ointment within 24 to 48 hours. Ointment is best applied to both eyes every 2 to 3 hours with the patient at rest in a darkened room. The patient should be informed that the eye ointment will not immediately relieve pain and that eye movements should be avoided. Therapeutic contact lenses are an additional option.

18.6.2 Burns

▶ **Etiology.** Flaring flames such as from a cigarette lighter, hot vapors, boiling water, and splatters of hot grease or hot metal cause thermal coagulation of the corneal and conjunctival surface. Because of the eye-closing reflex, the eyelids often will be affected as well.

Injuries due to explosion or burns from a starter's gun also include particles of burned powder (powder burns). Injuries from a gas pistol will also involve a chemical injury.

▶ **Symptoms and diagnostic considerations.** Symptoms are similar to those of chemical injuries (epiphora, blepharospasm, and pain).

A topical anesthetic is administered, and the eye is examined as in a chemical injury. *Immediate opacification of the cornea* will be readily apparent. This is due to scaling of the epithelium and tissue necrosis, whose depth will vary with the severity of the burn. In burns from metal splinters, one will often find cooled metal particles embedded in the cornea.

▶ **Treatment.** Initial treatment consists of applying cooling antiseptic bandages to relieve pain, after which necrotic areas of the skin, conjunctiva, and cornea are removed under local anesthesia. Foreign particles such as **embedded ash and smoke particles in the eyelids and facial area** are removed in cooperation with a dermatologist by brushing them out with a sterile toothbrush under general anesthesia. This is done to prevent them from growing into the skin like a tattoo. **Superficial particles in the cornea and conjunctiva** are removed under local anesthesia together with the necrotic tissue. The affected areas are then treated with an antibiotic ointment.

▶ **Prognosis.** The clinical course of a burn is usually less severe than that of a chemical injury. This is because burns, like acid injuries, cause superficial coagulation. Usually they heal well when treated with antibiotic ointment.

18.6.3 Radiation Injuries (Ionizing Radiation)

▶ **Etiology.** Ionizing radiation (neutrons, gamma-rays, or X-rays) has high energy that can cause ionization and formation of radicals in cellular tissue. The penetration depth in the eye varies with the type of radiation—i.e., the wavelength—resulting in characteristic types of tissue damage (▶ Fig. 18.13). This tissue damage always manifests itself after a latency period, often only after a period of years (see also Symptoms and clinical picture). Common sites include the lens (radiation cataract) and retina (radiation retinopathy). This tissue damage is usually the result of tumor irradiation in the eye or nasopharynx. Radiation disorders have been observed in patients from Hiroshima and Nagasaki and, more recently, in those from Chernobyl and Fukushima.

▶ **Symptoms and clinical picture.** Loss of the eyelashes and eyelid pigmentation accompanied by blepharitis are typical symptoms. A dry eye is a sign of damage to the conjunctival epithelium (loss of the goblet cells). Loss of visual acuity due to a radiation cataract is usually observed within 1 to 2 years of the irradiation. Radiation retinopathy in the form of ischemic retinopathy with bleeding, cotton-wool spots, vascular occlusion, and retinal neovascularization usually occurs within months of irradiation.

▶ **Treatment and prophylaxis.** Care should be taken to cover the eyes prior to planned radiation therapy in the head and neck. Radiation cataract can be treated surgically. Radiation retinopathy can be treated with panretinal photocoagulation with an argon laser.

18.7 Indirect Ocular Trauma

18.7.1 Purtscher's Retinopathy

▶ **Etiology.** Arterial and venous circulatory disruption in the retina characterized by a sudden increase in intravascular pressure may occur following severe chest injuries (compression trauma such as in a seat-belt injury) or fractures of long bones (presumably due to fat embolisms or vascular spasms).

▶ **Symptoms and diagnostic considerations.** Acute retinal ischemia with impaired vision and loss of visual acuity will occur either immediately or within 3 to 4 days of the injury. Examination of the fundus will reveal cotton-wool spots and intraretinal bleeding indicative of focal retinal ischemia. Lines of bleeding will also be observed.

▶ **Treatment.** Fundus symptoms will usually disappear spontaneously within 4 to 6 weeks. Reduced visual acuity and visual field defects may occasionally persist. Occasionally treatment is attempted with high doses of systemic steroids and prostaglandin inhibitors.

18.7.2 High-Altitude Retinopathy

▶ **Etiology.** Increased concentrations of hematocrit and hemoglobin are frequent findings in high-altitude climbers. They are caused by excessive fluid loss (up to 8 liters of water a day) as a result of the required moistening of the extremely dry, cold air that is breathed and due to sweating (as a result of strenuous climbing).

Raised hematocrit levels and hypoxia are dangerous for climbers, as they lead to:

• Altitude sickness (dizziness, disorientation).
• Cerebral edema.

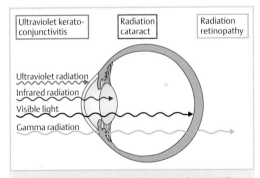

Fig. 18.13 Possible radiation damage to the eye. The penetration depth of radiation in the eye varies depending on its wavelength. Any radiation injury therefore causes characteristic tissue damage.

- Pulmonary edema.
- Thromboembolism.
- High-altitude retinopathy.

▶ **Symptoms.** Bilateral intraretinal hemorrhage with loss of vision and scotomas.

▶ **Treatment and prophylaxis.** Normalization of hematocrit and hemoglobin readings with isovolu-metric hemodilution and treatment with pentoxi-fylline.

Appropriate training for high-altitude exercise includes practicing climbing and descending stages beforehand and ensuring the required fluid intake. As extremely high altitudes can compromise the microcirculation, prophylactic hemodilution after a descent may be able to prevent the high-altitude complications listed above.

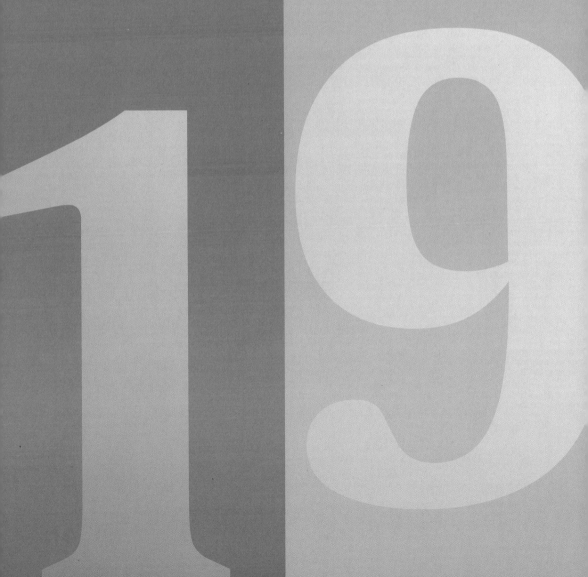

Chapter 19

Cardinal Symptoms

19 Cardinal Symptoms

Stefan Lang and Gerhard K. Lang

The following list of cardinal symptoms (▸ Table 19.1) is included to provide the medical student, intern, or ophthalmology resident with a concise overview of the range of possible underlying clinical syndromes. This compilation of cardinal symptoms cannot and does not represent a complete and comprehensive listing. However, it may be helpful for recalling the most important clinical pictures in ophthalmology and providing a review of the material. The page references indicate where individual topics are discussed in detail.

Table 19.1 Cardinal symptoms, associated symptoms/findings, tentative diagnosis, and diagnostic work-up

Cardinal symptoms	Possible associated symptoms and findings	Tentative diagnosis	Further diagnostic work-up
Burning sensation and	• Reddening of the eyelids • Adhesion of the eyelashes • Scales on the eyelids and bases of the eyelashes • Itchy eyelid margins • Common in fair-haired patients	**Common:** • Blepharitis (see p. 20) • *Demodex folliculorum*	Exclude refractive anomaly as possible cause
	• Sensation of pressure, dryness, and sand in the eyes • Occasionally excessive tearing in response to dry eyes • Dryness of other mucous membranes	• Dry eyes (keratoconjunctivitis sicca) (see p. 40) • Sjögren's syndrome	Evaluate tear secretion with Schirmer tear testing and tear break-up time (TBUT)
	• Reddened conjunctiva • Purulent, mucoid, or watery discharge • Sticky eyelids in the morning	• Conjunctivitis (see p. 49) • Epidemic keratoconjunctivitis (see p. 56)	Obtain smear for microbiological examination. Hygiene: risk of contagion
	• Usually segmental, livid reddening of the conjunctiva. • Nodular mobile swelling that is tender to palpation	**Rare:** • Episcleritis (see p. 97)	Unequivocal diagnosis
	• Circumscribed reddening at the pinguecula. • Thickened conjunctival vessels	• Irritated pinguecula (see p. 47)	Unequivocal diagnosis
	• Circumscribed reddening at the pterygium	• Irritated pterygium (see p. 47)	Unequivocal diagnosis
	• Reddening in the upper circumference near the limbus	• Keratitis of the upper limbus	Unequivocal diagnosis
Tearing (epiphora) and	• Buphthalmos • Increased glare and squinting • Unilateral or bilateral • Corneal opacification	**In children most likely:** • Congenital glaucoma (see p. 169)	**Risk of blindness!** Measure intraocular pressure immediately
	• Red eye • Severe foreign-body sensation • Pain causing blepharospasm • Photophobia • Eyelid swelling • Decreased visual acuity	• Subtarsal or corneal foreign body (see p. 322) • Corneal erosion (see p. 322)	• Full eversion of the eyelids to localize subtarsal foreign body • Apply fluorescein dye to evaluate cornea where corneal erosion is suspected

Table 19.1 Cardinal symptoms, associated symptoms/findings, tentative diagnosis, and diagnostic work-up (continued)

Cardinal symptoms	Possible associated symptoms and findings	Tentative diagnosis	Further diagnostic work-up
Tearing (epiphora) and	• No pain • Nearly constant purulent watery discharge • Sticky eyelids in the morning • No itching or reddening of the eye and no visible eyelid deformity	Dacryostenosis (valve of Hasner)	Irrigate lacrimal system to locate the stenosis
Tearing (painless or nearly painless) and	• Reddening of the conjunctiva • Ectropion develops from constantly wiping away tears • Epidermization of the exposed conjunctiva	• Ectropion (see p. 18)	Unequivocal diagnosis
	• Sandy, dry feeling • Eye often free of irritation • Oral, nasal, and genital mucous membranes often also dry	• Dry eyes • Dry eyes in conjunction with keratoconjunctivitis sicca (see p. 40)	Evaluate tear secretion with Schirmer tear testing and tear break-up time (TBUT)
Tearing (painless) and	• Purulent discharge of thickened tear fluid and pus is common (expressed from the punctum by pressing on the lacrimal sac) • Recurrent dacryocystitis	Obstructed drainage through the lower lacrimal system, possibly with inflammation (see p. 34)	Irrigate the lower lacrimal system to localize the stenosis
	• Clear tear fluid • Punctum is covered by connective tissue or projects from the eye	Obstruction or eversion of the punctum lacrimale	Unequivocal diagnosis
Tearing (painful) and	• Severe foreign-body sensation • Eyelid swelling • Blepharospasm and photophobia • Reddened eye • Decreased visual acuity	• Corneal erosion (see p. 322) • Subtarsal corneal foreign body (see p. 321)	• Apply fluorescein dye to evaluate cornea where corneal erosion is suspected • Evert eyelid to localize subtarsal corneal foreign body
	• Foreign-body sensation (eyelashes scratch cornea) • Inward deformity of the eyelashes, eyelid turned inward	Trichiasis, entropion (see p. 16)	Unequivocal diagnosis
Increased glare and	• Gray to white pupillary reflex • Gradual progressive loss of visual acuity	Cataract (see p. 105)	Slit lamp examination. Diagnosis is unequivocal where the opacity is visible under retroillumination
	• Wide pupil (mydriasis) • Little or no pupillary response to light • Pupil width is different from fellow eye	Traumatic or drug-induced paralysis of the sphincter pupillae	Slit lamp examination. Iris and pupillary response may be evaluated under retroillumination
	• Pigmentation deficiency in iris • Skin and hair pigmentation deficiency	• Albinism (see p. 128) • Ocular albinism	Unequivocal diagnosis; VEP if necessary
	• Trauma history • Pupil is not round • Complete or partial aniridia	Iris defects such as avulsion of the root of the iris (see p. 322) or aniridia (see p. 322)	Unequivocal diagnosis

Table 19.1 Cardinal symptoms, associated symptoms/findings, tentative diagnosis, and diagnostic work-up (continued)

Cardinal symptoms	Possible associated symptoms and findings	Tentative diagnosis	Further diagnostic work-up
Increased glare and	• Enlargement of the cornea and unilateral or bilateral opacification • Increased glare with squinting	**Only in children:** • Buphthalmos (see p. 169)	**Risk of blindness!** Measure intraocular pressure immediately
Diplopia (binocular) and	• No eye pain • Neurologic symptoms depending on cause • Trauma history	Cranial nerve palsy (e.g., in central ischemia or apoplexy, intracranial tumors, or cerebral trauma)	Neurologic and neuroradiologic diagnostic studies are indicated
	• Eye pain	Painful oculomotor palsy	Eliminate possible aneurysm
	• Trauma history (always in cases of ocular contusion; when eyelid is swollen shut, diplopia will not be apparent to the patient) • Limited ocular motility in elevation and depression • Enophthalmos (posteriorly displaced eye)	Fracture of the floor of the orbit (see p. 323)	CT to precisely localize the fracture
	• Pain during eye motion • Reddening and swelling of the eyelid and conjunctiva	Ocular myositis (see p. 266)	Ultrasound scan of the muscles
	• Severe swelling of the eyelid and conjunctiva • Severe malaise • Affected eye is often immobile ("cemented" globe) • Exophthalmos (in children, this is a sign of orbital cellulitis)	Orbital cellulitis (see p. 263)	• **Risk of blindness (optic nerve atrophy)!** • **Cavernous sinus thrombosis is a life-threatening sequela!** • Consult ENT specialist: orbital cellulitis originates in the paranasal sinuses in 60% of cases, and in 84% of cases in children
	• Associated hyperthyreosis (in 60% of cases) and keratoconjunctivitis sicca • Unilateral or bilateral exophthalmos may be present • Characteristic eyelid signs (see ▶ Table 15.3)	Graves's disease (see p. 262)	• Ultrasound and/or CT is indicated to determine whether muscles are thickened • Thyroid diagnostic studies by endocrinologist
	• Patient suddenly experiences diplopia vision (often at the age of 2 to 6 years) • Patient closes one eye to suppress diplopia	Late strabismus with normal sensory development (see p. 302)	Unequivocal diagnosis
	• Scarring limits ocular motility • Diplopia in temporal gaze • Pterygium clearly visible with the naked eye	Pterygium (see p. 47)	Unequivocal diagnosis

Table 19.1 Cardinal symptoms, associated symptoms/findings, tentative diagnosis, and diagnostic work-up (continued)

Cardinal symptoms	Possible associated symptoms and findings	Tentative diagnosis	Further diagnostic work-up
Diplopia (monocular) and	• Gray to white pupillary reflex • Gradual loss of visual acuity • Increased glare	Cataract (see p. 105) (multiple focal points in a single lens)	Slit lamp examination. Diagnosis is unequivocal where the opacity is visible under retroillumination
	• Alternating diplopia (dislocated lens changes its position in the eye and may fall back into place in the plane of the pupil when the patient bends forward)	Dislocation or subluxation of the lens (see p. 120)	Unequivocal diagnosis. Equator of the lens is visible in the plane of the pupil under retroillumination
	• History of trauma (avulsion of the root of the iris) • Congenital or traumatic aniridia	"Double" pupil due to an iris defect (e.g., avulsion of the root of the iris or aniridia) (see p. 322)	Unequivocal diagnosis
	• Conical or hemispherical protrusion deformation of the cornea	Keratoconus (see p. 72) or keratoglobus (see p. 74). Diplopia results from multiple focal points of the deformed cornea	Unequivocal diagnosis. Condition may be visible with the naked eye or verified by standard keratoscopy or video keratoscopy
Enophthalmos (eye recedes into orbit) and	• Trauma history (signs of ocular contusion) • Diplopia • Eyelid swelling • Limited ocular motility in elevation and depression	Fracture of the floor of the orbit (see p. 323)	• Obtain radiographs • In difficult cases, CT is indicated for precise localization of the fracture
	• Triad of ptosis, mitosis, enophthalmos (unilateral findings)	Horner's syndrome (see p. 141)	Neurologic examination
	• Blind eye • Phthisis (shrinkage of the eyeball) • Pseudoenophthalmos (severe trauma, surgery, or retinal detachment) and chronic inflammation (uveitis or retinitis)	Ocular atrophy with shrinkage of the globe	Unequivocal diagnosis
	• Loss of orbital fatty tissue in advanced age (eyes recede into the orbit) • Always bilateral	Senile sunken eye	Unequivocal diagnosis
Exophthalmos (projecting eye) and	• Associated hyperthyreosis (in 60% of cases) • Often in association with diplopia • Often in association with keratoconjunctivitis sicca	Graves's disease (see p. 262)	• Ultrasound and/or CT is indicated to determine whether muscles are thickened • Thyroid diagnostic studies by endocrinologist are indicated
	• Metamorphopsia • Retinal impression folds are visible under ophthalmoscopy	Retrobulbar tumor (see p. 267) (exophthalmos due to posterior pressure on the globe)	CT scan
	• History of trauma • Eyelid hematoma (black eye) • Eyelid swelling	Orbital bleeding (see p. 267)	Radiographs to exclude injury of the bony structures of the orbit

Table 19.1 Cardinal symptoms, associated symptoms/findings, tentative diagnosis, and diagnostic work-up (continued)

Cardinal symptoms	Possible associated symptoms and findings	Tentative diagnosis	Further diagnostic work-up
Exophthalmos (projecting eye) and	• Pseudoexophthalmos due to long globe • Occasionally unilateral • Difference in refraction (anisometropia) • Poor distance vision; good near vision	Severe myopia (see p. 278)	Refraction testing
	• Pain during eye motion • Diplopia • Reddening and swelling of the eyelid and conjunctiva	Ocular myositis (see p. 266)	Ultrasound scan of the muscles
	• Patients are often children • Severe swelling of the eyelid and conjunctiva • Severe malaise • Affected eye is often immobile ("cemented" globe)	Orbital cellulitis (see p. 263)	• **Risk of blindness (optic nerve atrophy)!** • **Cavernous sinus thrombosis is a life-threatening sequela!** • Consult ENT specialist: orbital cellulitis originates in the paranasal sinuses in 60% of cases, and in 84% of cases in children
	• Other developmental anomalies may accompany exophthalmos, which is usually bilateral	Craniosynostosis (see p. 262)	Unequivocal diagnosis
Hypopyon and	• Deep eye pain that hardly responds to analgesics at all • Reddening and swelling of the eyelids and conjunctiva • Acutely decreased visual acuity • Prior intraocular surgery, penetrating injury, or corneal ulceration	Acute endophthalmitis (see p. 180)	**Risk of blindness within hours!** • Microbiological diagnostic studies
	• Reddening of the conjunctiva • Corneal ulcer • Eyelid swelling • Pain	Serpiginous corneal ulcer (see p. 76)	**Rapid progression of the ulcer can threaten the eye!** • Microbiological diagnostic studies
	• No ocular pain • Iritis or iridocyclitis	Sterile hypopyon	• Diagnostic studies for uveitis • Systemic, immunologic, and rheumatologic examinations are required
Headaches and	• Unilaterally red, hard eye • Pupil fixed and dilated • Corneal opacification • Severe pain • Frequent vomiting	Acute glaucoma (see p. 164)	**Risk of blindness!** • Measure intraocular pressure immediately

Table 19.1 Cardinal symptoms, associated symptoms/findings, tentative diagnosis, and diagnostic work-up (continued)

Cardinal symptoms	Possible associated symptoms and findings	Tentative diagnosis	Further diagnostic work-up
Headaches and	• Sudden unilateral loss of visual acuity • Patients are usually over 60 years • Headache pain in temples • Temporal artery tender to palpation	• AION: anterior ischemic optic neuropathy due to arteritis • Giant cell arteritis (see p. 241) in temporal arteritis	**Risk of blindness!** • Circular or segmental swelling of the optic disc will be visible upon ophthalmoscopy
	• Pain when chewing, weight loss • Poor overall health • Myalgia • Stiff neck		• Arterial biopsy and histologic examination are indicated • Determine erythrocyte sedimentation rate and level of C-reactive protein (precipitous drops occur in temporal arteritis)
	• Poor vision • Need for eyeglasses or change of eyeglass • Rapid fatigue (for example when reading) • Burning sensation	Asthenopic symptoms	Test visual acuity, Refraction test
	• Papilledema on ophthalmoscopy. Possibly visual field defects	Papilledema (see p. 237)	Measurement of cerebral pressure
	• Obesity	Idiopathic intracranial hypertension	
Flashes of light and	• Often in older patients • Flashes of light and shadows seen when moving the eyes, even in the dark • Floaters	Posterior vitreous detachment (see p. 175)	• Essentially harmless age-related disorder • Examine fundus to exclude retinal tears or detachment
	• Patient sees shadows (a "wall" from below or a "curtain" from above)	Retinal detachment (see p. 208)	**Risk of blindness!** • Ophthalmoscopy
	• Often without any other symptoms	Retinal tear (see p. 209)	**Risk of retinal detachment!** • Ophthalmoscopy
	• Often encountered in patients with consumptive systemic disorders such as AIDS	Retinitis (see p. 224)	Consult specialist for internal medicine for diagnosis of cause
Eyelid swelling, inflammatory and	• Clear vesicles on the eyelids • Eyelid swelling • Inflammatory ptosis	Herpes-simplex virus infection (see p. 21)	Unequivocal diagnosis
	• Painful pressure point on the eyelid • Circumscribed swelling and reddening of the eyelid • Often severe pulsating pain • Spot of yellow pus • Pseudoptosis	Hordeolum (see p. 24)	Unequivocal diagnosis
	• Sting is often visible • Clear swelling • Unilateral • Itching	Insect sting	Unequivocal diagnosis

Table 19.1 Cardinal symptoms, associated symptoms/findings, tentative diagnosis, and diagnostic work-up (continued)

Cardinal symptoms	Possible associated symptoms and findings	Tentative diagnosis	Further diagnostic work-up
Eyelid swelling, inflammatory and	• Red eye • Often few symptoms • Sticky eyelids in the morning • Purulent or watery discharge	Conjunctivitis (see p. 49)	Microbiological diagnostic studies
	• Large, hard swelling and reddening with edema are often present • Pain • Ptosis	Eyelid abscess (see p. 22)	Unequivocal diagnosis
	• Severe swelling of the eyelid and conjunctiva • Severe malaise • Affected eye is often immobile ("cemented" globe)	Orbital cellulitis (see p. 263)	• **Risk of blindness (optic nerve atrophy)!** • **Cavernous sinus thrombosis is a life-threatening sequela!** • Consult ENT specialist: orbital cellulitis originates in the paranasal sinuses in 60% of cases, and in 84% of cases in children
	• Severe pain • Bleeding vesicles • Pattern of lesions follows trigeminal nerve	Herpes zoster ophthalmicus (see p. 21)	Refer patient to dermatologist
Eyelid swelling, noninflammatory and	• Painless, circumscribed swelling of the eyelid • No reddening • Hard palpable nodules on the eyelid • Pseudoptosis	Chalazion (see p. 24)	Unequivocal diagnosis
	• Occurs in older patients (aging skin) • Limp, drooping eyelid • Drooping eyebrows	• Cutis laxa senilis (see p. 13) • Blepharochalasis (see p.13)	Unequivocal diagnosis
	• S-shaped upper eyelid • No reddening • Palpable mass	• Eyelid tumor (see p. 25) • Lacrimal gland tumor (see p. 42)	Biopsy
	• No other ocular symptoms	Systemic cause (heart, kidney, or thyroid disorder)	Refer patient to specialist for internal medicine
	• Yellowish prolapsed fat under the eyelids, easily mobile under the connective tissue and the eyelids	Orbital fat hernia	Unequivocal diagnosis

Table 19.1 Cardinal symptoms, associated symptoms/findings, tentative diagnosis, and diagnostic work-up (continued)

Cardinal symptoms	Possible associated symptoms and findings	Tentative diagnosis	Further diagnostic work-up
Eyelid swelling, noninflammatory and	• Enophthalmos • History of trauma (ocular contusion) • Diplopia may be present	Fracture of the floor of the orbit (see p. 323)	• Obtain radiographs • In difficult cases, CT is also indicated for precise localization of the fracture
Pseudoptosis and	• In older patients (aging skin) • Limp eyelid skin • Drooping eyebrows	• Cutis laxa senilis (see p.13) • Blepharochalasis (see p. 13)	Unequivocal diagnosis
	• History of trauma (signs of ocular contusion • Diplopia may be present • Eyelid swelling • Enophthalmos	Fracture of the floor of the orbit (see p. 323)	• Obtain radiographs • In difficult cases, CT is also indicated for precise localization of the fracture
	• Pseudoenophthalmos • Often secondary to severe trauma, surgery, or chronic inflammation (uveitis or retinitis) • Blind eye	Phthisis (shrinkage of the eyeball)	Unequivocal diagnosis
	• Palpable, immobile swelling	Eyelid tumors (see p. 25)	Biopsy
Ptosis and	• History of trauma or older patient	**Likely common cause:** • Tear in the levator palpebrae	Unequivocal diagnosis
	• Secondary to intraocular surgery	Elongation of the levator palpebrae	Unequivocal diagnosis
	• Bilateral; present at birth	Congenital ptosis (see p. 15)	Unequivocal diagnosis
	• Paralysis of one or of all extraocular muscles	**Rare:** • Chronic progressive external ophthalmoplegia	Refer patient to neurologist
	• Eyelid swelling • Pain • Foreign-body sensation • Blepharospasm	• Corneal erosion (see p. 322) • Corneal foreign body (see p. 322) • Subtarsal corneal foreign body (see p. 322)	• Examine cornea • Fully evert the eyelids where subtarsal foreign body is suspected • Apply fluorescein dye to evaluate cornea where corneal erosion is suspected
	• Secondary to application of antiglaucoma medications containing guanethidine	Drug side effects	Unequivocal diagnosis
	• Triad of ptosis, miosis, and enophthalmos	Horner's syndrome (see p. 141)	Refer patient to neurologist
	• Severity of ptosis can vary from day to day	Myasthenia gravis (see p. 15)	Refer patient to neurologist
	• Accompanied by dilated pupil and diplopia	Oculomotor nerve palsy (see p. 314)	Refer patient to neurologist

Table 19.1 Cardinal symptoms, associated symptoms/findings, tentative diagnosis, and diagnostic work-up (continued)

Cardinal symptoms	Possible associated symptoms and findings	Tentative diagnosis	Further diagnostic work-up
Pupillary dysfunction, miosis, and	• Secondary to application of pilocarpine • Secondary to use of morphine	• Drug-induced miosis • Toxic miosis	Unequivocal diagnosis
Pupillary dysfunction, ptosis and enophthalmos, and	• Iritis/Iridocyclitis • Red eye • Pain	Horner's syndrome (see p. 141)	Refer patient to neurologist
		Reactive miosis	Unequivocal diagnosis
Pupillary dysfunction, mydriasis, and	• Secondary to administration of atropine or mydriatics	Drug-induced mydriasis	Unequivocal diagnosis
	• Ischemia • Tumor • History of trauma	Lesion of the optic nerve or optic tract	Refer patient to neurologist
	• Pupil does not respond to light	Following sudden blindness	Unequivocal diagnosis
Rings around light sources and	• Gradual progressive loss of visual acuity • Increased glare • Grayish-white pupillary reflex	Cataract (see p. 105)	Slit lamp examination. Diagnosis is unequivocal where the opacity is visible under retroillumination
	• Corneal edema	Increased intraocular pressure	Measure intraocular pressure
Red eye and	• Conjunctival injection • Full visual acuity • Purulent or watery discharge • Swelling of the eyelid and conjunctiva • Sticky eyelids in the morning	Conjunctivitis (see p. 49)	Obtain smear for microbiological examination
	• Combined injection • Reduced visual acuity • Intraocular structures obscured • Pain	Scleritis (see p. 97)and/or episcleritis (see p. 97)	Unequivocal diagnosis
	• Eye hard to palpation • Pupil fixed and dilated • Head and eye pain • Loss of visual acuity • Nausea, possibly with vomiting	Glaucoma attack (see p. 164)	**Risk of blindness!** • Measure intraocular pressure immediately

Table 19.1 Cardinal symptoms, associated symptoms/findings, tentative diagnosis, and diagnostic work-up (continued)

Cardinal symptoms	Possible associated symptoms and findings	Tentative diagnosis	Further diagnostic work-up
Red eye and	• Spontaneous (normal history) • Secondary to exercise (such as lifting heavy objects, pressing, defecation of hard stool) and coughing or sneezing • Secondary to trauma or surgery • Due to arteriosclerosis (may be recurrent in older patients) • With impaired coagulation (hemophilia or medication such as coumarin derivatives)	Subconjunctival hemorrhage (see p. 48)	Diagnosis is unequivocal where confirmed by patient's history
Black spots ("floating around before the eyes"), so-called "mouches volantes" or "floaters," and	• Usually no other ocular symptoms • Decreased visual acuity only in severe cases	Vitreous opacification (see p. 175)	Unequivocal diagnosis
	• Patients are often older • Patient perceives veils and curtains in the eye, even in the dark • Floaters move with the eye, most noticeable when looking against a white wall • Flashes of light	Posterior vitreous detachment (see p. 175)	Isolated findings are harmless • Examine fundus to exclude retinal defects
	• Inflammatory debris in the vitreous body	Posterior uveitis (see p. 128)	Examine fundus
Decreased visual acuity; transient (visual acuity improves within 24 h, usually within 1 h), and	• Lasts a few seconds • Darkening that may include amaurosis	Amaurosis fugax (such as in ipsilateral stenosis in the internal carotid artery)	No abnormal ocular findings **Fundus examination is indicated where visual acuity is decreased!** Neurological examination
	• Poor general health • Visual acuity improves with improvement in general health	Circulatory failure	No abnormal ocular findings
	• Visual field defects • Scintillating scotoma for 10 to 20 minutes • Vertigo and vomiting	Ocular migraine (see p. 254), visual aura with or without headache pain	Unequivocal diagnosis, based on the patient's description of symptoms
	• Blurred vision • General feeling of fatigue	Hypoglycemia	**Risk of blindness!** • Administer glucose. diagnosis is unequivocal where visual acuity returns to normal as blood glucose level increases
Decreased visual acuity persisting longer than 24 h, sudden onset, painless, and	• Unilateral loss of visual acuity • Headache is possible	AION: anterior ischemic optic neuropathy (see p. 241)	Determine erythrocyte sedimentation rate and level of CRP (precipitous drops occur in temporal arteritis)
	• Mobile shadows before the eyes • Clear when eyes immobilized so that blood will settle	Vitreous hemorrhage (see p. 179)	Examine fundus. Diagnosis is unequivocal where fundus is obscured Ultrasound: rule out retinal detachment

Table 19.1 Cardinal symptoms, associated symptoms/findings, tentative diagnosis, and diagnostic work-up (continued)

Cardinal symptoms	Possible associated symptoms and findings	Tentative diagnosis	Further diagnostic work-up
Decreased visual acuity persisting longer than 24 h, sudden onset, painless, and	• Severe loss of visual acuity • Flashes of light	Retinal detachment (see p. 208)	**Risk of blindness!** • Ophthalmoscopy (clearly visible retinal detachment)
	• Pain from posterior swelling and with eye motion • Increasing loss of visual acuity following exercise • Central scotoma • Normal findings upon ophthalmoscopy (patient sees nothing; examiner sees nothing)	Retrobulbar optic neuritis (see p. 239)	Neurologic examination

	• Intraretinal linear hemorrhages
	  ○ In one quadrant
	  ○ In two quadrants
	  ○ In four quadrants
		• Branch retinal vein occlusion (see p. 202)
		• Hemispherical occlusion (see p. 202)
		• Central retinal vein occlusion (see p. 202)
			• Ophthalmoscopy (linear hemorrhages)
			• Fluorescein angiography to differentiate ischemic from nonischemic type

	• Segmental or total visual field defects • Sudden unilateral blindness	Central retinal artery occlusion (see p. 203)	Ophthalmoscopy: whitish retinal edema, visible "cherry red spot" (macula)
	• Patient is usually over 60 years • Unilateral decrease in visual acuity • Headaches • Temporal artery is tender to palpation • Cervical myalgia • Pain when chewing • Weight loss	AION (see p. 241): anterior ischemic optic neuropathy due to arteritis in giant cell arteritis (see p. 241) or temporal arteritis	**Risk of blindness!** • Arterial biopsy and histologic examination are indicated • Circular or segmental swelling of the optic disc will be visible upon ophthalmoscopy • Determine erythrocyte sedimentation rate and level of CRP (heightened levels in temporal arteritis) • Unequivocal diagnosis
Decreased visual acuity, slowly increasing over a period of weeks, months, or years; painless, and	• Gray to white pupillary reflex • Loss of contrast • Increased glare	Cataract (see p. 105)	Slit lamp examination Diagnosis is unequivocal where the opacity is visible under retroillumination
	• Corneal opacification • Corneal scarring	Chronic corneal degeneration, keratopathy (see p. 86)	• Unequivocal diagnosis • Slit lamp examination will reveal corneal degeneration and scarring
	• Central visual field defect • Patient is usually over 65 years • Blurred vision, micropsia, and macropsia may be present	Age-related macular degeneration (see p. 214)	Fluorescein angiography

Table 19.1 Cardinal symptoms, associated symptoms/findings, tentative diagnosis, and diagnostic work-up (continued)

Cardinal symptoms	Possible associated symptoms and findings	Tentative diagnosis	Further diagnostic work-up
Decreased visual acuity, slowly increasing over a period of weeks, months, or years; painless, and	• Increased intraocular pressure • Visual field defects	Primary chronic open angle glaucoma (see p. 153)	**Risk of blindness!** • Measure intraocular pressure
	• Decreased visual acuity is typically more severe in the morning than in the evening	Fuchs's endothelial dystrophy (see p. 86)	Slit lamp examination
	• Specifically decreased visual acuity in near or distance vision	• Myopia (see p. 277) • Hyperopia (see p. 280)	Test visual acuity
	• Asymmetry • Optic disc pallor	Mass in the area of the optical nerve or visual pathway	MRI
	• Disorder of night and twilight vision • "Bone spicules" on ophthalmoscopy	Retinal dystrophy	Genetic work-up
Deterioration of vision, painful, acute, and	• Whitish corneal opacification	Acute keratoconus (see p. 72)	Typical conical projection of the cornea is visible under slit lamp examination
	• Red eye, hard to palpation • Pupil fixed and dilated • Nausea, possibly with vomiting	Acute glaucoma (see p. 164)	**Risk of blindness!** • Measure intraocular pressure immediately
	• Central scotoma. • Increasing loss of visual acuity following exercise; pain from posterior swelling and with eye motion • Normal findings upon ophthalmoscopy (patient sees nothing; examiner sees nothing)	Retrobulbar optic neuritis (see p. 239)	Neurologic examination
	• Combined injection • Eye pain • Fibrin and cells in the anterior chamber • Vitreous infiltration • Anterior and posterior synechiae	Uveitis (see p. 128)	Slit lamp examination
Blurred or distorted vision, especially when fixating close or remote objects, and	• Older patients (65 years and older) • Gradual progressive loss of visual acuity	• Refraction anomaly (myopia (see p. 277) or hyperopia (see p. 280), astigmatism (see p. 282) and presbyopia (see p. 214)	Refraction testing
		• Age-related macular degeneration (see p. 214)	Ophthalmoscopy

Table 19.1 Cardinal symptoms, associated symptoms/findings, tentative diagnosis, and diagnostic work-up (continued)

Cardinal symptoms	Possible associated symptoms and findings	Tentative diagnosis	Further diagnostic work-up
Distorted vision, blurred vision, and	• Patient under emotional or physical stress • Men in their thirties and forties are most commonly affected • Objects appear enlarged or reduced in size • Central relative visual field defects (patients see a dark spot)	Central serous chorioretinopathy (see p. 213)	Ophthalmoscopy
	• Headaches, possibly with nausea; scintillating scotoma, transient	Migraine (see p. 254), aura with or without headache	Unequivocal diagnosis
	• Permanent or worsening • Possibly with diplopia • Increased glare • Gray to white pupillary reflex	Cataract (see p. 105)	Slit lamp examination will reveal obvious lens opacity where a cataract is present
	• Narrowed or dilated pupil	Following administration of eye drops (miotics or mydriatics)	Unequivocal with corresponding medical history
	• Fundus reflex absent or weak • Patient sees shadows (a "wall" from below or a "curtain" from above)	Retinal detachment (see p. 208)	Unequivocal diagnosis
	• Headache • Visual field defect • Diplopia • Ophthalmoplegia • Prominent, edematous optic disc	Cerebral cause (tumor or increased intracranial pressure)	• Neurologic work-up • CT scan
White pupillary reflex (leukocoria) in children, unilateral or bilateral Often first noticed in photographs, and		Cataract (see p. 105)	Slit lamp examination. Diagnosis is unequivocal where lens opacity is visible under retroillumination
	• Up to 90% of patients are male among children and teenagers • Unilateral leukocoria (occasionally combined with strabismus) • Exudative retinal detachment visible upon ophthalmoscopy	Coats's disease (see p. 206)	Unequivocal diagnosis
	• Retinal detachment visible upon ophthalmoscopy	Retinal detachment, for example in retinopathy of prematurity (see p. 208)	Unequivocal diagnosis
	• Usually unilateral • Congenital (leukocoria manifests itself at birth) • Microphthalmos is usually present	PHPV (persistent hyperplastic primary vitreous) (see p. 177)	Ultrasound scan
	• Usually unilateral (two-thirds of all cases) • May be accompanied by red eye • Child is usually below the age of 3 years • Globe is normal size	Retinoblastoma (see p. 226) (whitish vitreous, retinal, or subretinal tumor) **Retinoblastoma should be excluded in leukocoria!**	• Ophthalmoscopy also in fellow eye to exclude a bilateral retinoblastoma • CT

20 Appendix

20.1 Topical Ophthalmic Preparations

Drug	Indications	Ocular effects and side effects	Systemic side effects
Acyclovir	• Herpes simplex keratitis • Herpes zoster ophthalmicus	Local irritation, keratitis, allergic reaction in eyelids and conjunctiva	No known systemic effects from topical use
Atropine	• Cycloplegia • Uveitis	Mydriasis, angle closure glaucoma, cycloplegia, decreased visual acuity, increased intraocular pressure	Confusion, tachycardia, dry mouth
Beta blockers	Glaucoma therapy	Decreased intraocular pressure, decreased visual acuity, dry eye	Bronchoconstriction, bradycardia
Carbachol	Glaucoma therapy	Decreased intraocular pressure, miosis, accommodation spasm, decreased visual acuity	Fever, syncope, nausea
Clonidine	Glaucoma therapy	Decreased intraocular pressure, decreased blood supply to the head of the optic nerve	Decreased blood pressure
Cyclopentolate	• Mydriatic • Cycloplegic	Mydriasis, angle closure glaucoma, decreased visual acuity, increased intraocular pressure	Central nervous system dysfunction, tachycardia, dry mouth, nausea
Chloramphenicol	Severe ocular bacterial infections	Local irritation, keratitis, allergic reaction in eyelids and conjunctiva, keratitis	Aplastic anemia (rare)
Dorzolamide (local carbonic anhydrase inhibitor)	• Glaucoma therapy • Prophylaxis against increased intraocular pressure following laser surgery	Local allergic reaction in eyelids and conjunctiva	Malaise, depression, metallic taste
Epinephrine	Glaucoma therapy	Decreased intraocular pressure, cystoid macular edema	Headaches, perspiration, syncope
Ganciclovir	Herpes simplex keratitis	Burning sensation Stabbing pain Superficial punctate keratitis	No known side effects
Gentamicin	Ocular bacterial infections, especially *Pseudomonas aeruginosa, Escherichia coli, Proteus* species, *Klebsiella pneumoniae*	Local irritation and allergic reaction in eyelids and conjunctiva, keratitis; intravitreous administration may cause retinal damage and atrophy of the optic nerve	No known systemic effects from topical use
Glucocorticoids	Anti-inflammatory therapy	Increased intraocular pressure, posterior subcapsular cataract	Decreased plasma cortisol levels
Idoxuridine, trifluridine, vidarabine	Herpes simplex keratitis	Local irritation, corneal damage, ptosis, and obstruction of the punctum lacrimale	No known systemic effects from topical use
Naphazoline	Symptomatic treatment of allergic or inflammatory reactions	Conjunctival vasoconstriction, local irritation, mydriasis, angle closure glaucoma, keratitis	Rare: headaches, increased blood pressure, nausea, cardiac arrhythmia
Neostigmine	Glaucoma therapy	Decreased intraocular pressure, local irritation, miosis, accommodation spasm, decreased visual acuity	No know systemic effects from topical use

Drug	Indications	Ocular effects and side effects	Systemic side effects
Penicillin	Ocular bacterial infections	Local irritations, allergic reactions in eyelids and conjunctiva	No know systemic effects from topical use
Phenylephrine	• Mydriatic • Vasoconstrictor	Mydriasis, angle closure glaucoma, vasoconstriction	Increased blood pressure, myocardial infarction, tachycardia
Pilocarpine	Glaucoma therapy	Decreased intraocular pressure, miosis, accommodation spasm, decreased visual acuity, retinal tears (rare)	
Prostaglandin analogues (latanoprost, travoprost, bimatoprost)	Glaucoma therapy	Increased iris pigmentation in 16% of patients Increased growth of lashes (thickness and length)	
Rifampicin	Ocular infections with *Chlamydia*	Conjunctival hyperemia, pain, tearing	
Scopolamine	• Therapeutic mydriasis • Uveitis	Decreased visual acuity, mydriasis, angle closure glaucoma, cycloplegia, increased intraocular pressure	Confusion, hallucinations
Sulfonamide	Ocular bacterial infections	Local irritation, allergic reaction, keratitis	No known systemic effects from topical use
Tetracycline	Ocular bacterial infections (including *Mycoplasma* strains)	Unspecific conjunctivitis, allergic reactions	No known systemic effects from topical use

20.2 Nonophthalmic Preparations with Ocular Side Effects

Drug	Indications	Ocular effects and side effects	Systemic side effects
Systemic cardiovascular medication			
Amiodarone	Ventricular arrhythmias that do not respond to treatment	Yellowish-brown deposits in the cornea, conjunctiva, and lens	Thyroid dysfunction, pulmonary fibrosis, photosensitivity
Atropine	• Bradycardic arrhythmia • Gastrointestinal spasms	Decreased visual acuity, mydriasis, angle closure glaucoma, visual hallucinations	Tachycardia, agitation, confusion
Beta blockers	• Arterial hypertension • Coronary heart disease • Cardiac insufficiency (in low doses)	Decreased visual acuity, visual hallucinations, decreased intraocular pressure, dry eye	Decreased blood pressure, bradycardia, dyspnea, stupor
Clonidine	Arterial hypertension	Decreased intraocular pressure, decreased visual acuity, allergic reaction in eyelids and conjunctiva	Sedation, bradycardia, dry mouth, depressive moods
Digitalis glycosides (digoxin, digitoxin, acetyldigoxin)	• Cardiac insufficiency • Cardiac arrhythmia	Color vision defects (xanthopsia)	Nausea, bradycardia
Systemic CNS medication			
Amphetamines	• Narcolepsy • Appetite suppression • Hyperkinetic child syndrome (pediatrics)	Decreased visual acuity, mydriasis, angle closure glaucoma, enlarged palpebral fissures, visual hallucinations	Agitated and restless states, tachycardia, insomnia

Continued ▶

Drug	Indications	Ocular effects and side effects	Systemic side effects
Barbiturates	• Epilepsy • Anesthesia • Tranquilizers and sedatives	Ocular motility disturbances (depressed convergence response, ophthalmoplegia, nystagmus), ptosis, and blepharoclonus from chronic use	Decreased blood pressure, suppression of REM sleep phases, respiratory depression, hyperalgesia
Benzodiazepines (alprazolam, diazepam, clonazepam, midazolam)	• Anxiety and agitated states • Epilepsy • Insomnia	Suppression of corneal reflex, depressed accommodation and depth perception, ocular motility disturbances, allergic conjunctivitis	Respiratory depression, fatigue, development of tolerance
Chloral hydrate	Sedative	Miosis, ptosis, depressed convergence response	Irritation of mucous membranes, liver toxicity
Chlorpromazine, thioridazine, perphenazine (group of phenothiazine neuroleptics)	• Schizophrenia • Psychomotor agitation • Manias • Chronic pain syndromes	Decreased visual acuity, pigment deposits on the surface of the lens and cornea, changes in the retinal pigment epithelium (especially with thioridazine)	Parkinson disease, early dyskinesia and tardive dyskinesia, liver damage
Carbamazepine	• Epilepsy • Neuralgia (trigeminal neuralgia)	Diplopia, blurred vision, sensation of heaviness in the eyelids	Fatigue, ataxia, blood count changes
L-dopa	Parkinson's disease	Mydriasis (angle closure glaucoma), eyelid retraction, ptosis	Orthostatic circulatory symptoms, nausea, dyskinesia, psychosis
Haloperidol (group of butyrophenone neuroleptics)	• Schizophrenia • Psychomotor agitation • Manias • Chronic pain syndromes	Mydriasis, decreased visual acuity	Parkinson's disease, early dyskinesia and tardive dyskinesia, liver damage
Lithium	• Manic phases • Prophylaxis against endogenous depression	Decreased visual acuity, nystagmus, exophthalmos (due to thyroid dysfunction)	Goiter, ataxia, diarrhea, tremor
Morphine	Severe pain	Miosis, decreased visual acuity, decreased accommodation and convergence reaction. During withdrawal: mydriasis, tearing, and diplopia	Respiratory depression, bronchoconstriction, constipation, euphoria (addictive)
Phenytoin	Epilepsy	Nystagmus, decreased visual acuity, mydriasis	Hypertrichosis, gingival hyperplasia, cerebral ataxia, osteopathy
Tricyclic antidepressants (amitriptyline, desipramine, imipramine)	Depression	Mydriasis, angle closure glaucoma, cycloplegia, dry eyes, diplopia	Tachycardia, constipation, micturition difficulties
Systemic medication for treating infection			
Chloramphenicol	Severe bacterial infections such as abdominal typhus, *Haemophilus influenzae* meningitis	Decreased visual acuity, visual field changes (scotomas or limitation), optic neuritis or retrobulbar optic neuritis, local allergic reactions	Aplastic anemia, gastrointestinal dysfunction, fever, "gray syndrome"
Chloroquine and hydroxychloroquine	• Malaria • Amebiasis	Deposits on the cornea, changes in the retinal pigment epithelium (bull's eye maculopathy), visual field changes	Nausea, headache, bleaching of the hair, blood count changes

Drug	Indications	Ocular effects and side effects	Systemic side effects
Quinine	Malaria infection	Decreased visual acuity including toxic amblyopia, mydriasis, retinal damage (edema or vascular constriction), optic disc edema, scotomas	Hemolytic anemia, allergic reactions, hearing loss
Ethambutol	Tuberculosis	Optic neuritis, visual field changes, color vision defects	Hyperuricemia, nausea
Isoniazid	Tuberculosis	Optic neuritis, atrophy of the optic nerve, visual field changes, optic disc edema, color vision defects	Polyneuropathy (vitamin B_6 metabolic dysfunction), allergic reactions, liver damage
Penicillin	Bacterial infections	Mydriasis, depressed accommodation, diplopia, optic disc edema with cerebral pseudo-tumor (secondary)	Nausea, allergic reactions
Rifampicin	Tuberculosis	Conjunctival hyperemia, blepharoconjunctivitis, color change (orange) of fluid is possible	Liver dysfunction, nausea, allergic reactions, hepatic enzyme induction
Streptomycin	Tuberculosis	Nystagmus, decreased visual acuity, toxic amblyopia, color vision defect, atrophy of the optic nerve	Ototoxicity, nephrotoxicity, allergy
Sulfonamides	Bacterial infections	Myopia, unspecific irritation	Allergic reactions, nausea, photosensitivity
Tetracycline	Bacterial infections	Myopia, optic disc edema with cerebral pseudotumor, decreased visual acuity, diplopia	Nausea, allergic reactions, liver damage
Systemic medication for treating rheumatic disorders			
Acetyl salicylic acid and salicylic acid	• Fever, pain • Rheumatoid arthritis • Thrombocyte aggregation inhibitor	Allergies, conjunctivitis, decreased visual acuity, transient blindness	Microscopic gastrointestinal bleeding, allergies, bronchospasm, ototoxic side effects
Chloroquine and hydroxychloroquine	Base medication in rheumatoid arthritis	Deposits on the cornea, changes in the retinal pigment epithelium (bull's eye maculopathy), visual field changes	Nausea, headache, bleaching of the hair, blood count changes
Gold salts	Base medication in rheumatoid arthritis	Deposits on the eyelids, conjunctiva, cornea (chrysiasis), and lens (rare). Ptosis, nystagmus, and diplopia are rare	Blood count changes, nephrotoxicity, mucous membrane damage
Ibuprofen	• Rheumatoid arthritis • Inflammation in degenerative joint disease	Blurred vision, diplopia, color vision defects, dry eyes, optic neuritis (rare)	Damage to gastrointestinal mucous membranes
Indomethacin	• Rheumatoid arthritis • Inflammation in degenerative joint disease	Decreased visual acuity, diplopia, color vision defects, corneal deposits	Damage to gastrointestinal mucous membranes, headaches
Hormone preparations			
Glucocorticoids	• Anaphylactic shock, immunosuppressive therapy (such as in ulcerous colitis or immunohemolytic anemia) • Bronchial asthma • Acute rheumatic fever	Decreased visual acuity, increased intraocular pressure, posterior subcapsular cataract	Increased blood glucose levels, Cushing's syndrome, osteoporosis, increased risk of thrombosis, increased susceptibility to infection

Continued ▶

Drug	Indications	Ocular effects and side effects	Systemic side effects
Oral contraceptives	• Contraception • Regulation of menstrual cycle	Decreased visual acuity, retinal vascular changes (occlusion, bleeding, spasm), retinal edema, visual field changes, optic neuritis, dry eye syndrome	Varicosis, migraine, edemas

Other important medications with ocular side effects

Coumarin derivatives (phenprocoumon, warfarin)	Thinning of blood as prophylaxis against and treatment of venous thrombosis	Subconjunctival or retinal bleeding, hyphema	Loss of hair, nausea, cerebral bleeding, spontaneous hematomas
Nicotinic acid	Fat metabolism disorders	Cystoid maculopathy, decreased visual acuity, local allergic reactions	Flush symptoms, restlessness, nausea, vomiting, diarrhea
Sildenafil (Viagra, Cialis)	Erectile dysfunction	Visual disturbances, increased glare perception, color vision defects, ERG changes	Headache pain, blood pressure drop, increased microcirculation of the skin (flush), dyspepsia and swelling of nasal mucosa
Vitamin A	• Vitamin A deficiency • Acne vulgaris	Loss of eyelashes, increased intracranial pressure (cerebral pseudotumor), diplopia, strabismus	Severe headaches, loss of hair, nausea, pruritus, rhagades, bone and joint pain
Vitamin D	• Vitamin D deficiency • Hypoparathyroidism	Strabismus, calcium deposits in the conjunctiva and cornea (calcific band keratopathy), atrophy of the optic nerve due to calcium occlusion of the optic canal	Calcification of parenchymal organs such as the kidneys

20.3 Ocular Symptoms of Poisoning

Toxic substance	Ocular effects and side effects	Systemic side effects
Atropine	Mydriasis, decreased visual acuity, angle closure glaucoma, cycloplegia, increased intraocular pressure	Dry mouth, dry skin, confusion, tachycardia, hyperthermia
Lead	Increased intraocular pressure	Fatigue, headache and pain in the extremities, paleness, intestinal colic, paralysis, lead halo on the gums
Quinine	Decreased visual acuity, retinal vascular spasms, atrophy of the optic nerve to the point of blindness	Allergic reactions, hemolytic anemia, vertigo, tinnitus, cyanosis, cardiac death
Digitalis	Scintillation; patient sees clouds, color vision defects	Cardiac arrhythmia, (AV conduction blocks, bigeminy), nausea, vomiting, headaches, confusion
Ethanol	Transient amblyopia, decreased intraocular pressure, nystagmus, diplopia, conjunctival hyperemia	Disturbed gait, disorientation including impaired consciousness, cramps, tachycardia
Methyl alcohol	Atrophy of the optic nerve to the point of blindness	Nausea, colic, acidosis, oliguria

20.4 Standard Values and Reference Dimensions in Ophthalmology

Structure/property/characteristic	Value
External dimensions	
Orbital diameter	Horizontal 40 mm
	Vertical 35 mm
Bulbar length	23.6 mm
Bulbar volume	6.5 mL
Exophthalmometry	>20 mm
Lateral difference	<2 mm
Muscle–limbus distance	
Medial rectus	5.5 mm
Inferior rectus	6.5 mm
Lateral rectus	6.9 mm
Superior rectus	7.7 mm
Scleral thickness	
Limbus	0.8 mm
Equator	0.5 mm
Attachment of rectus muscles	0.3 mm
Posterior pole	1.0 mm
Palpebral fissures	
Palpebral fissure (vertical)	9 mm
Palpebral fissure (horizontal)	28–30 mm
Pupillary distance (PD)	
Birth	39 ± 3 mm
Adult	62 ± 3 mm
Pupillary diameter	
Miosis	0.5 mm
Mydriasis	8 mm
Iris diameter	12–13 mm
Anterior chamber depth	3 mm
Cornea	
Corneal refractive power	42–43 dpt.
Corneal diameter	
Adult	Horizontal 11.7 mm
	Vertical 10.6 mm
Child <1 year	9.5–10 mm (at 2 years = adult value)
Corneal thickness	
Center	0.52–0.54 mm
Limbus	0.8 mm

Structure/property/characteristic	Value
Epithelium	50–100 µm
Stroma	90% of total thickness
Corneal radius	Horizontal 7.8 mm
	Vertical 7.7 mm
Corneal endothelial cells	
Youth	2,500–5,000/mm^2
Advanced age	1,500–2,750/mm^2
Lens	
Lens diameter	9 mm
Refractive power of lens	21 diopters
Lens thickness	
Birth	3.5 mm
Advanced age	5 mm
Interior of eye	
Surface area	1.5–2.8/mm^2
Neuroretinal rim volume	0.3 mm^3
Neuroretinal rim surface area	1.5 mm^2
Optic nerve length	35–55 mm
Number of axons	1,000,000
Retina	
Retinal surface area	1,206 mm^2
Diameter of posterior retinal pole	5–6 mm
Macular diameter	3 mm
Foveola diameter	0.35 mm
Foveal diameter	1.5 mm
Location of macula	3.4 mm temporal to papillary rim, 0.8 mm below the papillary center
Number of rods	110–125 × 10^6
Number of cones	6.3–6.8 × 10^6
Distance from ora serrata to Schwalbe line (±0.8 mm)	5.8 mm nasal 6.1 mm superior 6.2 mm inferior 6.5 mm temporal
Thickness ora serrata	0.11 mm
Perifoveal thickness	0.23 mm
Foveal thickness	0.1 mm

Continued ▶

Structure/property/characteristic	Value
Various standard values	
Tear film break-up time	<15 s
Schirmer test	After 5 min <15 mm
Outer limits field of view	Nasal and superior 60°, inferior 70° temporal 90° to fixation point
Blind spot in visual field	Medial margin 12° Temporal margin 17°, situated 1° below the horizontal

Structure/property/characteristic	Value
Anomaly quotient (AQ)	Normal AQ: 1.0 (0.8–1.3) Protanomaly: 0.1–0.65 Deuteranomaly: 1.75–20 Propanopia AQ: 0–∞ Deuteranopia AQ: 0–∞
Arm-retina time (fluorescence angiography)	15–20 s

20.5 Clinical Images and Examples

20.5.1 Clinical Images and Corresponding Optical Coherence Tomography (OCT) Images in Retinal Diseases

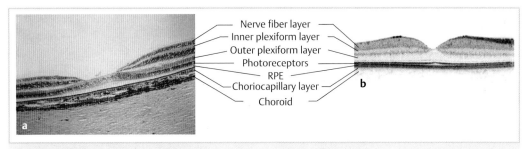

Nerve fiber layer
Inner plexiform layer
Outer plexiform layer
Photoreceptors
RPE
Choriocapillary layer
Choroid

a b

Fig. 20.1 (a, b) Normal macula. Comparison of histologic image and OCT.

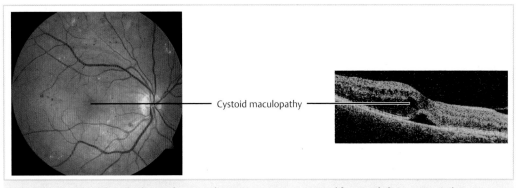

Cystoid maculopathy

Fig. 20.2 Cystoid maculopathy, hemorrhages and microaneurysms in nonproliferative diabetic retinopathy.

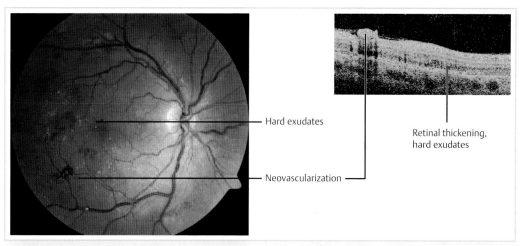

Hard exudates

Retinal thickening, hard exudates

Neovascularization

Fig. 20.3 Clinically significant macula edema with retinal thickening and hard exudates in proliferative diabetic retinopathy.

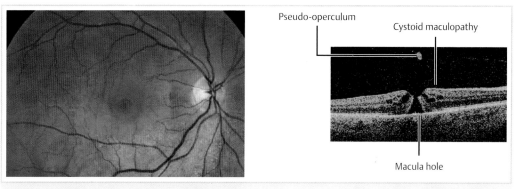

Pseudo-operculum

Cystoid maculopathy

Macula hole

Fig. 20.4 Macular hole with cystoid maculopathy and pseudo-operculum.

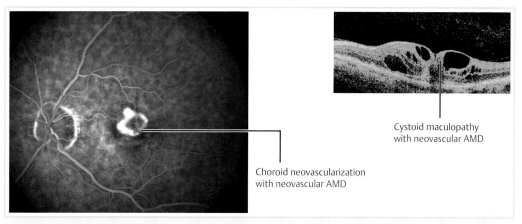

Cystoid maculopathy with neovascular AMD

Choroid neovascularization with neovascular AMD

Fig. 20.5 Late age-related macular degeneration (AMD) (neovascular). Fluorescein angiography.

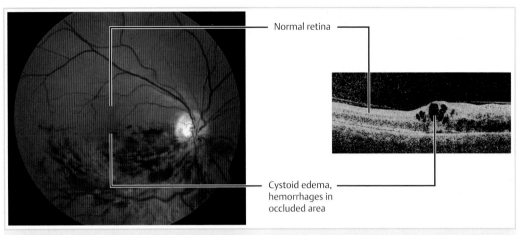

Normal retina

Cystoid edema,
hemorrhages in
occluded area

Fig. 20.6 Branch vein occlusion with hemorrhages.

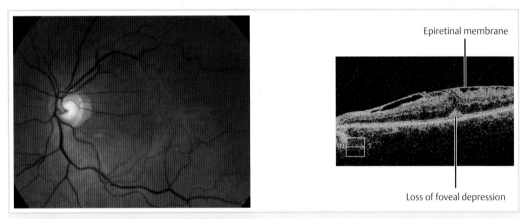

Epiretinal membrane

Loss of foveal depression

Fig. 20.7 Epiretinal membrane (synonym "macular pucker"). Due to a contracted membrane the retina is detached, leading to the loss of the foveal depression.

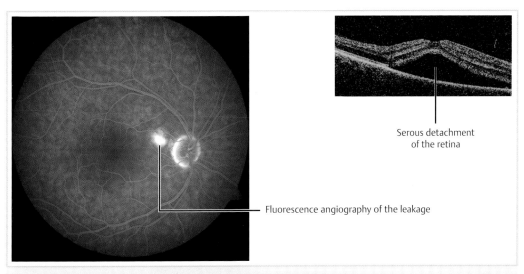

Serous detachment
of the retina

Fluorescence angiography of the leakage

Fig. 20.8 Central serous chorioretinopathy with serous detachment of the retina.

20.5.2 Typical Visual Field Defects in Certain Diseases

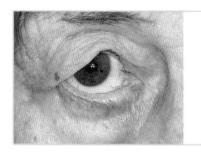
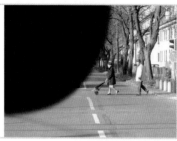

Fig. 20.9 Blepharoptosis.

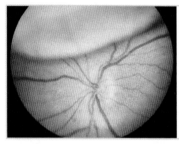
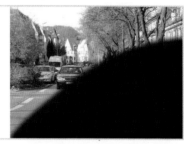

Fig. 20.10 Retinal detachment.

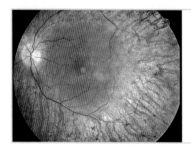
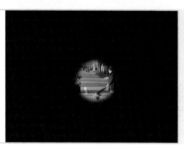

Fig. 20.11 Retinitis pigmentosa (tunnel vision).

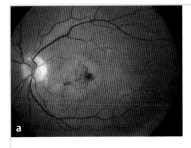
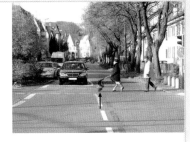

Fig. 20.12 Age-related macular degeneration (AMD). (a) Exudative AMD—distortion in the center of the field of vision (arrow). (b) Fibrous retinal scar in age-related macular degeneration (AMD).

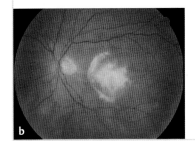
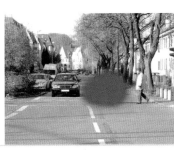

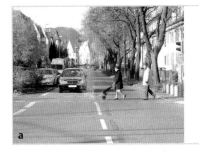
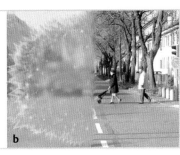

Fig. 20.13 Migraine with aura. (a) Visual defect initially. (b) The full picture.

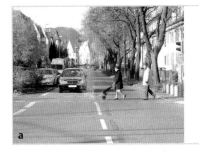
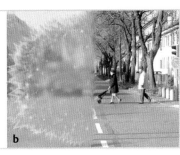

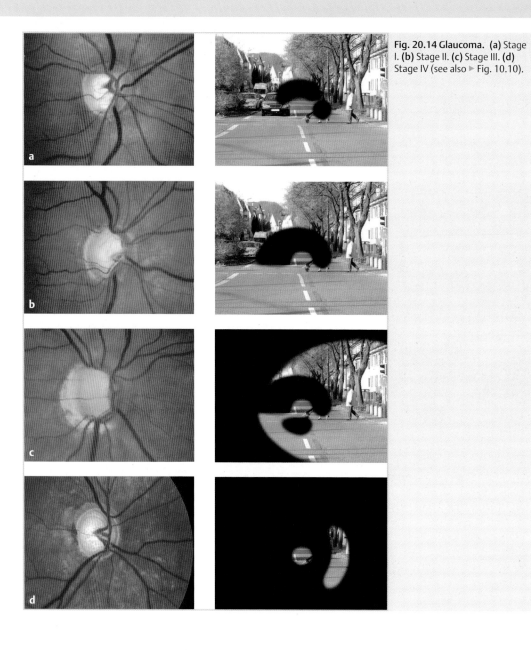

Fig. 20.14 Glaucoma. (a) Stage I. **(b)** Stage II. **(c)** Stage III. **(d)** Stage IV (see also ▶ Fig. 10.10).

Chapter 21
Glossary

Glossary

This glossary is limited to the most important ophthalmologic terms that will not necessarily be familiar to medical students. The list does not include basic anatomical terms (wherever necessary, these are explained in the text) or examination methods (please refer to the text).

Abducens nerve palsy Paralysis of the lateral rectus muscle.

Abduction Lateral rotation of the eye.

Ablatio retinae Retinal detachment.

Accommodation Increase in the refractive power of the eye's natural lens to allow visualization of near objects with sharp contours.

Adduction Medial rotation of the eye.

AION Anterior ischemic optic neuropathy due to a vascular process.

ALT Argon laser trabeculoplasty; laser treatment of the trabecular meshwork to manage glaucoma.

Amaurosis Blindness.

Amaurosis fugax Monocular loss of visual acuity lasting from several minutes to several hours that may result in retinal or cerebral embolism.

Amblyopia Monocular or binocular reduction in visual acuity lacking an organic cause, for example, in uncorrected poor vision.

Ametropia A refractive error in the eye.

Anisocoria Unequal pupil size.

Anisometropia A difference in refractive power between the two eyes (one eye is farsighted, the other nearsighted).

Anopsia Failure to see, as in visual field defects.

Asthenopia Pain and burning sensation in the eyes in the presence of uncorrected poor vision.

Astigmatism Varying refractive power in different corneal meridians.

Blepharospasm Involuntary spasmodic closing of the eyelids.

Buphthalmos Increase in the size of the globe in juvenile glaucoma.

Cataract Lens opacity.

Chemosis Conjunctival edema.

Coloboma A gap resulting from incomplete closure of the embryonic choroidal fissure.

Conjunctivitis Inflammation of the conjunctiva.

Cotton-wool spot Infarction of the layer of optic nerve fibers of the retina.

Cycloplegia Paralysis of the ciliary body.

Diplopia Double vision.

Ectopia lentis Displacement of the lens.

Ectropion Condition in which the margin of the eyelid is turned away from the eyeball.

Emmetropia Normal vision.

Enophthalmos Recession of the eyeball within the orbital cavity.

Entropion Condition in which the margin of the eyelid is turned inward toward the eyeball.

Enucleation Removal of the eye.

Epiphora Excessive tearing.

Episcleritis Inflammation of the surface of the sclera.

Esophoria Latent inward deviation of the visual axis.

Esotropia Manifest inward deviation of the visual axis.

Exophoria Latent outward deviation of the visual axis.

Exophthalmos Protrusion of the globe from the orbital cavity.

Exotropia Manifest outward deviation of the visual axis.

Gonioscopy Examination of the angle of the anterior chamber with special lenses.

Hemianopsia Loss of vision for one-half of the visual field.

Heterochromia Difference in coloration between the left and right iris.

Hyperopia Farsightedness.

Hyphema Bleeding in the anterior chamber.

Hypopyon Collection of pus in the anterior chamber.

Hyposphagma Blood between the conjunctiva and sclera.

Iridodialysis Separation of the iris at its peripheral base.

Iridocyclitis Inflammation of the iris and ciliary body.

Iris coloboma A gap in the iris.

Iritis Inflammation of the iris.

Keratitis Inflammation of the cornea.

LASEK Laser-assisted epithelial keratomileusis.

LASIK Laser-assisted in-situ keratomileusis.

Leukocoria White pupil, such as can occur in a cataract.

Meibomianitis Inflammation of the meibomian glands of the eyelids.

Metamorphopsia Perception of distorted images.

Microphthalmos Congenital anomaly in which the eye is abnormally small and deformed.

Miosis Constriction of the pupil.

Mydriasis Dilation of the pupil.

Myopia Nearsightedness.

Nanophthalmos Congenital anomaly in which the eye is abnormally small but otherwise normal.

Nystagmus Rhythmical oscillation of the eyeballs.

Oculomotor nerve palsy Paralysis of the eye muscles supplied by the oculomotor nerve; it may be *complete* (involving all intraocular and nearly all extraocular muscles) or *partial* (isolated paralysis of the intraocular *or* extraocular muscles supplied by the oculomotor nerve).

Ophthalmoplegia Paralysis of the extraocular muscles.

Ophthalmoscopy Visualization of the fundus of the eye.

Optic disc edema Swelling of the head of the optic nerve.

Orbital exenteration Removal of the entire contents of the orbital cavity including the eye.

Phoria A latent deviation of the visual axis.

Photophobia Sensitivity to light with a sensation of pain.

Photopsia Perception of light sensations, such as flashes of light.

Presbyopia Age-related loss of accommodation.

Ptosis Drooping of the upper eyelid.

Refraction The refractive power of the eye; its ability to deflect light.

Retinitis Inflammation of the retina.

Rhegmatogenous retinal detachment Detachment resulting from a break in the retina.

Rubeosis iridis Neovascularization in the iris.

Scleritis Inflammation of the sclera.

Scotoma A visual field defect.

Staphyloma A bulging of the cornea or sclera containing uveal tissue.

Strabismus Misalignment of the eyes.

Tarsorrhaphy Surgical procedure in which the temporal margins of the eyelids are sutured together to compensate for incomplete closure of the eyelids, as can occur in facial nerve palsy.

Trichiasis Rubbing of the eyelashes against the surface of the eyeball.

Trochlear nerve palsy Paralysis of the superior oblique muscle.

Uveitis Inflammation of the iris, ciliary body, and choroid.

Visual acuity Sharpness of vision.

Further Reading

Axenfeld T, Pau H. Lehrbuch der Augenheilkunde. Stuttgart: Fischer, 1992.

Fraunfelder FT, Roy FH, eds. Current ocular therapy. 5th ed. Philadelphia: Saunders, 2000.

Gramberg-Danielsen B. Rechtliche Grundlagen der augenärztlichen Tätigkeit. Stuttgart: Enke, 1986.

Gramberg-Danielsen B, Meve L. Augenärztliche Begutachtung im Versicherungswesen. Stuttgart: Enke, 1995.

Heimann H, Kellner U, Foerster MH. Atlas of Fundus Angiography. Stuttgart: Thieme, 2006.

Kanski JJ. Klinische Ophthalmologie. Munich: Urban & Fischer, 2004.

Kaufmann H. Strabismus. Stuttgart: Thieme, 2004.

Keith NM, Wagener HP, Barker MW. Some different types of essential hypertension: their course and prognosis. Am J Med Sci 1939;197:332–343.

Krause K. Methoden der Refraktionsbestimmung. Münster, Germany: Regensberg & Biermann, 1985.

Kritzinger EE, Beaumont HM. Farbatlas der Papillenbefunde. Hanover, Germany: Schlütersche, 1990.

Levin LA, Arnold AC. Neuro-Ophthalmology. Stuttgart: Thieme, 2005.

Naumann GOH. Pathologie des Auges. Heidelberg: Springer, 1997.

Ryan SJ, ed. Retina. 4th ed. St. Louis: Mosby, 2006.

Scheie HG. Evaluation of ophthalmoscopic changes of hypertension and arteriolar sclerosis. Arch Ophthalmol 1953;49:117–124.

Schuman JS, Puliafito C, Fujimoto JG, eds. Optical Coherence Tomography of Ocular Diseases. Thorofare, New Jersey: Slack, 2004.

Tasman W, Jaeger EA, eds. The Wills Eye Hospital atlas of clinical ophthalmology, 2nd ed. Philadelphia: Lippincott-Raven, 2001.

Index

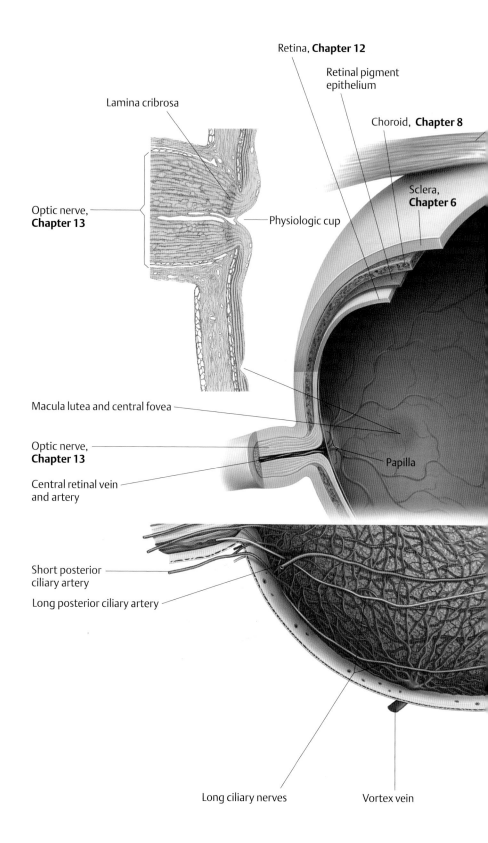

Retina, **Chapter 12**

Retinal pigment
epithelium

Choroid, **Chapter 8**

Lamina cribrosa

Sclera,
Chapter 6

Optic nerve,
Chapter 13

Physiologic cup

Macula lutea and central fovea

Optic nerve,
Chapter 13

Papilla

Central retinal vein
and artery

Short posterior
ciliary artery

Long posterior ciliary artery

Long ciliary nerves

Vortex vein

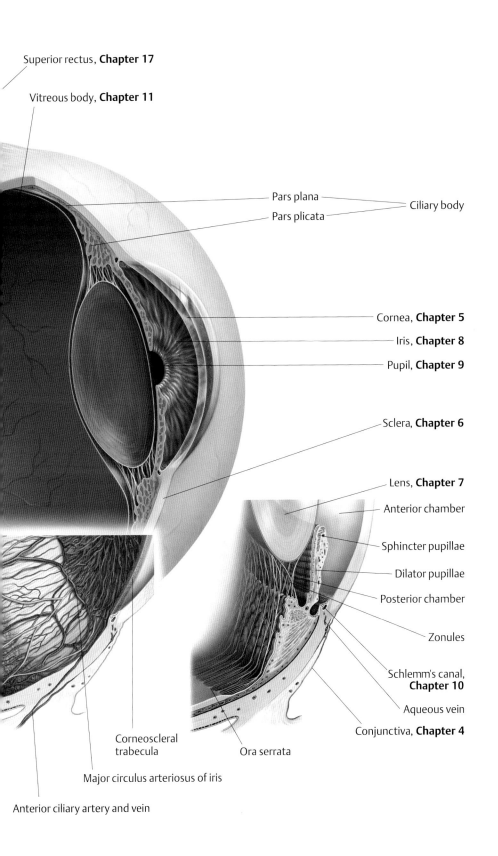

Superior rectus, **Chapter 17**

Vitreous body, **Chapter 11**

Pars plana

Pars plicata

Ciliary body

Cornea, **Chapter 5**

Iris, **Chapter 8**

Pupil, **Chapter 9**

Sclera, **Chapter 6**

Lens, **Chapter 7**

Anterior chamber

Sphincter pupillae

Dilator pupillae

Posterior chamber

Zonules

Schlemm's canal,
Chapter 10

Aqueous vein

Conjunctiva, **Chapter 4**

Corneoscleral
trabecula

Ora serrata

Major circulus arteriosus of iris

Anterior ciliary artery and vein